# Temperament Based Therapy with Support
# for Anorexia Nervosa

# Temperament Based Therapy with Support for Anorexia Nervosa

A Novel Treatment

**Laura L. Hill**
The Ohio State University
University of California, San Diego

**Stephanie Knatz Peck**
University of California, San Diego

**Christina E. Wierenga**
University of California, San Diego

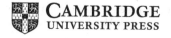

CAMBRIDGE
UNIVERSITY PRESS

# CAMBRIDGE
## UNIVERSITY PRESS

University Printing House, Cambridge CB2 8BS, United Kingdom

One Liberty Plaza, 20th Floor, New York, NY 10006, USA

477 Williamstown Road, Port Melbourne, VIC 3207, Australia

314–321, 3rd Floor, Plot 3, Splendor Forum, Jasola District Centre,
New Delhi – 110025, India

103 Penang Road, #05–06/07, Visioncrest Commercial, Singapore 238467

Cambridge University Press is part of the University of Cambridge.

It furthers the University's mission by disseminating knowledge in the pursuit of
education, learning, and research at the highest international levels of excellence.

www.cambridge.org
Information on this title: www.cambridge.org/9781009016803
DOI: 10.1017/9781009032063

First published 2022

*A catalogue record for this publication is available from the British Library.*

*Library of Congress Cataloging-in-Publication Data*
Names: Hill, Laura (Psychiatry) author. | Knatz, Stephanie Peck, author. | Wierenga, Christina, author.
Title: Temperament based therapy with support for anorexia nervosa / Laura Hill, Ohio State University,
Stephanie Peck Knatz, University of California, San Diego, Christina Wierenga, University of California,
San Diego.
Description: Cambridge, United Kingdom ; New York, NY : Cambridge University Press, 2022. | Includes
bibliographical references and index.
Identifiers: LCCN 2021024720 (print) | LCCN 2021024721 (ebook) | ISBN 9781009016803 (paperback) |
ISBN 9781009032063 (ebook)
Subjects: LCSH: Anorexia nervosa – Treatment. | Eating disorders. | Brain – Diseases – Treatment. |
Therapist and patient. | BISAC: MEDICAL / Mental Health
Classification: LCC RC552.A5 H55 2022  (print) | LCC RC552.A5  (ebook) | DDC 616.85/262–dc23
LC record available at https://lccn.loc.gov/2021024720
LC ebook record available at https://lccn.loc.gov/2021024721

ISBN 978-1-009-01680-3 Paperback

Cambridge University Press has no responsibility for the persistence or accuracy of
URLs for external or third-party internet websites referred to in this publication
and does not guarantee that any content on such websites is, or will remain,
accurate or appropriate.

..............................................................................................................................................

Every effort has been made in preparing this book to provide accurate and up-to-date information that
is in accord with accepted standards and practice at the time of publication. Although case histories are
drawn from actual cases, every effort has been made to disguise the identities of the individuals involved.
Nevertheless, the authors, editors, and publishers can make no warranties that the information
contained herein is totally free from error, not least because clinical standards are constantly changing
through research and regulation. The authors, editors, and publishers therefore disclaim all liability for
direct or consequential damages resulting from the use of material contained in this book. Readers are
strongly advised to pay careful attention to information provided by the manufacturer of any drugs or
equipment that they plan to use.

We dedicate this book to
**Walter H. Kaye, MD**
"Walt"
The visionary behind this
novel and emerging treatment:
Temperament Based Therapy with Support
(TBT-S)

# Contents

## Section 3  TBT-S Treatment Interventions

# Section 4 TBT-S Augmenting Eating Disorder Treatments

# Figures

# Tables

# Contributors

**Dr. Laura L. Hill** is Adjunct Associate Professor of Psychiatry and Behavioral Health, The Ohio State University, and Voluntary Assistant Clinical Professor in the Department of Psychiatry at the University of California, San Diego. Dr. Hill is one of the original founders of the Academy for Eating Disorders and was Director of the National Eating Disorder Organization, now known as the National Eating Disorder Association (NEDA), from 1990 to 1994. She was also Founder, President, and Chief Executive Officer of The Center for Balanced Living from 2000 to 2017. Dr. Hill is the recipient of the Muskingum University Distinguished Service Award and the NEDA 2011 Lori Irving Award for Excellence in Eating Disorders Prevention and Awareness. She is a 2012 TEDx presenter, titled "Eating Disorders from the Inside Out," and has spoken internationally and conducted eating disorder research for more than forty years.

**Dr. Stephanie Knatz Peck** is Associate Clinical Professor at the University of California, San Diego (UCSD). She is Director of Intensive Family Treatment (IFT) Programs at the UCSD Eating Disorders Treatment and Research Program, an internationally known eating disorders treatment program emphasizing family involvement, peer support, and brain-based treatment. In addition to her clinical work, Dr. Peck co-developed Temperament Based Therapy with Support (TBT-S) and is responsible for the development and evaluation of the Young Adult version of TBT-S. In addition to program development and oversight, she

continues to pursue her passion for helping others by providing direct clinical care for clients and family members affected by eating disorders. Dr. Peck has directly treated hundreds of clients and families over her career.

Dr. Peck has presented nationally and internationally on her work related to brain-based treatments and the Intensive Family Treatment Programs with world-renowned experts. She frequently conducts continuing education seminars for professionals and has presented clinical workshops and intensive trainings for lead organizations in the field, including the Academy of Eating Disorders/International Conference of Eating Disorders (ICED), the National Eating Disorder Association (NEDA), and the International Association of Eating Disorder Professionals (IAEDP). Additionally, she co-runs biannual two-day intensive trainings at the UCSD Eating Disorders Center for invited professionals. Dr. Peck has coauthored nine book chapters and various original scientific articles on topics related to eating disorders, including brain-based treatment.

**Dr. Christina E. Wierenga** is Professor of Psychiatry and Clinical Neuropsychologist at the University of California, San Diego (UCSD), and Co-director of the Research Program at the UCSD Eating Disorders Treatment and Research Program. She received her PhD in clinical psychology with a specialization in neuropsychology, neuro-rehabilitation, and clinical neuroscience from the University of Florida and completed an NIH postdoctoral fellowship at UCSD in biological psychiatry and neuroscience. She is an expert in the neurobiology of eating disorders, in particular related to the neural circuitry supporting cognition and behavior. She conducts neuroimaging and neuropsychological research examining the brain basis of disordered eating, with an emphasis on key constructs that contribute to altered motivation to eat, including cognitive control, reward processing, learning, and interoception. She is also heavily involved in treatment development efforts for eating disorders guided by a neurobiological understanding of temperament based behavior, as well as treatment outcome studies. Through close collaboration with Drs. Peck and Hill, she has developed and continues to test the Temperament Based Therapy with Support (TBT-S) approach for individuals with eating disorders. She is a Fellow of the American Psychological Association, a Fellow of the Academy for Eating Disorders and a member of the Eating Disorder Research Society and has published more than 100 peer-reviewed papers and received research funding from multiple agencies (e.g., National Institutes of Health, National Eating Disorders Association, the Department of Veterans Affairs).

# Foreword

## Walter H. Kaye, MD

Distinguished Professor of Psychiatry, University of California, San Diego Department of Psychiatry, and Founder and Executive Director, UCSD Eating Disorder Treatment and Research Program

Anorexia nervosa is often a chronic behavioral disorder with a high rate of medical complications and risk of dying. However, there has been limited progress in developing more effective treatments for this disorder. In part, a lack of a mechanistic understanding of anorexia nervosa has thwarted efforts to develop powerful evidence-based interventions. In recent years, innovations in genetic and biobehavioral research on anorexia nervosa have shed light on the neurobiological contributions to disease risk and chronicity. Temperament Based Therapy with Support (TBT-S) offers insights into how this knowledge can be translated into effective clinical interventions.

There has been a growing realization that people with anorexia nervosa tend to have certain personality and temperament traits. These traits, such as drive for achievement, perfectionism, anxiety, or risk or harm avoidance, tend to occur first in childhood, well before the onset of an eating disorder. These traits tend to become exacerbated when the individual is ill but persist in a mild to moderate form after recovery. These traits may create a vulnerability to developing anorexia nervosa and play a role in restricted eating.

For most people, not eating for a few days is uncomfortable, whereas hunger makes food more motivating and rewarding. In contrast, for those with anorexia nervosa, eating is anxiety producing, whereas not eating reduces anxiety or may even be empowering. New brain imaging research is revealing that primitive systems in the brain that we share with lower animals may miscode reward and anxiety signals in those with anorexia nervosa, resulting in anxious messages about food.[1] That is, the anxious temperament in many with anorexia nervosa may flood the brain and overwhelm motivating and reward messages about food.

It is very difficult to change temperament. Several years ago, we raised the question, in a paper called "Temperament-Based Treatment for Anorexia Nervosa,"[2] that people could learn compensatory skills to better understand and manage temperament in anorexia nervosa. This concept was tested and published in several papers.[3–5] How is this possible? Humans are remarkably adaptable to learning to compensate for deficits. For example, if you are blind, you can learn to use touch and sound to navigate the world. As we begin to understand more about these temperaments, which are hardwired into the brain, we can help people with anorexia nervosa, and their families, develop compensatory skills and strategies to manage their anxiety and facilitate eating.

I am very grateful that I have been fortunate to have worked with Laura, Stephanie, and Christina in developing these concepts and treatment. They are extremely talented, clever, and smart and have shown outstanding imagination and skill in transforming biological concepts into treatment applications. Laura has constantly amazed me in regard to her insights into behavior of those with anorexia nervosa and her creativity in developing interactive approaches that get the attention and participation of those with this disorder. Stephanie is one of most brilliant therapists I know in terms of her ability to explain the symptoms of anorexia nervosa to families and guide them in conceptualization of effective interactions. I am in awe of Christina's outstanding ability to demystify complex, cutting-edge science and translate these constructs in terms that both laypeople and therapists can understand and use. I am delighted to see them bring to life this comprehensive and detailed book that describes neurobiology, core principles, and a range of applications of TBT-S. I have witnessed the enthusiasm of patients and families who use and benefit from TBT-S because it explains their puzzling symptoms and, most importantly, gives them strategies that are effective. Moreover, Laura, Stephanie, and Christina make this treatment interesting, and even fun, and build an alliance between those with anorexia nervosa and their Supports.

I am particularly proud of the work that has contributed to the development of TBT-S. As I get older, it is reassuring to know that Laura, Stephanie, and Christina will continue this work, expand the reach of TBT-S, and continue to generate data that will demonstrate efficacy – and that TBT-S improves communication with those with anorexia nervosa, who often lack motivation to change or insight into their behaviors, and provides tools that they are more willing to employ and skills that help them recover.

# References

1. Kaye WH, Wierenga CE, Bischoff-Grethe A, et al. Neural insensitivity to the effects of hunger in women remitted from anorexia nervosa. Am J Psychiatr. 2020;177 (7):601–10.

2. Kaye WH, Wierenga CE, Knatz S, et al. Temperament-based treatment for anorexia nervosa. Eur Eat Disord Rev. 2015;23 (1):12–8.

3. Marzola E, Knatz S, Murray S, et al. Short-term intensive family therapy for adolescent eating disorders: 30-month outcome. Eur Eat Disord Rev. 2015;23(3):210–18.

4. Knatz S, Wierenga CE, Murray S, et al. Neurobiologically-informed treatment for adults with anorexia nervosa: A novel approach to a chronic disorder. Dialogues Clin Neurosci. 2015;17(2):229–36.

5. Wierenga CE, Hill L, Knatz Peck S, et al. The acceptability, feasibility, and possible benefits of a neurobiologically-informed 5-day multifamily treatment for adults with anorexia nervosa. Int J Eat Disord. 2018;51 (8):863–9.

# Preface

I (Laura Hill) was formally introduced to the work by the artist Henri Matisse in the house of Matisse, in Nice, France. Until that time in my early life, I had thought art was not "real art" unless the subject matter looked like illustrations, such as paintings by Norman Rockwell. The day I walked into the Matisse Museum, my appreciation for art turned around 180 degrees.

The rooms were laid out chronologically. The first room was filled with portraits. At first I thought they were black-and-white photographs. Upon closer examination, I realized they were pencil drawings – hundreds of lines portraying a face, a shadow, and light, hundreds of lines detailing a woman's eyes, nose, mouth, chin, and hair. I was mesmerized by the exactness of the images.

The next room continued to display Matisse's portraits of various subjects, but the drawings had fewer lines. Lines were removed, yet the essence of the image remained strong and clear. In each consecutive room, lines were removed from the images. Some portraits displayed great detail of half of the subjects' faces; the other half was blank, allowing the viewer to perceptually complete the images. The essential lines defined the image as they simultaneously opened the viewer to the expanse of their potential.

The rooms culminated in the upstairs loft area, where Matisse's cutouts filled the space. His flowers, leaves, shapes, and figures were simply portrayed, yet they vibrantly expressed the essence of the overall image. A transformative new technique was developed in art making. I stood in that space, looking at the work of an artist who presented the viewer with less, and yet so much more.

A few years later, I was in the Metropolitan Museum of Art in New York City, walking down a hallway looking ahead at a colorful depiction of chaos in a large painting by Jackson Pollock. I became aware of a sensation that I was swimming. I looked to my right, and there on the hallway wall was a continuous flow of blue paper, cut in wave-like shapes. One line flowed throughout the image. I stopped. The title of the piece was *The Swimmer*. It was by Matisse.

This book introduces you to a new treatment approach, Temperament Based Therapy with Support (TBT-S). We originally wrote the book by using hundreds of lines to depict an illustrative understanding of the treatment. We portrayed in detail its development, its interactive process, and the biological nature of the illness and treatment. However, each draft contained so many lines that it became difficult to see the core principles illustrated throughout the book. The challenge became, how do we present the reader with a novel treatment, without writing every line and describing every aspect?

We decided less is more. This manual describes the essential points of TBT-S. We share the key point of each topic and simultaneously open the reader to the expanse of its potential. This is harder than it appears. We have removed sections, lines, dimensions, and details. It has taken many versions to maintain the clear and strong fundamental nature of the treatment, while leaving it open for the reader to realize the breadth of its ability to augment other treatments and to intervene in other diagnoses. Whether the reader is new to eating disorder treatment or an expert, this book is a manual of the essential themes of TBT-S. The intent of this style of writing is to influence clinicians as they enter a treatment session to detect client traits flowing through their thoughts, feelings, and actions and realize the traits are "cut out" from the client's temperament.

The manual practices what TBT-S preaches: to actively move toward a solution, allowing one's natural tendencies (temperament) to drive and determine what works best to reach that destination. The ongoing neurobiological findings of anorexia nervosa are complex. Eating disorder symptom reduction is complex, difficult, and counter to dominant eating disorder trait tendencies. Yet, people with anorexia nervosa can and do get better. How? What has been missing that could help ongoing treatment processes become more succinct in the short term and have better long-lasting outcomes? This book provides a novel temperament based approach that fills in a significant therapeutic gap by integrating research findings on the neurobiological bases of AN with clinical interventions.

We hope you find this manual helpful to your practice. Young adult (YA) clients with anorexia nervosa and those with severe-and-enduring anorexia nervosa (SE-AN) have repeatedly told us that TBT-S has turned them around 180 degrees. They reported that they understood their illness better and realized what they could and could not do to move forward on their own. This manual is to be used to augment ongoing eating disorder therapies, as a classroom guide to instruct emerging professionals and for research studies. It addresses how to approach the essential nature of anorexia nervosa. A key point is that TBT-S treats to the traits – the core substance that delineates one's potential.

# Acknowledgments

We, Laura, Stephanie, and Christina, acknowledge and offer our deep gratitude to the nonprofit organization Eating Disorder Families of Australia (EDFA). EDFA was developed to ensure that Supports are included in the treatment of anorexia nervosa, to help increase treatment outcomes and improve collaboration among clinicians, clients, and Supports. Their goal overlaps with a core principle of Temperament Based Therapy with Support, to include Supports (any person to whom the client turns for support) in portions of the treatment process. EDFA led the hosting of extensive TBT-S training programs across Australia, collaborating with other eating disorder organizations. The authors of this book led face-to-face trainings for clinicians and Supports from coast to coast. This book was conceived during this tour of trainings in 2019.

## Laura Hill

I offer my sincere appreciation for input, feedback, suggestions, and encouragement from

- Kitty Soldano, PhD
- Kamryn Eddy, PhD
- Jim Mitchell, MD
- Erica Temes, ABD
- Janie Drake
- Krista Crotty, PhD,
- Kristin Stedal, PhD, in Norway
- Jodi Sark, PhD, in Canada
- Juana Poulisis, MD, in Argentina
- Maria Tsiaka, PhD, in Greece
- My dearest and beloved, Nicholas Hill

## Stephanie Knatz Peck and Christina E. Wierenga

We share our sincere gratitude to the clinical research team and the amazing clinical staff at the UCSD Eating Disorders Treatment and Research Program. We personally acknowledge the following for their input, help with development and evaluation, and encouragement:

- Ivan Eisler, PhD
- Terra Towne, PhD
- Hannah Patrick, LMFT
- Roxie Rockwell, PhD
- Salma Soliman, LCSW
- Taylor Perry, BA
- McKenzie Miller, M.A.
- Emily Han, B.S.
- Stuart Murray, PhD

- ○ Diane Mickley, MD
- ○ Global Foundation for Eating Disorders (GFED)

## Stephanie Knatz Peck

I personally dedicate this book to my parents, Kenneth and Marilyn Knatz, and my husband, Colby Peck, who supported me through my own recovery as a young adult and were my earliest inspirations for this work.

## Christina E. Wierenga

I thank my early mentors, Drs. Bruce Crosson and Leslie Gonzalez Rothi, for teaching me the power of the principles of neuroplasticity to promote recovery of function. I am grateful to the National Eating Disorders Association (NEDA) Feeding Hope Fund for their financial support of early development and testing of TBT-S. Lastly, I acknowledge my parents, Edward and Wilma Wierenga, for their unwavering support.

# Introduction

Temperament is the biologically based facet of personality that contributes to defining who a person is. Temperament can be shaped and refined to shift destructive trait expressions to productive expressions of strength and well-being. Temperament is an underlying cause of anorexia nervosa (AN).

Temperament Based Therapy with Support (TBT-S) is a novel treatment approach that addresses underlying genetic, neurobiological, and trait bases of anorexia nervosa. It is applied in modules. Novel treatments are needed because anorexia nervosa has one of the highest mortality rates among all mental illnesses and a low treatment efficacy over time. TBT-S was developed to augment ongoing eating disorder treatments. This manual addresses what TBT-S is and how to apply its wide range of temperament based modules in all levels of care and treatment settings. It offers a plethora of treatment tools and skills for clinicians, dietitians, medical professionals, and educators. Scripts are in *italics* throughout the manual. Clinicians are encouraged not to read the scripts verbatim but instead to learn the points and share them in their own voices.

The treatment name, Temperament Based Therapy with Support, uses the word "Support." Adult clients with anorexia nervosa chose this word. They shared that they did not want people to whom they turned for support to be labeled as "caregivers," because they did not want to be "taken care of." Adult clients requested that they be referred to as "Supports." In many cases, these support persons extend far beyond their parents and family of origin. "Family" in family-based therapy is descriptive for adolescents with an eating disorder (ED). Adults with ED, however, reported they preferred a broader descriptor for people that they turn to for support. They chose the word "Supports" to describe both the people and the actions they need from them. Support becomes a two for one term. "Supports" is capitalized throughout the manual, referring to the *persons to* whom adult clients turn for support.

The manual is divided into four sections. Section 1 provides an overview of TBT-S. TBT-S is launching as a new mental health intervention. This book focuses on AN, recognizing that TBT-S holds the potential to be applied to the temperamental bases of all mental illnesses. The manual focuses on the adult AN population, offering two sub-approaches, one for young adults (YA), and one for clients with severe-and-enduring anorexia nervosa (SE-AN). The two TBT-S approaches allow treatment providers to draw upon young adult developmental needs, while also offering intervention tools that align with chronic AN symptoms.

Section 1 has five chapters introducing TBT-S as a treatment intervention. Chapter 1 describes TBT-S as a novel treatment approach that centers on temperament. It explains how TBT-S is grounded in neurobiological research that identifies common, altered brain circuits underpinning ED symptoms. Chapter 2 explains TBT-S core principles, while Chapter 3 introduces intervention strategies that apply those principles. Chapter 4 describes the state of TBT-S evidence and the need for randomized controlled trials. This manual is a treatment resource for such studies. Chapter 5 closes Section 1 by clarifying how the manual can be used.

Section 2 addresses integrating TBT-S within the ongoing ED treatment context. How to initiate TBT-S treatment is described in Chapter 6. How to include Supports (friends, spouses, colleagues, family) in adult treatment is discussed in Chapter 7. Chapter 7 also addresses why Supports are a necessary part of the treatment team for adults with anorexia nervosa, recognizing interdependence as an essential developmental stage. Chapter 8 offers the "nuts and bolts" of how to set up a temperament based approach preparing clinicians to weave TBT-S modules into their ongoing treatment approaches.

Section 3 takes treatment providers and educators into the depths of TBT-S interventions for YA and SE-AN clients. Chapters 9–13 present treatment providers with neurobiological psychoeducational modules to integrate into ongoing ED therapies. Chapters 14–17 describe TBT-S strategies designed specifically for YA clients and their parents. Chapters 18–19 introduce the primary TBT-S experiential activities, tools and skills that can be inserted as modules into ongoing ED therapies.

Chapter 20 is the TBT-S dietary module. It provides strategies for integrating meal plans into a process that is congruent with client traits. It details a portion of the Behavioral Agreement (BA) that provides the dietitian with a structure to work within when treating YA and SE-AN clients that is conducive to AN temperament. This chapter guides dietitians to include Supports in selected sessions to ensure dietary understanding and intervention continuity inside and outside of treatment sessions.

Chapters 21–23 cover the central TBT-S Behavioral Agreements (BA), one for YA and one for SE-AN clients, and their Supports. The BA offers clinicians and clients a structure to identify practical and tangible plans regarding what needs to be done, by whom, when, and how. The BAs are grounded in client traits.

Section 4 offers methods to integrate TBT-S modules into ongoing ED therapies to augment ED treatment. Chapter 24 offers examples of TBT-S treatment schedules. The examples range from the 5-day, 40-hour TBT-S treatment schedules for YA and SE-AN clients (the format in which the TBT-S open trials were studied) to examples of TBT-S modules added to outpatient therapy sessions. Chapter 25 offers ways to apply TBT-S in diverse treatment settings. Chapter 26 addresses how to interface TBT-S with ongoing ED treatment providers and programs. Chapter 27 summarizes TBT-S Matisse style, in one line.

The book chapters are half of the manual. The other half are the appendices. Each appendix details a different experiential TBT-S activity, tool, or handout of psychoeducational information. They are provided for clinicians and educators to learn the information and apply it to ongoing ED treatment and educational settings.

# What Is Temperament Based Therapy with Support (TBT-S)?

## Why TBT-S Began by Focusing on Anorexia Nervosa

Anorexia nervosa (AN) is a serious, life-threatening condition that has one of the highest death rates of all mental illnesses.[1–4] It is diagnostically defined as having extremely low body weight, an intense fear of weight gain, and disturbance in how one's body weight and shape are experienced.[5] It occurs primarily in females,[6] usually taking form during puberty with the potential to develop acute and chronic impairment over one's lifetime.[7] The illness places a considerable strain on families, friends, and work settings. While progress has been made in understanding the psychosocial and behavioral mechanisms responsible for the development and maintenance of the illness, there is an urgent need to optimize treatment approaches to reduce chronicity and improve outcomes.[7] This necessitates new and innovative treatments that contribute to long-term symptom reduction and incorporate contemporary neurobiological findings such as those covered in TBT-S.

> Key Point: TBT-S has focused on AN because of its high mortality rate and low treatment efficacy over time.

## TBT-S Description

Temperament Based Therapy with Support (TBT-S) is an emerging neurobiologically informed treatment approach designed to augment existing treatments. This book describes how and why TBT-S has been developed for adults with AN, recognizing it has the capacity to be applied to other psychological disorders. TBT-S fills the gap between research and clinical practice by acknowledging and treating underlying brain-based factors. TBT-S recognizes that there is a biological basis to psychological illnesses that involves temperament and altered brain function. This affects the regulation of eating and emotion for those with AN. TBT-S applies neurobiological research findings to inform treatment targets.

TBT-S combines psychoeducation and experiential activities that emphasize the key role of neurobiological factors in the development and maintenance of AN to increase insight and recognize temperament patterns. Skills-based training is used to teach clients and Supports age-appropriate strategies to manage these neurobiological factors to reduce problem thoughts and behaviors. TBT-S treatment targets include common AN temperament traits (e.g., anxiety, cognitive inflexibility, harm avoidance) and related brain processes such as altered reward and punishment sensitivity, interoception, inhibitory control, and decision-making.

The focus of TBT-S is to work *with* clients who have AN *and* their Support persons to acknowledge, understand, and utilize their own temperament as a primary source for strength and change. Supports can include members of one's family of origin (such as parents, siblings, grandparents, adult children) and of one's "family" of choice (such as spouses, partners, friends, housemates, or colleagues). The TBT-S approach was developed and refined over a 10-year period, integrating AN research with ongoing client and Support feedback to assure the intervention strategies accurately reflect client experiences and temperaments.[8, 9] TBT-S was originally developed and studied in an intensive 5-day, 40-hour program with groups of clients and their Supports.[9]

> Key Point: Temperament Based Therapy with Support (TBT-S) is an emerging and novel neurobiologically based treatment that works *with* clients' temperament to motivate change and to manage and reduce symptoms.

## What Is Temperament, and Why Is It Important?

*Temperament* is the biological basis of our personality, influenced by genetics, brain circuit development and function over one's life span. *Character* is the external shaping of one's temperament. Temperament is to nature as character is to nurture (Figure 1.1).

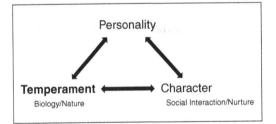

**Figure 1.1** Temperament in relation to personality and character
Source: Cloninger (2014).

Temperament has been studied for more than 70 years with a primary focus on children.[10] In the late 1980s Chess and Thomas led interventions for parents and educators to incorporate children's "reactive patterns" into classroom and parenting responses.[11] They countered the trend that children were solely "products of the environment," advocating that they bring their own tendencies to the picture. Subsequently temperament researchers began to acknowledge that traits can be disadvantageous in one situation and advantageous in others.[11] Educational and parental interventions encouraged a "goodness of fit" framework for children.[12] However, therapeutic interventions that focus on shaping adults' "natural" thoughts, feelings, and behaviors have been left off the therapeutic table in the area of eating disorders.[13, 14] Working *with* clients' temperaments acknowledges who they are and what they bring of themselves to the therapeutic experience (Figure 1.2).

### What is Temperament?

- The biological foundation to our personality

- Our innate (natural) features

- The genetic and neurobiological underpinnings that influence our thoughts, feelings, and behaviors *over a lifetime*.

**Figure 1.2** What is temperament? Source: Cole (2020); Mitchell (2018).

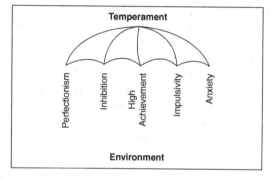

**Figure 1.3** Traits are distinguishing *features* of temperament that interact with environment

Temperament is expressed through traits, as shown in Figure 1.3, which affect our thoughts, feelings, and behaviors. Temperament traits are observed in infancy and are relatively preserved across the lifespan, suggesting that personality is hardwired and consistent across life. Importantly, temperament is strongly related to most psychopathologies, especially those involving anxiety and mood disturbance. People have varying levels of vulnerabilities to develop a psychological disorder based on the traits they inherit. In fact, growing evidence indicates that temperament traits are uniquely associated with specific brain systems linked to various psychopathologies, including those involved in eating disorders (ED).[15–19] This suggests that temperament traits are genetic and brain based and have a powerful influence on ED and thus should be included in treatment approaches. See Figure 1.4.

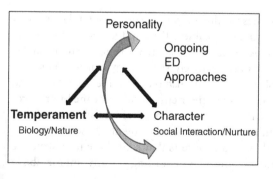

**Figure 1.4** Current ED therapies focus on personality and character

> **Key Point:** Temperament is the biological foundation of personality and consists of traits that are fundamental expressions of each person.

Accumulating behavioral and neuroimaging evidence points to a neurobiologically based AN temperament that increases risk and contributes to the development and maintenance of the disorder.[20–36] This AN temperament is characterized by anxiety, altered sensitivity to reward and punishment, altered interoceptive awareness, difficulty with decision-making, and cognitive inflexibility and rigidity.[30, 32, 37–42] Individuals with AN also tend to be high achieving, perfectionistic, inhibited, and rule abiding. These temperament and personality traits are related to altered insula and fronto-striatal neural circuit function, highlighting their neurobiological basis.[43–47] In addition to predating the disease, these traits often persist in a mild to modest degree after recovery, offering evidence they are biologically based traits and not behavioral symptom expressions.[30, 37–40, 48]

This AN temperament profile serves as a framework that identifies the neurobiological constructs and traits targeted in TBT-S; and guides the interventions designed to address symptoms specific to AN. TBT-S has been developed to fill a gap in ED treatment (Figure 1.5). It features AN temperament, focusing on the traits that make a person vulnerable to AN, why AN symptoms emerge and are maintained, and how to shift trait expressions or construct environmental modifications to reduce symptoms to impact positive change. See Figure 1.5.

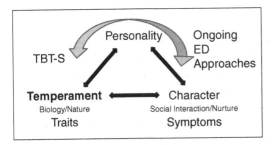

**Figure 1.5** TBT-S augments other treatments by focusing on temperament

> **Key Point:** AN has common traits creating a temperament profile that guides TBT-S interventions to work *with* client traits as natural resources for lifelong changes.

The theoretical model of TBT-S approaches the illness from the inside out. It begins with genes. Environmental factors (such as life stresses, malnutrition, and trauma) can modify gene expression and temperament via epigenetic processes (e.g., gene × environment interactions), suggesting that although traits are relatively stable, they can be shaped by experience and treatment.[49] Figure 1.6 shows the relationship between temperament and environmental influences on symptoms. Genes, the center circle, code how the brain wires its circuits impacting thoughts, perceptions, feelings, and actions. Traits develop from brain circuits structured by genes which are influenced by the environment. Persons with AN have specific alterations in the wiring of these brain circuits that contribute to destructive AN trait expressions. Other circuits function normally, affording healthy and/or above

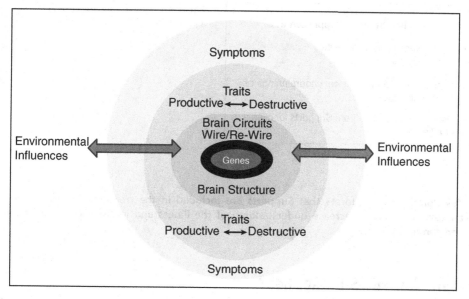

**Figure 1.6** The relationship between traits and environmental influences on symptoms

average productive trait expressions. Altered trait expressions impact the type of symptoms that develop. For example, elevated harm avoidance is related to dietary restriction and reduced social interactions. TBT-S focuses on acknowledging and utilizing one's trait expressions to modify, shape, and promote recovery. For example, TBT-S prescribes structure and routine, in alliance with a rule-bound trait, to reduce anxiety and intolerance of uncertainty around meals. The inside-out approach of TBT-S complements ongoing therapies that are grounded in environmental and behavioral models.

> **Key Point:** The TBT-S theoretical model approaches treatment from the inside out, targeting traits and underlying biology that complements other treatment approaches which work from the outside in.

## Who Are the Intended Participants?

TBT-S was designed to be administered to adult clients and their Supports. Thus, both clients and Supports participate with the clinical team. Conducting TBT-S with clients and their Supports is a powerful and effective way to ensure information is relayed, experienced, and processed similarly. We have focused our research and this book on adults with AN and their broad range of Supports in response to the higher chronicity and mortality within this subpopulation. The TBT-S focus is on improving client-Support relationships and communication to facilitate recovery. See Figure 1.7.

| **TBT-S is a treatment approach that:** |
| --- |
| • Works *with* clients' nature, their temperament/traits |
| • Explains the neurobiological underpinnings of client trait expressions |
| • Draws on assistance from Supports for clients of *all ages*. |

**Figure 1.7** Temperament Based Therapy with Support (TBT-S)

Key Point: TBT-S endorses that Supports are included in the treatment of adults with anorexia nervosa to increase understanding of the illness and improve communication and continuity in care.

## Where Can TBT-S Be Applied?

TBT-S core principles and modules could be applied in (a) one-on-one, (b) client with Support person, and(c) client and/or Support group sessions either (d) virtually or face-to-face, (e) ranging from outpatient through day hospital levels of care. When TBT-S core principles are described in therapy sessions, clients learn about the neurobiological underpinnings of their temperament expressions and skills to help shape their traits. The therapeutic change process is enhanced when additional components include virtual or face-to-face: (a) Support person(s), and (b) the act of practicing the skills together. The learning and change process can be further enhanced by providing TBT-S interventions in group settings through the power of client and Support interactions.[183]

TBT-S was originally developed in a 5-day group intensive format to maximize efficacy, build on skill development intensively, minimize attrition, and provide a practical and accessible approach for adult clients and Supports to work together in a discrete amount of time. Increased treatment frequency and intensity are critical components needed to elicit behavior change.[50, 51] Treatment models for anxiety indicate that intense, repeated, and focused *in vivo* practice is key to altering biologically driven avoidance behaviors by maximizing learning through massed practice and allowing close monitoring of compliance.[52–59]

Intensive treatment formats also show an increase in initial efficacy.[60, 61] This appears to be critical in treating AN, as evidence suggests that adolescents with AN who gain weight in the first four sessions of family-based treatment (FBT) have significantly better outcomes than those who do not gain weight early in treatment.[62] An intensive treatment format offers several additional advantages, including reduced burden on the adult client and Support(s) of having to commit to treatment over long periods of time, thus likely improving accessibility, acceptability, and compliance. An initial intensive model may also be a cost-effective "jump-start" to shorten residential or partial hospital treatments and augment outpatient ED treatments.

In the studied TBT-S 5-day model, multiple adult clients and Supports are treated together in a group structure, commonly known as a multi-family group in adolescent treatment. Group settings enable and facilitate peer-to-peer consultation, a powerful method of learning that can improve outcomes. Having multiple adult clients and their Supports together can improve participants' understanding of the illness by allowing them to learn from similar and diverse perspectives during group activities. Working with groups of clients and Supports broadens viewpoints on effective ways to manage recovery and generates new ideas. The TBT-S focus is on improving client-Support relationships and communication to facilitate recovery.

> **Key Point:** TBT-S was studied in a 5-day group format to intensify treatment intervention, unify clients and Supports, and increase accessibility to treatment.

## TBT-S Modular Structure

TBT-S is implemented as a modular treatment, meaning that it has multiple, individual, complementary treatment interventions that have been studied in different combinations as part of the 5-day TBT-S program. TBT-S treatment modules were designed to target symptoms using a broad array of intervention strategies (e.g., psychoeducation, experiential learning, skills training, meal coaching and behavioral agreements) that include both the client and Supports. Each TBT-S treatment module is described in Section 3 and includes a variety of treatment activities. Clinicians can select activities from each module deemed to be most relevant depending on the clinical presentations and developmental stage of the clients and their Supports present in treatment.

Many clinicians may not have the infrastructure to deliver TBT-S in its tested 5-day format. Individual treatment modules or activities can be administered independently across multiple treatment settings, including outpatient through partial hospitalization settings, and in multiple formats, such as group, individual, or family therapy settings (See Section 4). The TBT-S multi-day design has also been administered in shorter intensive formats over 2 to 4 days in outpatient and higher level of care settings in the United States, Canada, Norway and Greece. Efforts to deliver the multi-day TBT-S program in a virtual format also appear promising. Section 4 of this manual provides examples of how to structure and organize modules by treatment target or temperament trait in multiple treatment settings.

> **Key Point:** Clinicians can flexibly apply TBT-S integrating its modular format with multiple treatment strategies to formulate unique stylized interventions.

## Two TBT-S Versions: Young Adult (YA) and Severe-and-Enduring Anorexia Nervosa (SE-AN)

Two versions of TBT-S have been developed and tested to date, YA and SE-AN. Both versions uphold TBT-S core principles (see Chapter 2) as central themes and adhere to the same structure, format of treatment and the level of Support involvement. They differ in how adults are approached when in young adult stages of life development compared to adults who have severe-and-enduring forms of AN.

## Young Adult TBT-S (YA TBT-S)

The Young Adult model of TBT-S (YA TBT-S) is designed for clients with AN and other restrictive-type ED between the ages of 17 and 27 and their parents, who are automatically nominated as primary Supports. This highly focused version of TBT-S was designed to enhance treatment by integrating important developmental considerations since many adults seeking treatment for AN often fall within this age range. Naturally, young adults with AN are undergoing developmental changes and growth that are central to this age and often have a primary impact on treatment and recovery, both individually and within the context of their family system. YA TBT-S is tailored to provide education on neurobiology, skills training, and a model of family assistance that takes into account these important developmental considerations.

Emerging adulthood is a developmental window that has gained more attention in recent years, in part because the incidence of mental illness is highest in this developmental stage. Young adults do not squarely fit into either adult or child/adolescent services because most in this age category are embarking on the launch to independence (versus being fully independent) and, increasingly so, continue to be embedded in their family system in important ways. Young adults are adjusting to significant life transitions during this developmental stage, including separation from family of origin, increasing autonomy and individual responsibility, and more commonly in this modern era, interdependence within their family of origin.

Developmentally, young adults are striving to individuate from their family, learning to make their own decisions, and increasingly focusing on carving their own path in life. This developmental backdrop is significant and imposing in the life of a young adult and thus deserves consideration when working with clients with AN in this age range. YA TBT-S brings these developmental dilemmas to the forefront of treatment and addresses them within the context of recovery and treatment. Themes touched on in treatment include the capacity for change within the context of the temperament framework due to neurodevelopment, how to assist a YA in recovery from AN, how to make use of continued parental involvement to positively impact recovery, how to strike a balance of autonomous and family-focused recovery and navigating an effective working relationship among YAs and their parents.

## Severe-and-Enduring Anorexia Nervosa TBT-S (SE-AN TBT-S)

The SE-AN version of TBT-S is designed for all adults with AN across the life span who have chronic AN. It recognizes that traditional adult therapy focuses on individuation. In contrast, TBT-S integrates interdependence within a neurobiological framework. In this model, Supports may be anyone the client designates as a "support person." The SE-AN version of TBT-S has been studied with clients of all ages, from newly graduated 18-year-old females and males to older clients in their 50s and 60s who have developed chronic AN tendencies. As SE-AN clients age, they tend to turn to a wider diversity of Support persons, with many of their primary family members having "burned out." Trait expressions continue throughout one's lifetime. When TBT-S is offered in a group format, the expertise from older clients offers lived wisdom informing younger clients of symptoms that can become ingrained over time, while the younger clients resurrect hope and motivation in the older clients to reshape trait expressions. TBT-S presents neurobiological information that is congruent with AN temperament, increasing awareness that there are tools that those with AN can utilize that align with their own temperament.

Clients tend to enter treatment assuming they have little within themselves that can be a part of the solution. They report having tried many behavioral interventions, but some have failed over time. In a TBT-S approach, the adult client educates, coaches, and clarifies with their Supports their own experiences of what it is like to have AN traits, how symptoms allow relief and lower anxiety, and what helps and does not help. Clients actively explore how to utilize the same traits that have been expressed destructively in more productive ways. The discovery that their authentic selves, that their own temperament, has worth and is a means toward health and well-being motivates change and empowers their strengths. The more SE-AN adult clients align with the biological bases of their personality, the sooner they can begin to identify how to use their own traits to impact change. SE-AN adults have engrained rule-bound rituals that have sustained their ED symptoms over years. TBT-S utilizes its trait-based approach to empower the rule-bound traits as solutions to step away from destructive tendencies, using tools to shift the same traits toward productive expressions.

**Key Point:** There are two versions of TBT-S. YA TBT-S is designed for ages 17–27 and integrates important developmental considerations into the TBT-S model. SE-AN TBT-S is designed for ages 18–60 who have chronic AN symptoms (over five years of illness). Both versions interrupt and shift AN symptoms by teaching clients to identify *their own* trait-based behavioral solutions.

### Summary Key Points

- Temperament Based Therapy with Support (TBT-S) is an emerging neurobiologically informed treatment approach designed to augment existing treatments.
- TBT-S has been developed for adults with anorexia nervosa (AN), recognizing it has the capacity to be applied to other psychological disorders.
- TBT-S fills the gap between research and clinical practice by acknowledging and treating underlying brain-based factors.
- TBT-S recognizes that there is a biological basis to psychological illnesses that involves temperament and altered brain function.
- It is developed as a modular treatment to be administered virtually or face-to-face. Clinicians can insert TBT-S modules into ongoing therapies ranging from one module in an outpatient treatment setting to a day of TBT-S to the 5-day, 40-hour, 1-week TBT-S program that was studied.
- The "S" of TBT-S means "Support," the word chosen by adults clients with AN to describe anyone who offers support.

# Chapter 2

# TBT-S Core Principles

TBT-S has five core principles derived from neurobiological research:

1. Eating disorders are brain and biologically based illnesses.
2. Treat to the trait or the temperament underpinnings.
3. Food is medicine.
4. Supports are a necessary part of the treatment process.
5. Action or movement is fundamental to change.

## Eating Disorders Are Brain and Biologically Based Disorders

TBT-S is grounded in the temperament based neurobiological etiological model of anorexia nervosa (AN) initially developed by Kaye et al.[35] and coined "When Good Traits Go Bad: Temperament and the Course of AN." This model, as shown in Figure 2.1, recognizes AN as a heritable illness with a strong genetic component.[6, 27, 28, 33, 63–66] Heritable risk is conferred through temperament traits that increase susceptibility to developing AN and also serve to maintain the illness. This neurobiological model has been updated to integrate findings from brain imaging studies showing altered function in brain systems regulating food intake in AN.

> Key Point: Temperament traits and altered brain responses inform the treatment targets of TBT-S, which include altered anxiety, interoception, reward and punishment sensitivity, decision-making, and cognitive or inhibitory control.

The updated neurobiological model shown in Figure 2.1 depicts that good traits can go bad, and then become good again. This is the TBT-S philosophy. More detail is provided in Chapter 9.

Approaching AN from a temperament based neurobiological perspective provides a biological foundation and conceptual framework from which to view symptoms and the underlying mechanisms that drive behavior. Temperament informs targeted interventions directed at the *cause of the behavior*, rather than the behavior itself. This is a paradigm shift for many. Treatment of AN has been thwarted by the lack of a mechanistic understanding of the disorder and recognition of the central role of temperament in its biological basis. This is similar to how treatments of medical illnesses (like diabetes) were ineffective until the underlying mechanisms (insulin production) were discovered. Similarly, by adopting a temperament based neurobiological etiological model of AN, the treatment emphasis shifts away from attempts to understand how behaviors developed and toward a focus on

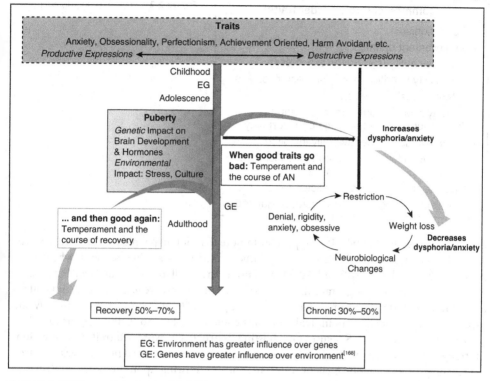

**Figure 2.1** TBT-S neurobiological model of AN

their *functional* impact to guide strategies to *redirect trait expressions* to achieve a reduction in eating disorder (ED) symptoms.

Key Point: TBT-S has emerged from a neurobiological model that identifies how "good" traits biologically shift to "bad" expressions and can become "good" again with trait-based intervention to promote recovery.

## Treat to the Trait: Targeting Temperament in Treatment

Individuals with AN often exhibit characteristic temperament traits (see Figure 2.2). Some AN traits are productive and serve as strengths throughout life. These traits can be utilized in the course of treatment to help clients manage destructive traits. For example, many persons with AN are highly achievement oriented, which is needed to reduce ED symptoms and accomplish recovery. On the other hand, some AN traits result from genetically induced altered neural circuit function that impacts the development and maintenance of the disorder. As indicated in the TBT-S neurobiological model, ultimately, the same traits that increase vulnerability to AN can be shifted from destructive expressions that exacerbate ED symptoms to productive expressions that become strengths in overcoming and maintaining a healthier

**Common eating disorder traits**

- Perfectionism
- Achievement oriented
- Obsessionality (symmetry, exactness)
- Sensitivity to criticism, punishment, mistakes
- Altered sensitivity to reward
- Anxiety, worry about what might happen (consequences), intolerance of uncertainty
- Harm avoidance, behaviorally inhibited
- Cognitive inflexibility, rule bound, difficulty with set shifting and decision-making
- Interoceptive awareness deficits
- Impulsive, emotionally reactive/dysregulated

**Figure 2.2** Common eating disorder traits

and more successful lifestyle. It is important to note that not all people with AN will identify with all of the traits associated with AN. Rather, these traits are like a menu, where most people with AN identify with at least a few, if not many or all, of these traits (see Figure 2.2). Rather than trying to change traits that are hardwired in the brain (e.g., it would be difficult for an introvert to naturally become an extrovert), the goal of "treat to the trait" is to identify and experientially explore how an individual's traits could contribute to their strengths to reduce their ED symptoms. TBT-S focuses on adjusting destructively expressed traits to expressions of strength by (a) clients experientially identifying their own trait-based productive responses, (b) teaching skills to endorse client solutions, and (c) drawing upon Supports' strategies to compensate for inherent difficulties.

The philosophy of TBT-S is to utilize "traits as strengths." Treatment modules and activities are specifically designed to target one or more of the destructive trait expressions and help clients realize how to shift them to strengths. This requires the clinician to adopt what may be a different framework for conceptualizing these traits as strengths. Table 2.1 provides an example of reconceptualizing traits as strengths and treatment strategies that are used when treating to the trait.

**Table 2.1** Reconceptualizing traits as strengths and strategies to treat to the trait

| Trait | Trait as strength (productively expressed) | TBT-S treatment strategy |
|---|---|---|
| Uncertainty Intolerance | Highly structured | • Structure treatment<br>• Structure meal plan<br>• Identify explicit rules |
| Altered sensitivity to reward/punishment | Motivated by having options/choices, planning, structure, and long-term goals | • Offer multiple options instead of open-ended questions<br>• Structure plans<br>• Contingency management/nonnegotiables |
| Obsessionality | High error detection<br>Attention to detail | • Specific, concrete rules<br>• Provide the details |

**Table 2.1** (cont.)

| Trait | Trait as strength (productively expressed) | TBT-S treatment strategy |
|---|---|---|
| Anxiety | Thinks about potential what-ifs, thinks through worst-case scenarios, ability to plan and prepare | • Redirect, re-attend<br>• Stop, reboot, reroute |
| Inhibition | Ability to delay gratification, cautious, and unlikely to impulsively enter into harmful situation | • Use long-term rewards and consequences via contingency management |

**Key Point: Traits can be expressed destructively or productively *and* clients can be taught to utilize their own traits as strengths throughout life.**

In discussing temperament, it is important to clarify differences between traits and symptoms, highlighted in Figures 2.3 and 2.4. Symptoms are thoughts, feelings, and behaviors that have become problematic, dysfunctional, or harmful for persons and/or those around them. They are often influenced by traits. For example, a person with a strong impulsive *trait* is more likely to develop a substance use disorder or engage in binge eating than a person with an inhibited trait, who is more likely to avoid eating. ED *symptoms*, such as food restriction, binge eating, purging, or excessive exercise, are behaviors that can and should be eliminated. Temperament and traits, however, *cannot* be eliminated.

**Symptoms**
• Are outward behavioral expressions
• Are indicators or reactions to illnesses
• Have the potential to be reduced and eliminated

**Traits**
• Are genetically programmed innate features
• Can be altered via *intentionally* shifting expressions
• Cannot be eliminated

**Figure 2.3** How traits relate to symptoms

| **Traits** | | **Symptoms** |
|---|---|---|
| Impulsive | Triggers | Binge Eating |
| Inhibited | | Restricts foods, activities |

**Figure 2.4** Example of trait impact on symptoms

**Key Point: Symptoms can be reduced or eliminated; traits are with us throughout life and vary in intensity.**

# Food Is Medicine

Drawing from a biological perspective, food is the natural and fundamental substance that "medicates" our bodies to be strong, healthy, and balanced. Food is energy. Like other ED treatments, TBT-S recognizes that appropriate nutrition and body composition stabilization are necessary and fundamental to recovery. To facilitate this, TBT-S includes comprehensive dietetic recommendations and meal plans "prescribed" by an ED dietitian.

The dietetic philosophy in TBT-S is that dosing energy for adults with AN is similar to dosing medicine. Clients and Supports attend dietary sessions and groups where they are "prescribed" foods and learn a meal plan tailored to the clients' needs alongside other basic dietary information. Biological tenets of TBT-S are woven into the dietary philosophy by prescribing a dietary approach that acknowledges core personality and temperament traits and the biologically based function of recommended foods. TBT-S emphasizes a highly structured meal plan in an effort to prioritize nutritional and weight rehabilitation in a way that honors the AN client's unique temperamental tendency toward structure and certainty.

Meal plans are organized to prioritize predictability and consistency. This can include adherence to highly scheduled meal and snack times and predictable (and, importantly, calorically sufficient) meals and snacks, among other things. In this way, the treatment prioritizes structure and certainty over flexibility and variety to cater to the clients' preferences for structure based on personality. TBT-S continues to acknowledge the need for dietary expansion, which may include incorporating additional foods or expanding food horizons in a variety of different ways. However, even this therapeutic endeavor toward variety is approached in a structured manner.

Alongside Supports and the dietary team, clients learn to plan out challenge foods in a structured format and, importantly, are the key stakeholders in deciding how and when, and even *if*, this therapeutic endeavor is undertaken. As such, TBT-S is unwavering in the need for abstinence from restriction and ensures that clients adopt and practice a meal plan that is calorically sufficient, includes major macronutrient groups, and upholds a more flexible approach with regard to variety. This allowance stems from acknowledging that the need for sameness and routine surrounding eating may be related to core personality styles and may in fact promote a more sustainable recovery practice in the long term. This structure and routine around meals compensate for altered interoception (e.g., altered hunger and/or satiety signaling that promotes food restriction or overeating, altered trust in body-related signals), decision-making (e.g., difficulty deciding what foods to eat), and reward sensitivity (e.g., reduced brain response for pleasure to motivate eating and affirm how much energy the body needs).

**Key Point: Food is framed as medicine for those with AN to integrate its biological purpose and "side effects" and is "prescribed" in a structured format that schedules food variety based on client traits.**

# Supports Are a Necessary Part of Treatment

TBT-S advocates that it is necessary to include Supports (spouses, parents, children of adult clients, roommates, partners, friends, colleagues, etc.) in the treatment process for adults of all ages. The term "Supports" was chosen at the request of clients participating in an open trial of TBT-S at The Center for Balanced Living in Ohio to reflect their preference for support rather than being cared for, which they believed the more common term "carer" connotes. TBT-S requires that a minimum of one Support person participate in treatment with each client in designated sessions. Family-based treatment (FBT) is the first-line treatment for adolescents with AN. It is effective because it teaches families strategies to understand, interact, and manage AN.[67–69] Similarly, TBT-S focuses on providing psychoeducation and skills training so that Supports learn about the causes of AN and effective ways to interact and manage symptoms.

Supports are appointed as part of the treatment team and are seen as an important asset to aid with recovery. The education, training, and practice that they receive in TBT-S sessions are intended to increase empathy and understanding by providing a biological understanding of AN and improving their ability to provide effective assistance. Supports in TBT-S sessions receive focused skills training on effective and age-appropriate assistance strategies that are practiced throughout the clients' treatment.

TBT-S takes the perspective that Supports play a critical role in recovery by providing accountability, assistance, leverage, and the potential to compensate for traits clients do not have. Supports learn tools that the client chooses as helpful to assist in the process of reducing ED symptoms. In addition to formal skills training, when TBT-S is offered in group settings, Supports also learn new skills by receiving feedback and consultation from both their loved one and other Supports, as part of the TBT-S group milieu. If TBT-S is offered in a 5-day program, upon completion, Supports are armed with what the adult clients deem to be the best practices for providing assistance, in the context of a biological and temperament perspective of the illness. TBT-S views clients as the experts. Experts, however, do not work and function alone.

> Key Point: A Support is any person who offers support/assistance in a client's life. Supports need the same information and tools as clients to offer consistency in reshaping altered trait expressions to promote recovery.

# Movement and/or Actions Are Fundamental to Change

TBT-S is a treatment of "doing." The tendency to be physically active is one of the first traits to be identified historically and is considered the most essential trait of one's temperament.[70] Behavioral change requires behavioral action. Learning occurs when "neurons that fire together, wire together."[50] Thus, our brains are fluidly flexible to change throughout life. The brain rewires through extensive practice of new ways of expression and behaviors, and TBT-S capitalizes on this through guiding *in vivo* practice of new skills during treatment. Clients and their Supports identify and practice the same phrases and actions that they have identified as helpful toward achieving a healthier lifestyle. Many of the TBT-S treatment interventions are movement driven; clients "try them on" to explore new behaviors that bring them closer to their goals. Active interventions are helpful because the brain learns through actions. Individuals are more likely to repeat what they have practiced. *In vivo* activities allow clients to refine their verbal and behavioral responses through corrective feedback via their own experience or from that of others. This iterative method of corrective feedback serves to enhance building new skills.

Movement is also needed to shift cognitive sets. Many ED behaviors represent rituals that have become automatic. Many individuals with AN have a trait-based tendency that causes their thoughts to become stuck on one topic. Movement can be used to interrupt destructive thoughts and behaviors to shift and move on to more productive thoughts and behaviors. TBT-S utilizes movement as a core part of the change process.

> **Key Point: TBT-S is an *active* intervention approach.**

> **Summary Key Point**
>
> TBT-S has five core principles that draw from neurobiological research to inform and direct treatment.

# Overview of TBT-S Intervention Strategies

## 3

TBT-S utilizes multiple intervention strategies to apply TBT-S principles. These strategies have been developed and adapted over a 10-year period through iteratively integrating client and Support feedback in the treatment development process to increase accuracy and acceptability. These intervention strategies follow:

1. Neurobiological Psychoeducation
2. Experiential Learning

    a. via Experiential Activities addressing (1) AN Neurobiology and Traits and (2) Problem Solving and Role of Supports
    b. via Multi-Family Therapy Activities (for Young Adult Version)

3. Client and Support Skills Training
4. Meal Coaching
5. Framework for Action via the Behavioral Agreement

## Neurobiological Psychoeducation

The primary goals of neurobiological psychoeducation are to educate clients and their Supports on relevant neurobiological constructs, temperament traits, and associated symptom expression and to provide a framework and rationale for TBT-S intervention strategies. In doing so, neurobiological psychoeducation serves as an intentional strategy to increase motivation for recovery and engagement in treatment, validate and reduce blame, and improve insight and awareness to inform skill use and drive behavior change. Psychoeducation materials include current genetic, neurobiological, and biological research findings that address causes of anorexia nervosa (AN) and introduce the neurobiologically based targets of treatment. These include the following temperament traits: anxiety, altered interoception, sensitivity to reward and punishment, inhibitory control, cognitive flexibility, and decision-making. This manual provides scripts to help clinicians communicate neurobiological research in a standardized manner without requiring that they independently become neuropsychologists. The manual describes relevant neurobiological information and key points for clinicians to share with clients and their Supports. The TBT-S handouts are designed to help clinicians therapeutically apply insights from neurobiological research. For example, see Appendix 1.

Key Point: Interactive psychoeducation identifies AN neurobiological underliers and offers a rationale for targeted interventions in a format all clinicians can utilize.

## Experiential Learning

TBT-S is a treatment of doing. This is accomplished through carefully constructed experiential activities and *in vivo* practice, conducted with clients, and Supports in various treatment formats. Learning by doing heightens retention of information and facilitates skill building. Practicing new skills and behaviors during treatment and developing solutions to problems rather than just talking about them increase the likelihood that clients and their Supports will continue to utilize the new skills and solutions in their daily lives.

## Experiential Activities

TBT-S includes a series of experiential activities that are designed to actively apply neurobiological information and elicit problem-solving strategies. They are intended to increase knowledge and empathy of eating disorder (ED) behaviors and motivate change. These clinician-led experiential TBT-S activities simulate AN experiences and temperament expressions through active metaphors to promote a better understanding of what it is like to live the illness, to experience and identify one's own traits, and to help clients and Supports identify and use methods congruent to their temperaments to solve problems. Using game-like approximations of their AN experiences is a less threatening and acceptable approach to help clients work through solutions and compensatory strategies that can be used to overcome and manage symptoms. Supports are included in the experiential activities sessions to learn about underlying causes and contributing factors of the illness at the *same time* as the clients. In addition, Supports are taught tools to develop skills that help their loved ones realize their potential outside of treatment and achieve success in symptom reduction.

> **Key Point:** Experiential treatment interventions provide frameworks for clients and their Supports to acknowledge and understand problems and explore solutions.

## Multi-Family Therapy (for Young Adult Version)

The Young Adult version of TBT-S includes approaches based on multi-family therapy (MFT), where multiple clients and their families are treated simultaneously in a group format. MFT has been shown to improve outcomes over single-family therapy.[71] In adult AN, family therapy shows promise.[71] Additionally, considerable evidence suggests that family interventions in adult mental health can be enhanced by using a multi-family treatment format[73–75] and is feasible in adult AN.[76, 77] MFT is a powerful approach because it can enhance learning and change among clients and their attending Supports because attendees have the benefit of learning from one another via sharing, feedback, modeling, and observation and comradery/group affiliation.

The Young Adult version of TBT-S considers the multi-family milieu as a powerful opportunity to enhance change and recovery. Multi-family activities are used to facilitate group cross-talk and sharing so that members have the opportunity to create a live assistance network consisting of others with lived experience. Exercises emphasize creating affiliation and relationships and, later, interfamily feedback and peer-to-peer consultation so that MFT group members have the opportunity to learn from one another. MFT strategies are described in Chapter 15.

Key Point: Multi-family therapy is a powerful treatment format that can enhance outcomes. TBT-S has been applied and tested in a multi-family format. The Young Adult version of TBT-S includes a variety of multi-family therapy activities.

# Client and Support Skills Training

Clients and Supports receive skills training to develop tools that can be used to reduce and manage symptoms and destructive or unhealthy trait expressions, such as obsessive pre-occupation with calories or food avoidance. Client coping skills focus on constructive, temperament-congruent strategies targeting symptom reduction. These include a variety of skills borrowed from other treatment modalities such as dialectical behavior therapy (DBT), as well as skills developed to target primary neurobiological targets such as anxiety and altered reward sensitivity. Supports receive training on effective tools to assist their loved one. These tools address a variety of factors that are common among Supports of individuals with AN, including tools that achieve a balance between providing emotional assistance and encouraging accountability. Support person skills also include a focus on developing effective communication, demonstrating client-identified effective responses to symptoms, reducing blame, increasing empathy, and managing Support burnout. In the 5-day program, clients and Supports are separated for skills training groups and receive training for effective management of ED symptoms in client-only or Support-only groups.

Key Point: Clients and Supports receive focused skills training that integrate their own traits into skills development to manage and reduce client eating disorder symptoms.

# Meal Coaching and Dietary Activities

As noted in the core principles, TBT-S emphasizes action as a central treatment component. Treatment encourages *in vivo* practice, including therapeutic meals in various treatment settings. Clients and Supports and/or TBT-S clinicians attend the meals throughout treatment. The dietitian provides feedback and coaching as necessary to navigate barriers to dietary success (See Chapter 20). The therapeutic meals may include the presence of ED behaviors such as restriction, skills deficits to manage anxiety and other challenging experiences, and/or client/Support conflict or ineffectiveness.

*In vivo* meal practice and observation are necessary and active treatment components. Clinicians and dietitians remain present to make an assessment of interventions and skills needed to increase success, and to observe client/Support patterns and any emerging problematic behaviors. The treatment team encourages clients and Supports to apply TBT-S skills learned during mealtimes and intervenes as necessary to ensure that clients and Supports alike are being skillful. Dietitians are also present to ensure that clients are practicing the prescribed meal plan. Clients are asked to make their meals and snacks, and dietitians "check off" on each meal and snack during treatment to ensure that they are adequate and to provide feedback, as necessary. Supports observe clients receiving feedback from dietitians. Additionally, they practice providing learned TBT-S assistance strategies as necessary during designated meals and snack sessions.

> Key Point: Eating within structures with active coaching allows adult clients and Supports to practice taking their "medicines" in "doses" and combinations to meet individual needs.

# Framework for Action via the Behavioral Agreement

During TBT-S, clients and their Support(s) develop a written Behavioral Agreement (BA) that establishes a mutually agreed upon framework for necessary action that the client has identified to achieve recovery. The Behavioral Agreement is a written document – a treatment plan – that includes daily commitments surrounding primary domains of recovery (such as eating or physical activity) and a detailed plan for Support involvement. There are two versions of the BA, the severe-and-enduring anorexia nervosa (SE-AN) and Young Adult (YA) versions. They take slightly different approaches addressing differing developmental stages and levels of Support involvement. The BAs are fundamental TBT-S clinician *and* client *and* Support structured tools to hold those with AN accountable and to develop and practice new client and Support skills. The BAs incorporate client temperaments to endorse congruence in client actions and client traits.

> Key Point: Behavioral Agreements are structured frameworks for treatment plans developed to align with AN temperaments.

> **Summary Key Point**
>
> TBT-S structures its interventions around Behavioral Agreements for young adults (YA BA) and those with severe-and-enduring anorexia nervosa (SE-AN BA) that integrate experiential learning, meal planning/coaching and skills training for clients and Supports.

# State of the Evidence Base for TBT-S

## Multi-Site Open Trial in YA and SE-AN Adults

The acceptability, feasibility, and possible benefits of the Adult Version of TBT-S were evaluated in a multi-center open trial administered in an intensive 5-day group format for adults with anorexia nervosa (AN) and their Supports conducted at the University of California San Diego Eating Disorders Treatment and Research Program and The Center for Balanced Living in Columbus, OH.[9] Each client was accompanied by at least one Support. Fifty-four adults with AN and 73 Supports received the 5-day treatment. Acceptability, feasibility, and attrition were measured posttreatment. Clinical outcome (body mass index [BMI], eating disorder (ED) psychopathology, family function) was assessed posttreatment and at >3-month follow-up. Results indicated the treatment had low attrition, with only one dropout due to medically needing a higher level of care.

Clients and Supports rated the intervention as highly acceptable, and clinicians reported good feasibility. At posttreatment, clients demonstrated significantly increased BMI, reduced ED psychopathology, and improved family function, in spite of the short amount of time that had passed. Benefits were maintained in the 39 clients who completed follow-up assessment, with 62 percent reporting full or partial remission. These preliminary results are encouraging and suggest this novel treatment is feasible and acceptable. To establish treatment efficacy, fully powered randomized controlled trials are necessary.

> Key Point: A 5-day, intensive group format of TBT-S has been evaluated in an open-trial design. Results suggest that the treatment is highly acceptable to both clients and Supports and may help reduce eating disorder symptoms.

## Single-Site Open Trial in YA AN

The acceptability, feasibility, and possible benefits of the Young Adult (YA) Version of TBT-S were evaluated in a single-site open trial administered in an intensive 5-day group format for young adults with an ED and their Supports conducted at the University of California San Diego Eating Disorders Treatment and Research Program.[9] Thirty-eight YA TBT-S participants ($m$ age = 19.58; SD 2.13) with anorexia nervosa (AN)–spectrum disorders (n = 24), bulimia nervosa (BN)–spectrum disorders (n = 8), and avoidant/restrictive food intake disorder (ARFID) (n = 6) participated in the trial. YA and Supports rated the treatment as highly acceptable with Client Satisfaction Questionnaire scores of 95.46/100 (YA) and 95.59/100 (Supports); 53.33 percent were in partial or full remission at 12-month follow-up.

Participants reported reductions in ED symptomatology (AN and BN), increases in BMI (AN and ARFID), and reductions in clinical impairment (AN and ARFID) at 12-month follow-up, suggesting that YA TBT-S may be an effective adjunctive treatment. Results endorse the Young Adult Version of TBT-S as a promising new treatment for young adults with restrictive eating disorders.

Key Point: Preliminary results of open trials of the SE-AN and Young Adult versions of TBT-S are promising and suggest this novel treatment is feasible and acceptable. To establish treatment efficacy, fully powered randomized controlled trials are necessary.

Summary Key Point

TBT-S has been studied in open trials to date. This book is the primary resource for TBT-S randomized controlled trials.

# How to Use This Manual

The manual is divided into four sections. Section 1 introduces clinicians to TBT-S, its fundamental philosophy and neurobiologically based principles upon which the treatment has been developed to augment other eating disorder (ED) therapies. Section 2 outlines the logistics to prepare for and apply TBT-S in multiple treatment settings. It describes the "how to" details for clinicians to initiate TBT-S with clients and prepare for inclusion of Supports at identified times. Many clinicians are not comfortable with including Supports in treatment. Strategies are offered to help provide focus and direction for client and Support interactions. TBT-S expands the treatment team to include the client as an expert of the illness, and Supports who know the client in unique ways. The clinician, dietitian, medical associate, and in many cases peer Supports are also a part of the treatment team. The actual and virtual settings for a multi-treatment team are described allowing clinicians to determine what space and resources are needed to provide TBT-S interventions. Section 3 details TBT-S treatment modules and activities, and Section 4 describes how TBT-S can be applied in various treatment settings and includes treatment schedules. Experiential TBT-S activities and client and Support handouts are provided in the Appendices.

As stated in the Introduction, TBT-S is a modular treatment that augments ongoing eating disorder therapies. Modules include temperament based psychoeducation, skills/tools, experiential activities, and Behavioral Agreements for young adults (YA) and adults with severe-and-enduring anorexia nervosa (SE-AN). Modules are like building blocks; one or more modules can be added into the ED treatment series at all levels of care, virtually or face-to-face. Module application could range from incorporating one module in treatment, to once a week, to delivering one full week of TBT-S. While most of the modules could be offered to clients individually, TBT-S strongly encourages including Supports in treatment for AN for adults of all ages. Clinicians choose the modules based on clinical presentation, concerns or treatment topics being addressed. The studied TBT-S program consisted of 40 hours of modules, back-to-back in a one-week period of time (see YA and SE-AN TBT-S one-week schedules in Chapter 24).

| Section and Summary Key Point |
| --- |
| This manual offers ED clinicians neurobiologically based modules to augment their treatment. |

Chapter

# 6 How to Introduce the Biological Bases of Eating Disorders at Initial Engagement

*Do you tend to experience little to no pleasure when eating a new food?* (Indicative of altered ventral striatal response.)

*Do you tend to act on an impulse* (impulsive trait) *or hold back* (avoidance trait) *when faced with new foods or social situations?*

Introducing eating disorders (ED) as brain-based illnesses during session one is ground zero. Assessing an adult client's temperament simultaneously with ED symptoms frames the illness within its biological structure. Evaluating traits during the initial assessment permits clinicians to discover temperament tendencies that sketch who the client is while identifying what the client's ED behaviors are. Integrating neurobiological information and trait-based questions with ongoing diagnostic assessment questions introduces adult clients to the biological underpinnings of their behavioral symptoms. Adult clients with severe-and-enduring anorexia nervosa (SE-AN) report that this approach is a game changer for them. Assessment becomes balanced by integrating inside-out trait bases with outside-in observed behavioral ED symptoms. Temperament frames what is possible for long-term cognitive and behavioral changes.

When clients are in crisis, it is indicative that their biological, psychological, and/or interpersonal assistance structures have collapsed. Crisis initiates the opportunity to introduce neurobiological explanations for ED symptoms with both young adults (YA) with AN and SE-AN clients. Realizing why their ED symptoms developed and have persisted from a temperament perspective removes unnecessary guilt that their illness is their choice. ED are not a choice. For example, administering the Trait Profile Checklist (Appendix 2) presents the opportunity for clients to recognize and reorganize their chaotic symptom expressions into a "good-fit" structure that utilizes clients' traits to transform symptoms.

Introducing temperament bases for AN and other EDs during assessments or crises or other times in therapy when new information could be introduced, can take place in all levels of care and formats:

- Outpatient therapy whether in one-on-one or group settings.
- Intensive outpatient treatment program groups (IOP).
- Partial day hospital program (PHP) assessments.
- Five-day, 40-hour TBT-S program. We refer to this format as "5-day TBT-S Program."

A temperament based approach can be "seasoned" throughout ongoing therapies at all levels of care starting with the first session. If attending a 5-day TBT-S Program, temperament-based neurobiological information is explained, tools/skills taught and practiced, and a Behavioral Agreement established by both adult clients and their Supports (friends, spouse, family, etc.) over 40 hours in one week. It serves to jump-start and recalibrate YA and SE-AN clients in understanding the biological nature of the illness and treats to the client's traits. TBT-S skills could continue to develop as clinicians integrate a temperament approach in day hospital through outpatient therapy settings.

The first treatment session, at all levels of care, holds a time for change that is new, yet fleeting, filled with potential regardless of whether clients are in crisis or enter therapy with less chaotic symptom expressions. The initial session is open to possibilities of innovative change. It is important not to waste these key moments.

### Introducing Temperament into an SE-AN Outpatient Assessment Session Script

*I am going to ask you questions about your symptoms, which seem to have triggered you to come to treatment.*

*You shared on your questionnaire that you eat* ... (insert clinician's summary of the client's responses to what, where and when they eat throughout the day). *Is there anything I said that is inaccurate?*

*Research is finding that* ... (insert a neuropsychological findings such as one of the ten research points summarized in Appendix 1).

*You have tendencies that are biologically based traits.* (Insert eating disorder traits the clinician is observing as the client responds to initial questions.) *Traits are lifelong but can vary in how they are expressed over time. Right now, some of your traits are working for you and others against you triggering your eating disorder symptoms. I suspect you actually feel better when you express your eating disorder symptoms. Is that in any way true for you?*

*The good news is that knowing why things go awry and what traits you have, opens the door for us to explore how you can work around the 'potholes' of problems. While you can't shed your traits, you can shift their expressions making them solutions for your symptoms.*

---

**Summary Key Point**

The first therapy session, or the beginning of a new treatment segment, holds the unique opportunity to introduce neurobiological underpinnings of identified ED symptoms while identifying client traits that can impact long-term change.

# How to Engage Supports in Treatment

## Introducing Supports at the Beginning of Treatment

Session one is the opportunity for new possibilities. It is an ideal session to introduce the need for ongoing support persons, referred to as "Support" (the "S" in TBT-S) for both young adults (YA) with anorexia nervosa (AN) and adults with severe and enduring AN (SE-AN), to enhance short- and long-term change. Adult clients may have many Supports who want to help and do not know how. Supports influence adult clients whether the client likes it or not. Acknowledging this dynamic during an initial session introduces the importance of including Supports while treatment plans are being established. This allows the clinician to include Supports with the client when providing information and skills/tools that the client identifies as needed. Adult clients working solo to reduce eating disorder (ED) symptoms in treatment is like swimming upstream. It may be possible for a short period of time, but exhaustion, becoming overwhelmed by social, work, and home currents contribute to clients drowning in their ED symptoms. The biological stream flows against clients as they try to reduce ED symptoms. If Supports are *not* brought into the therapeutic stream, the current could be intensified by Supports responding in unhelpful ways, preventing the adult client from making better progress. When Supports learn how to swim with the client, progress can improve exponentially.

Supports are typically present when there is a crisis. However, including Supports in outpatient therapy for adults is rare due to developmental models that promote individuation for persons entering adulthood. However, interdependency, although often ignored, is considered an ultimate stage of female adult development, both psychologically and interpersonally.[183] For those with AN, interdependency outweighs individuation.

However, many SE-AN clients have "burned their bridges" with family members and friends. Supports such as parents, spouses, and close friends may have become exhausted and disappointed that their help had not resulted in symptom reduction for their loved ones. Guilt often reigns, a feeling they should have done more, with no energy remaining to invest time and resources in additional treatment.

In addition, outpatient clinicians who provide one-on-one therapy often exclude Supports due to training, preference, and systemic structures. Adult clients with ED *often prefer one-on-one therapy*, seeking a more isolated setting that could enable AN avoidance tendencies. The interpersonal dynamic in one-on-one therapy forces the clinician to hold the support role. This prevents needed backup assistance outside of therapy. If at least one Support is not identified to be a part of identified treatment sessions, outside assistance may be based on uninformed ED myths and lack of clarity on what to do. It works against the client.

> **Key Point:** Introduce the need for Supports during session one when the opportunity is ripe to actualize interdependency, consistency, and biological information inside and outside of treatment.

## Including Supports in Treatment Segments

Including Supports in identified portions of treatment is a core principle of TBT-S. While resistance to include Supports is usually present, it is recommended that clinicians set the expectation that including Support(s) is required and continue moving forward, asking questions that help the client identify one or more people who could offer assistance in various ways. Possible Supports may not be obvious to clients, especially those with SE-AN. Clinicians could expand questions to a wider range of interpersonal connections and geographical areas, to identify at least one Support. Supports look different for different people. For example, the client may need a Support to talk with, another Support to eat with during specified times, or a Support to walk or do an action together virtually or face-to-face. In addition, Supports may offer financial, emotional, and accountability assistance.

During the initial session in a segment of treatment, the clinician sets a date to have a Support(s) identified. If a date is not set, the inclusion of Supports can be avoided or delayed endlessly. If the need for Supports is introduced in the second or third session, the "cement has begun to dry" with resistance hardening, making it exceedingly difficult to shift perspectives. The clinician determines which sessions to include Supports based upon when relevant neurobiological psychoeducation, treatment planning as a part of a Behavioral Agreement (BA), and teaching skills/tools will be introduced. Temperament based interventions are active when both adult clients and Supports are learning, practicing, and revising their skills together.

For young adults, clinicians should attempt to engage their parents and/or other members of their family of origin during initial sessions in treatment. Like older adults, YAs may be reluctant to do this because they are expecting individual treatment. It is important that clinicians orient YAs to treatment by informing them that their parents will be included in *aspects* of treatment focused on providing education on the brain basis of AN and learning ways to help. It is important that YAs are educated on the nature of parent involvement in the TBT-S method, especially if the YA is reluctant or has a history of family-involved treatment during their younger years.

Clinicians can emphasize that parent involvement does not replace individual treatment; instead, it serves to augment the process. It is also important to emphasize that parents will be brought in to be educated on the causes and effects of eating disorders and learn ways to assist the client based on the YA's instruction and feedback, thus maintaining the YA as an expert and key decision-making agent in treatment. Orienting the client to the parent-involved model *while also* making parental involvement nonnegotiable will set the YA up for success and establish expectations for parent involvement.

Virtual therapy has become the new norm for outpatient levels of care. Having Supports present virtually for both YA and SE-AN clients, from multiple locations during specified sessions is easier than when all outpatient sessions were in-person. This offers new opportunities to include Supports that may not live close to the client.

Key Point: One or more Supports are identified in the first few sessions of treatment to learn neurobiological information and participate in designated sessions that address treatment goals and skills development to promote consistency outside of treatment.

### Identifying Supports and Explaining Why Supports Are Needed in AN Treatment Script

*"I am going to ask you questions about those with whom you interact at work, home, your family and virtually. Sometimes those we feel closest to are those who live farther away."*

*"You may have burned some bridges with different friends or family members. Do you feel close to anyone at this time? With whom do you communicate even if it is not frequently, or whether they live close or far away?"*

*"It takes two of us to establish a treatment process. You need me to explain the biological nature of your illness and your traits to help you better manage or reduce your ED symptoms. I cannot be your Support outside of treatment. At least one person is needed for a period of time to hold that role. I can help you during sessions and the Support person can learn and practice tools with you and me during specified sessions to assist you outside of the therapy sessions."*

## How to Ask Supports to Join the Adult Client in Designated Sessions

The clinician should matter-of-factly *move forward*, just as a physician may instruct a patient to ask a family member or friend to come daily to the hospital to walk with the client to increase movement after heart surgery. The clinician moves through client hesitancy and avoidant tendencies by first stating that it is important to include a Support person in designated sessions. Then asking how (not if) the client wants to invite the Support(s) to join them in the identified therapy sessions. If the client does not know how to ask their Support(s) to be a part of identified treatment sessions, the clinician moves forward by offering structured questions with two-to-three options. See the Script that follows.

Supports are often more motivated than the adult clients to participate in treatment to learn what to do, versus continuing to guess and find their actions are ineffective. The TBT-S approach advocates that adult clients and Supports identify what they need from one another in joint sessions to ensure information, goals, and tools are consistent. (See Behavioral Agreements in Appendices 6 and 26.)

Key Point: A key time for change to occur is when something commences, such as the first treatment session, or the beginning of a new segment of treatment. This becomes the opportunity for the clinician to work with the adult client to identify, invite and then include needed Support.

### How to Ask Supports to Join the Client in Designated Sessions Script

The following is a suggested *script* to which clinicians can refer when inviting Supports into treatment. Clinicians are encouraged to offer multiple-choice questions, instead of open-ended questions, to respond empathically to AN temperament.

*"Every client has different ways to invite Supports to participate in therapy. It is not easy, but necessary, just as it is not easy to reduce ED symptoms, but it is necessary.*

*I'll offer some options. You may have ideas to add. The only option that doesn't work is to not ask."*

*"What do you think about texting, or emailing, or directly asking each Support?*

*If they ask questions that you cannot answer, I will be glad to set up a joint phone meeting to answer their questions. I think it would help if you listen in and add your own questions and comments, so all information goes through you."*

*"Here are some scheduled times I can offer for a phone meeting. Will you agree to make contact and request that they join us for a phone Q and A?"*

---

**Summary Key Point**

TBT-S encourages clinicians to move forward through client resistance by setting a structure and use 2–3 options, instead of open-ended questions when addressing how to ask Supports to join them in designated treatment sessions.

# Nuts and Bolts of TBT-S

## Who Is Involved in the TBT-S Treatment Team, and What Are Their Roles?

TBT-S mirrors multidisciplinary eating disorder (ED) research by utilizing a multidisciplinary treatment team. The ED treatment team is traditionally composed of a primary clinician (often a clinician or psychologist), a dietitian, and a medical professional. TBT-S brings the recipients of treatment, the client and their Supports, into the treatment team, recognizing their unique roles and critical input for effective progress and change over time.

The TBT-S treatment team is expanded from other ED approaches by including the adult client and their Support(s). Figure 8.1 describes the team members and their roles. Table 8.1 shows the relationship among team members.

Key Point: The TBT-S treatment team acknowledges the adult client as the expert, and at least one Support with the clinician, dietitian, a medical professional, and at times a psychiatrist.

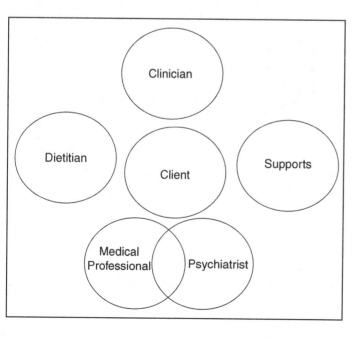

**Figure 8.1** Treatment team

**Table 8.1** TBT-S treatment team members and roles

| Team member | Role |
| --- | --- |
| Primary Clinician | • Implements TBT-S core principles and treatment components such as experiential activities and skill development.<br>• Introduces and frames treatment around client temperament and the neurobiological underpinnings of the illness.<br>• Forges forward when the client may want to hold back.<br>• Coordinates Behavioral Agreements for young adults (YA BA) and severe-and-enduring adults with anorexia nervosa (SE-AN BA). |
| Dietitian | • Establishes the meal plan with the adult client.<br>• Includes Supports in designated meal practice and dietary Q and A sessions.<br>• Approaches food as medicine, recognizing that foods have "side effects" in the AN brain that increase anxiety and "noise" (constant ED thoughts) that provoke body image disturbances. See Chapter 20 on "TBT-S Strategic Dietary Approach." |
| Psychiatrist | • Administers psychiatric evaluation.<br>• Provides psychiatric follow-up for those prescribed medications. |
| Medical professional | • Evaluates the physical stability of the client with ED.<br>• Establishes a baseline of the body systems such as cardiac, electrolyte and blood levels, renal function, and hormonal levels.<br>• Evaluates body mass.<br>• At times one professional holds both psychiatric and medical professional roles. |
| Adult client | • Core member of the treatment team.<br>• Expert on the experience of their illness, knowing what has worked, and what has not worked.<br>• Holds keys to solutions brought forth through their temperament. |
| Support(s) | • May be the spouse, parents, sibling, children of the client, grandparents, aunts, coworkers, friends living near or far, pastor, etc.<br>• Contribute their expertise to inform decisions based on their knowledge and experience of the client. |

# Where TBT-S Treatment Takes Place

A TBT-S approach could be implemented face-to-face in treatment settings or virtually ranging from outpatient to day-hospital levels of care. Open trial studies have been conducted in-person for the TBT-S 5-day program, showing significant impact for both the Young Adult (YA) and Severe-and-Enduring Anorexia Nervosa (SE-AN) versions.[9] See Chapter 9 for details on how to apply TBT-S in diverse settings.

> Key Point: TBT-S could be applied in all levels of care from outpatient to partial hospital levels of care. It has been studied in open trials on a 5-day, 40-hour treatment program both virtually and face-to-face.

# Food Considerations

The TBT-S model advocates that meal plans are developed by the dietitian and adult client with a Support present to listen and ask questions. The structure to approach food and food considerations is identified by the client and dietitian using the Young Adult Behavioral Agreement (YA BA) or the Severe-and-Enduring Anorexia Nervosa Behavioral Agreement (SE-AN BA) with the Support person participating during invited sessions. The Behavioral Agreements are structured to incorporate anorexia nervosa and other eating disorder traits into the process to enhance working with clients' temperaments, not against them.

Eating meals and snacks is a part of TBT-S treatment at all levels of care. Change is achieved through the act of eating together, not simply talking about food intake. TBT-S encourages Supports and the clinician and dietitian to eat *with* the adult client during treatment so the client and Supports practice together during therapy to work through problems and influence more success outside of the therapy setting. The client and Supports learn, observe, and practice dietary recommendations from the dietitian who assesses and coaches them on food combinations and portion sizes. During designated sessions, the clinician and/or Supports observe the client working with the dietitian with whom the client asks questions to monitor meal portions during ongoing treatment and outside of therapy. TBT-S recommends that dietitians align recommendations with the client's temperament when making dietary suggestions.

> Key Point: Dietitians acknowledge and work *with* a client's traits and include Supports when making dietary recommendations on food combinations, accessibility, and preparation to restore and maintain a healthy body strength.

# How TBT-S Meals Are Conducted at All Levels of Care

If treatment is provided in face-to-face settings, adult clients and their Supports bring their "prescribed" food combinations and prepare recommended portion sizes during meal treatment sessions. Prepackaged meals are often utilized on site for meals or snacks during treatment sessions. This could occur in outpatient (OP), intensive outpatient (IOP), or partial day hospital (PHP) level of care.

TBT-S advocates that every aspect of food intake is repeatedly practiced during and outside of treatment. The clinician may allocate one or more sessions in OP treatment over a specified period of time for meal/snack procedures to be practiced and productive habits initiated. New actions stimulate the brain to rewire the new responses. Meal sessions are initially refined with dietitian recommendations. The client and Support experiment to make the process efficient. When food intake occurs during the IOP level of care, a portion of the time is spent preparing and eating the foods, and another portion of the treatment addresses TBT-S and other ongoing ED therapeutic interventions. In a PHP level of care or the 5-day TBT-S Program, meals and snack times are scheduled and interspersed daily with other TBT-S interventions that include neurobiological psychoeducation, Behavioral Agreement development, experiential problem-solving activities, and skills/tools training. See Chapter 20 for dietary strategies.

If treatment is conducted virtually, it allows food access, preparation, and consumption to be practical and *in vivo*. It promotes productive habit formation by allowing clients to be in their home and work settings. Due to the COVID pandemic, internet capabilities have expanded for all treatment team members. Now the clinician can come to the client's setting instead of the client to the clinician's office or treatment setting. Food does not have to be carted into treatment settings. Clinicians, dietitians, and Supports are now better able to eat in different settings simultaneously with the adult client.

The clinician and dietitian can work with the client virtually, at home or work. Supports may virtually shop for groceries with the client or eat together in different settings. Access to and preparation of foods become *in vivo* interventions whether with the Supports, dietitian, or clinician.

---

**Section and Summary Key Point**

TBT-S face-to-face or virtually advocates that food intake is practiced with Supports during designated treatment sessions at all levels of care to stimulate brain rewiring of productive habit formation.

# TBT-S Treatment Modules

Temperament Based Therapy with Support (TBT-S) is made up of modules. A module is a distinct unit of treatment that can be combined with other, interrelated modules to create a program, or it can be selected singularly and inserted into a different treatment to augment ongoing eating disorder (ED) treatment approaches. TBT-S modules include (a) psychoeducation, (b) experiential activities (which are subdivided into experiential neurobiological training and problem-solving activities, and multi-family therapy activities), (c) skills training and tools, (d) dietary TBT-S strategies, and (e) Behavioral Agreements. Modules are like building blocks. Clinicians can choose which modules to insert into their ongoing treatment approach and when.

As explained in Chapter 4, TBT-S has been studied in open trials, applying selected modules back-to-back over 1 week for 40 hours (see also Chapter 24).[9, 78, 79] There is amazing power and momentum to this treatment format, having clients and Supports work together hour after hour over 1 week. However, many clinicians cannot provide a multi-day treatment. TBT-S has been designed so that clinicians can choose TBT-S modules based on factors such as (a) intent to include selected ED neurobiological psychoeducational information, (b) level of care, (c) clinicians' treatment approach, (d) individual or group settings, (e) the introduction of interactive problem-solving interventions, (f) practicing tools and skills, and (g) method of delivery such as virtual or face-to-face.

TBT-S modules have a wide range of variation. For example, combining TBT-S modules in a 3- to 5-day TBT-S program, selecting modules to insert into segments of outpatient weekly therapy (OP), intensive outpatient programs (IOP), or partial hospital programs (PHP) and ED residential programs. Chapters 9–23 describe the TBT-S modules, with detailed application instructions in Appendices 1–28. For example, a TBT-S Behavioral Agreement Module could be inserted into a specific number of outpatient weekly therapy sessions, or it could be incorporated into ED programs' treatment planning sessions at all levels of care.

> **Key Point:** TBT-S incorporates neurobiologically based modules as the treatment format to augment ongoing ED therapies at all levels of care.

**Chapter**

# How to Deliver Neurobiology Psychoeducation as a Motivational Strategy

**9**

### Neurobiological and Trait Targets

- Motivation

## Objective

The purpose of the Neurobiology Psychoeducation Modules is to provide research evidence on anorexia nervosa (AN) as a neurobiological and brain-based disorder. This evidence provides the neurobiological foundation, framework, and rationale for the neurobiologically based intervention strategies that have evolved into a novel treatment approach called Temperament Based Therapy with Support (TBT-S).

Its specific goals follow:

- Introduce and provide educational information on relevant neurobiological constructs, temperament traits, and associated symptom expression.
- Offer a biologically based reason for hope and increase motivation for recovery.
- Motivate engagement in treatment.
- Validate client/Support experience and reduce self/other blame.
- Improve client/Support insight and awareness of their own destructive/productive trait expression to inform skill use.

The Neurobiology Psychoeducation Modules are organized by neurobiological and temperament targets that are specifically addressed with temperament based interventions. Clinicians can provide these modules whenever deemed appropriate. This manual includes four psychoeducation modules addressing the primary neurobiological targets of TBT-S: (a) Neurobiological Overview, (b) Anxiety and Interoception, (c) Reward and Punishment Processing, and (d) Decision-Making and Cognitive Control.

## Who Is Involved

These psychoeducation modules are designed to be shared with clients and/or their Supports in a range of settings, including outpatient individual and group settings through higher levels of care, to educate clients and/or their Supports on the neurobiological underpinnings of AN. Delivering psychoeducation in group settings offers the advantage of fostering discussion and sharing of experiences and knowledge among group members to facilitate communication and shared understanding.

## What Is Needed

It is helpful to provide visual aids, either via handouts or a formal presentation (e.g., PowerPoint presentation), that may necessitate a computer, monitor, screen, and/or projector. Some visual aids are provided in Chapters 10–13 and the Appendices.

## Content

Content for each module on specific neurobiological constructs and traits is provided in the following chapters.

## What Does the Research Say?

Several studies show benefits of providing psychoeducation to clients, their family members, and the community.[80–82] Importantly, this research suggests that psychoeducational messages emphasizing "malleable biology" and "cognitive-behavioral factors" tend to produce more optimism and self-efficacy in recovery, and perceived credibility of therapy compared with "biologically reductionist" messages that communicate that one's psychological and emotional experience is nothing more than the result of brain or biological functions.[81–85] In anxious individuals, biologically based psychoeducation has also been shown to reduce self-blame.[86]

However, clinicians should also be aware that studies have identified factors associated with poor outcomes following psychoeducation. These include psychoeducation that takes an overly narrow and reductionist biological etiological stance, and psychoeducation that is delivered solely via written text or recorded videos or involves assigning educational materials individually or online.[87, 88]

To maximize benefits, TBT-S psychoeducation is designed to be conducted by a clinician during a therapeutic session with clients and/or Supports, encouraging questions and discussion, generating real-life examples, and providing validation of the clients' experiences. TBT-S emphasizes neurobiological malleability and neuroplasticity. The brain can be re-wired through behavioral practice and skill use to manage AN traits and move toward recovery. As such, TBT-S psychoeducation modules are used to increase understanding and motivation for recovery, validate client experience when clinicians encourage clients to compare their own experiences with research evidence, reduce Support blame and criticism, and gain trust of and commitment to the TBT-S therapeutic interventions. Clients report this increases their motivation to change their eating disorder (ED) symptoms.

## Psychoeducation Module Instructions

Neurobiological psychoeducation in TBT-S is designed to be delivered in an informal interactive lecture-style format. The content is included in the following chapters. The clinician role is to engage discussions about individual experiences and knowledge in relation to the research findings. This provides an opportunity for the clinician to correct misunderstandings about ED such as inaccurate beliefs about the causes of AN (e.g., AN is a choice or the parents' fault) and misattributions of the function of ED behaviors (e.g., food refusal is willful). This is best done by the clinician sharing the research findings objectively and validating client/Support experiences. The clinician can highlight the damage that misinformation causes (e.g., blame, stigma). This also serves to position the client as expert (consistent with TBT-S philosophy) and facilitates open communication regarding knowledge and beliefs about AN to align understanding and improve the client-Support relationship.

Clinician techniques and *scripts* (in italics) that can be used with all psychoeducation modules follow:

1. Clinicians are encouraged to ask questions of the client and Support or group members to facilitate discussion and sharing of experiences.
   - *How do these findings compare with your own experience?*
   - *Can you relate to these findings? How or what specifically resonates with your experience? What does not resonate for you?*
   - *Is there an example in your life that reflect these findings?*

2. Clinicians solicit questions to tailor information to the specific needs and interests of the clients/Supports.
   - *How does this make sense, or not make sense to you?*
   - *Do you have any questions about what has been covered today?*
   - *What is your take-home message of this information in relation to your experience?*

3. Clinicians acknowledge when they do not know an answer to a question.
   - Full transparency is modeled by clinician authenticity and scientific humility. This builds trust and fosters collaboration between clinicians and clients/Supports.
   - Clinicians do not need to be experts in neurobiology to share neurobiological research findings. Research is constantly growing.
   - This manual provides basic neurobiological information informing the TBT-S approach. It is not exhaustive. If a clinician does not know an answer, then the answer is, *I will look into that and find out.*
   - A handout on Ten Biological Facts about Anorexia Nervosa is provided in Appendix 1. The reference list at the end of the book may be helpful for clinicians who would like to take a deeper dive into the scientific literature to share with clients/Supports.

4. Clinicians are encouraged to acknowledge limits to existing research and validate when the study findings do not match with an individual's experience. If the clinician is sharing research findings that they have read independently of the findings reported in this manual, study limitations should be acknowledged. The findings described in this manual take the limitations into account. Some common research limitations include the following:
   - Results report averages across people in the study. It is expected that individual client experiences may vary from the average findings reported.
   - Many studies include a small number of clients in a homogenous group that is not representative of the clients who are present for treatment. For example, many studies are expected to not include clients who have comorbid diagnoses, when in reality most clients have comorbid diagnoses such as depression, anxiety disorders, trauma history, or substance abuse.
   - Some studies do not differentiate between AN-restricting type and AN–binge purge type.
   - Studies may address people at different states of illness (e.g., malnourished, weight-restored but symptomatic, recovered), which can impact results.

5. Clinicians use neurobiological research as a foundation to engender hope that recovery is possible

  - Clinicians validate that treatment is difficult, and that clients may feel counter to what they want to feel, due to their biological predisposition.
  - *You have to work harder than people who don't have eating disorders to eat in a healthier way. It is counter to the way you are hardwired. Your brain signals are telling you not to eat, yet the best way to re-wire your brain is through practice of eating specified foods. You are swimming upstream and you are stronger by doing so.*

**Summary Key Points**

- Research indicates that providing biologically informed psychoeducation is beneficial to clients and their families.
- Psychoeducation that communicates that biology both contributes to AN and that biology can change to promote recovery is more effective than messages that only focus on the causative role of biology.
- TBT-S uses interactive psychoeducation as an interventional strategy to increase motivation for treatment and recovery, validate client/Support experience, reduce stigma and blame, and raise awareness of the role of temperament and neurobiology in maintaining eating disorder symptoms.

# 10 TBT-S Neurobiology Psychoeducation Module
## Overview of the Neurobiology of Anorexia Nervosa

**Neurobiological and Trait Targets**
- Overview of the Neurobiological and Temperament Model of AN

## Objective

The purpose of the Overview of the Neurobiology of Anorexia Nervosa (AN) Psychoeducation Module is to introduce clients and/or Supports to the scientific evidence that describes AN as a neurobiological and brain-based disorder, and to establish how that information can be placed within the neurobiological treatment framework of TBT-S. This module introduces the neurobiological concepts that have informed the TBT-S interventions.

### When Is This Module Provided

This module could be applied any time the clinician or treatment program decides is best during the treatment process. It is recommended that the educational module precede a temperament based intervention skill or experiential activity so that clients can understand how the research applies or does not apply to their own lives. In the 5-day TBT-S Programs that were studied, this overview was the first psychoeducation module applied.

### Who Is Involved

This module can be offered to clients only and/or Supports only, individually or in a group. It was tested in a 5-day, 40-hour format with a group of clients and their Supports to foster discussion and sharing of experiences among the group.

### What Is Needed

It is helpful to provide visual aids, either via handouts or a formal presentation (e.g., PowerPoint presentation) during this module. This may necessitate a computer, monitor, screen, and/or projector. Some visual aids are provided in this chapter and the Appendices.

# Content

The following six talking points and additional evidence are offered for clinicians to share with clients and Supports. Clinician scripts (which can be said verbatim) and notes are provided to help guide discussion.

## Point 1: AN Has a Genetic Basis [23, 25, 49, 65, 89–91]

1. Family studies show an increased rate of eating disorders in first degree relatives; for example, females who have a relative with AN are 11 times more likely to develop AN than those without a relative with AN.
2. Twin studies indicate approximately 50 percent to 80 percent of the risk of developing an eating disorder is due to heredity.
3. Genome-wide association studies (GWAS) identified genetic correlations in AN with psychiatric disorders, physical activity, and metabolic function, suggesting a reconceptualization of AN as a "metabo-psychiatric" disorder. (See Ten Biological Facts about Anorexia Nervosa, Appendix 1.)

### Clinician *Scripts*

It is useful for the clinician to pose questions at the beginning of the module, before discussing Point 1, to help the clinician gauge the level of knowledge of the clients and/or Supports, and to set the stage for facilitating dialogue.

The primary goal of this discussion is to bring awareness to the detrimental effects of misinformation regarding the cause of AN (e.g., stigma, blame, invalidation, lack of funding for research to better understand the illness), and to appreciate the utility of viewing AN from a biological lens (e.g., reduce stigma and blame, validate experience, inform targets of treatment).

- *In your understanding, what causes anorexia nervosa?*
- *What are some societal and family messages about the causes of anorexia nervosa?*
- *What are some myths about the cause of anorexia nervosa?*
- *What is a benefit to viewing anorexia nervosa through a medical or biological lens?*

After presenting the material, the clinician may ask the following questions:

- *How do these findings compare with your experience?*
- *What is a bottom-line message you have learned that explains viewing anorexia nervosa through a medical or biological lens?*

### Notes for the Clinician

- People are increasingly familiar with the biological basis of AN.
- It can be helpful to question the sources of clients' and Supports' responses to obtain a broad sense of their level of understanding.
- Other common responses include sociocultural influences and the need for control. The neurobiological research finds that while sociocultural influences may contribute to the onset of AN and contribute to maintaining disordered eating,

social media messages and pressures and culture alone are not likely to be a sufficient cause of AN.

- Most people in industrialized societies are exposed to the "thin ideal" messaging in society and most people have tried and failed to diet. This suggests there is something unique about those who develop eating disorders.
- TBT-S incorporates scientific data that have consistently found that a biologically determined vulnerability increases susceptibility to developing AN.
- Viewing AN through a biological lens reduces blame and stigma associated with the misconception that AN is a choice.

# Point 2: Role of Temperament in AN [30, 32, 37–40, 92–95]

1. Genes cause childhood (premorbid) traits that are thought to make someone more susceptible to developing an eating disorder.
2. Traits that are common in childhood in individuals who later developed AN include
   - Perfectionism
   - Achievement oriented
   - Obsessionality
   - Sensitivity to criticism, punishment, errors (high error detection)
   - Altered sensitivity to reward
   - Anxiety, anticipatory anxiety (worry about what might happen; consequences), intolerance of uncertainty
   - High harm avoidance (cognitive inflexibility, inhibition, anxiety)
   - Difficulty with set shifting and decision-making, rule bound
   - Impulsive, emotionally reactive/dysregulated

### Clinician *Scripts*

To introduce Point 2 material:

- To all: *What temperament or personality traits are common in anorexia nervosa?*
- To parents (in YA version): *Do you share any of these traits?*
- To parents (in YA version): *Did your child exhibit any of these traits as children, before the eating disorder?*
- To Supports (in SE-AN version): *Can you see any of these traits in the client? How do you see them to be expressed?*
- To clients (in YA and SE-AN versions): *Can you give examples of how these traits play out in your lives?*

  After presenting Point 2 material (in SE-AN version):
- *I would like you to take the Trait Profile Checklist. (See Appendix 2.)*
- *What traits have you identified on the Trait Profile Checklist that are on the List of Common AN Traits handout?*
- *Which of your traits are productive? Which of your traits are you currently expressing destructively?*

**Notes for the Clinician**

It is common for individuals to identify with one or more of the traits listed earlier or on the Trait Profile Checklist handout.

- It is important to note that this is a list of common traits, and not everyone experiences all of these traits.
- It is also important to validate when clients indicate that they do not identify with certain traits. Use the opportunity to solicit additional information about the traits they identified during discussion or on the Trait Profile Checklist to inform treatment modifications tailored to the clients' trait profiles.
- Asking whether these traits are currently being expressed "productively" or "destructively" begins the practice of gaining awareness of the beneficial and maladaptive expressions of these traits on behavior.

# Point 3: TBT-S Treatment Philosophy

1. TBT-S harnesses the positives of the AN temperament.
2. Traits can be strengths as well as weaknesses.
3. TBT-S works *with* clients' traits to shift their expression from destructive to productive.
4. TBT-S does not attempt to change temperament but to use temperament to reduce problematic behaviors.

**Notes for the Clinician**

All traits can be expressed productively and destructively.

- Treatment usually approaches traits from a pathological perspective.
- A goal of TBT-S is to help clients/Supports recognize that effectively using their traits can set them up for success.
- Clinicians can take an affirming stance that instills hope and motivates clients to identify which of their traits help equip them to achieve recovery.

# Point 4: Temperament and Neurobiological Developmental Model of AN [35]

"When good traits go bad, and then good again":

1. Childhood risk: Genetically determined temperament traits that increase susceptibility to develop AN are often present in childhood.
2. Adolescent risk (aka, a perfect storm): Changes that often occur in adolescence further increase the risk of developing AN. These include brain development (including a shifting balance between early-emerging reward circuits and later emerging cognitive control circuits), hormonal and body changes related to puberty, stress, and interpersonal and environmental factors. These may exacerbate existing traits, leading to increased anxiety and/or negative mood.
3. One way this happens is through epigenetics, or gene-environment interactions. Environmental factors (e.g., stress, malnutrition) influence neurocircuit and genetic

expression and can result in the overexpression of genes that code for traits that contribute to AN. Thus, genes are thought to have greater influence than environmental factors during this stage.[96, 97] In this way, traits that were appearing good during childhood shift and "go bad" during adolescence triggering AN to emerge.

4. Weight loss (either intentional or not) reduces anxiety/dysphoria. However, it results in neurobiological changes and increases destructive trait expression (e.g., depression, obsessionality, cognitive rigidity) that serves to perpetuate food avoidance/dietary restriction. This ultimately triggers a vicious cycle (See Figure 10.1).

5. Research indicates about 50 percent to 70 percent of individuals with AN eventually recover, though often after a prolonged illness with relapsing/remitting course; 30 percent to 50 percent develop a chronic illness, and ~10 percent die from complications associated with AN.

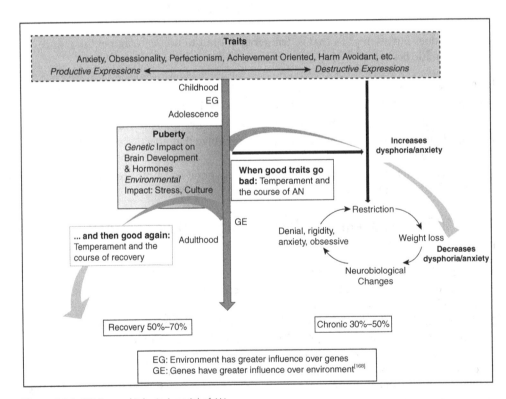

**Figure 10.1** TBT-S neurobiological model of AN

**Clinician** *Scripts*

- To introduce Point 4: *Research findings have informed a temperament and neurobiological model of AN that serves as the framework for TBT-S.*

**Notes for the Clinician**

- Clinicians are encouraged to present the model depicted in Figure 10.1 and stress the urgency of intervening to prevent a chronic course of AN.
- Clinicians can help clients acknowledge their once productive or "good" trait expressions, and with the use of tools and structure and the help of Supports, the temporary destructive expressions, or "bad traits," can shift to become productive again.

# Point 5: Revisiting the Neurobiological Model with Brain Systems Included

1. Several brain systems and associated cognitive functions are involved in the regulation of appetite and eating behavior:

   - *Interoception*, or the sense of one's physiological state (e.g., body-related experiences, including hunger, fullness, pain, touch), which is localized to the insula.
   - *Reward and punishment processing* and *emotion/anxiety*, which are aided by the reward (limbic) circuit.
   - *Executive control and decision-making*, which are localized to the frontal cortex.

2. Brain imaging studies of individuals with AN suggest that these systems are disrupted in AN and may contribute to AN symptoms and disordered eating behaviors. This will be discussed in greater detail in other neurobiology psychoeducation modules. These studies inform the treatment targets and interventions in TBT-S.

**Clinician** *Scripts*

- To introduce Point 5 material: *"New insights into brain functions and systems involved in regulating eating, and evidence of their disruption in AN, further informs the biological basis of AN and identifies neurobiologically-based targets for treatment."*

**Notes for the Clinician**

- It can be helpful to present the model depicted in Figure 10.2 and to visualize that interoception, reward and punishment processing, anxiety/emotion, and inhibitory and decision-making are encoded in brain circuits and implicated in AN.

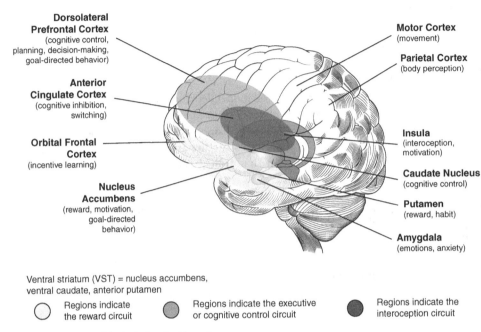

**Figure 10.2** Areas of the brain involved in eating

# Point 6: How Does TBT-S Apply This Information to Treatment?

1. TBT-S leverages principles of neural plasticity to promote behavior change. Neural plasticity suggests that the brain is "plastic" and *is able* to re-wire to promote new behaviors.
2. Learning occurs when "neurons that fire together wire together."[50]
3. The brain is malleable and can be changed via behavioral practice.
4. Repeated practice of healthy behavior is needed to re-wire the brain. Thus, TBT-S is a treatment of "doing" and involves practicing new behaviors and routines.

### Clinician *Scripts*

• To introduce Point 6 material: *Neuroplasticity can change or re-wire the brain with repeated, intensive practice of new skills to manage recovery.*

### Notes for the Clinician

It can be helpful to give examples of neuroplasticity. For instance, the motor cortex changes when musicians learn new finger sequences, and brain networks regulating attention change following mastery of mindfulness practice.

> **Summary Key Points**
>
> • Studies show that eating disorders tend to run in families. This suggests genes contribute to eating disorders.

- Genes cause traits. Several studies show people with eating disorders share traits that existed before the disorder and may help maintain the disorder. For example, this includes perfectionism, obsessionality, high achievement orientation, and anxiety.
- Brain imaging studies show differences in the parts of the brain involved in eating in individuals with eating disorders compared with those who do not have eating disorders.
- Together, research shows there are strong genetic and neurobiological causes of eating disorders.

# TBT-S Neurobiology Psychoeducation Module
## Anxiety and Interoception

**Neurobiological and Trait Targets**

- Anxiety
- Interoception
- Prediction Error (i.e., a mismatch between what is expected and what is experienced)

## Objective

The purpose of the Anxiety and Interoception Psychoeducation Module is to introduce clients and Supports to the scientific evidence addressing the role of anxiety and altered interoception in disordered eating behavior and other symptoms of anorexia nervosa (AN). This module also provides the justification and rationale for intervention strategies aimed at managing anxiety and compensating for altered interoception by reducing reliance on internal (interoceptive) signaling to promote healthy eating behavior.

### When Is This Module Provided

This module is provided early in treatment to set the stage for a trait-based approach. However, it can be provided whenever the clinician wishes to introduce this topic. In the studied 5-day TBT-S Programs, it was offered on the second day.

### Who Is Involved

This module can be offered to clients only and/or Supports only, individually or in a group. It was tested in a 5-day, 40-hour format with a group of clients and their Supports to foster discussion and sharing of experiences among the group.

### What Is Needed

It is helpful to provide visual aids, via either handouts or a formal presentation (e.g., PowerPoint presentation), that may necessitate a computer, monitor, screen, and/or projector. Some visual aids are provided in this chapter and the Appendices.

## Content

The following six talking points and additional evidence are offered for clinicians to share with clients and Supports. Clinician *scripts* (which can be said verbatim) and notes are provided to help guide discussion.

# Point 1: Individuals with AN Often Have High Anxiety[37, 104]

1. Anxiety can be cognitive (e.g., anxious thoughts, worry), physiological (e.g., stomachache, nausea, difficulty breathing, racing heart), and/or anticipatory (fear of upcoming event).
2. Anxiety can be a state or a trait. If anxiety occurs rarely and only in a specific situation, it tends to be state anxiety. If the person experiences anxiety over various stages of life and has a tendency to feel overwhelmed and anxious over things, anxiety tends to be a trait.
3. Forty percent of adults with AN had childhood anxiety disorders.
4. In AN, eating is associated with anxiety; food restriction or avoiding meals often serves to reduce anxiety.
5. Anxiety in AN is associated with

   o Lower BMI and greater caloric restriction
   o More intense symptoms
   o Poor outcome
   o "Anxiety" genes (i.e., genes linked to anxiety are also associated with AN)

6. Anxiety management is necessary to reduce symptoms of AN; TBT-S teaches skills to effectively manage state and trait anxiety.

# Point 2: Role of Interoception in AN

1. AN fundamentally involves disturbances in the experience of physical sensations inside one's body, referred to as *interoception*.
2. Interoception includes internal physical body-state experiences, such as hunger and fullness, taste, pain, touch, heartbeat, breathing, and gastrointestinal (GI) sensations.
3. Many symptoms of AN relate to altered interoceptive experience, such as increased GI discomfort/distress, a disconnect between hunger/satiety and eating behavior, and excessive exercise without experiencing much pain.
4. Some of the earliest clinical descriptions of patients with AN are by Hilde Bruch, who in 1962 acknowledged "a failure of recognizing bodily states" as an important characteristic of the disorder, with disturbed perception of bodily sensations and distrust or inability to accurately identify feelings and sensations.
5. Recent research indicates individuals with AN have reduced trust in their body signals, and this distrust is related to worse eating disorder symptoms.[117]

## Clinician *Scripts*

- *Can you sense if you are hungry?*
- *Can you sense when you are full most of the time?*
- *Do you have a high pain threshold? Or, does it take intense pain before you tend to feel discomfort?*

## Notes for the Clinician

It can be helpful to discuss what the patient quote communicates, including difficulty making sense of internal signals. Poor interoception leads to a sense of blindness or absence of guiding information. This makes it difficult to know what to expect of one's self, and what the client needs from others (aka, Supports).

- Clarifying what to do when interoception is faulty is necessary. Clients and Supports can collaboratively set expectations and serve as guides. (A TBT-S structure to do this is through the Behavioral Agreements. The YA BA is in Appendix 27, and the SE-AN BA is in Appendix 28.)

## Point 3: The Insula Is Responsible for Interoception

1. The insula is the area in the brain that receives and evaluates interoceptive signals from the body (taste, hunger, fullness, pain, touch) and integrates these signals with motivational/emotional information to indicate if a person should approach or avoid various situations at any given time.
2. The insula also includes the "gustatory cortex" or the region of the brain involved in processing taste.
3. Brain imaging studies show that the insula functions differently in individuals with AN, often with reduced response to interoceptive stimuli like taste and stomach sensations.[35, 45–47, 107]

### Notes for the Clinician

- It can be helpful to present Figure 11.1.

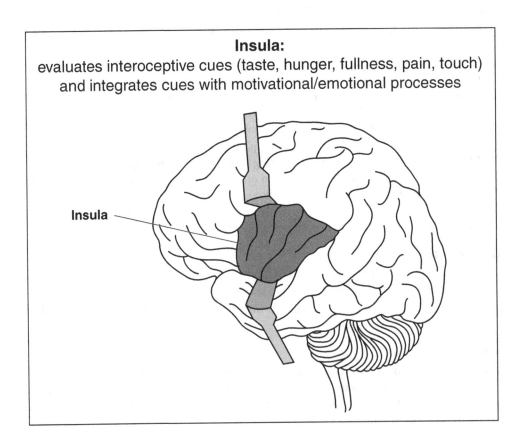

**Figure 11.1** Insula

# Point 4: Individuals with AN Also Tend to Experience Interoceptive Prediction Errors

1. A prediction error is the mismatch between what is expected and what is experienced.
2. The ability to learn and adapt to one's environment depends on the ability to accurately predict outcomes using environmental cues.
3. Learning occurs through modifying expectations to meet experience (i.e., use feedback from the experience to modify the next prediction and ultimately reduce the prediction error).
4. An inability to make accurate predictions may impair learning from experience, explaining persistent engagement in maladaptive behavior.
5. Several brain imaging studies show larger differences in the brain response during anticipation versus receipt of an interoceptive experience (e.g., touch, restricted breathing, taste, pain). This suggests there is a brain basis for interoceptive prediction errors.[105, 106, 118–120] An example of a neural interoceptive prediction error is shown in Figure 11.2

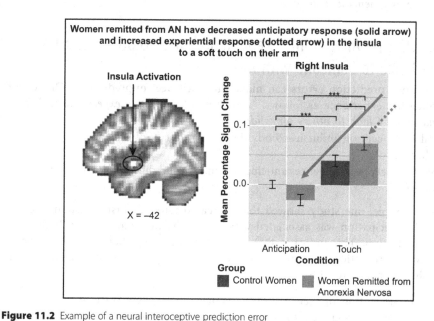

**Figure 11.2** Example of a neural interoceptive prediction error

### Clinician *Scripts*

- *Can you think of some real-world events in which what you expected did not match what you experienced? (Prediction Error).*
- *How did this impact your behavior? Did this trigger anxiety? Did it contribute to being unsure of what to do?*
- *How has this caused you to modify your behavior?*

### Notes for the Clinician

- It can be helpful to provide examples of real-world prediction errors if the client or group has difficulty generating examples. Some examples follow:

  o A person did not study for a test because they expected it to be easy and then failed it.
  o A person feels nervous about getting an injection only to experience it was not painful.
  o A person worries about a meal and it is not as bad as expected.

- It is also helpful to discuss how this interoceptive mismatch or expectancy error informs future behavior. For example, does this cause someone to modify their behavior (i.e., learn from experience)? If so, why?

## Point 5: What Do Altered Interoception and Interoceptive Prediction Errors Feel Like to Someone with AN?

1. Interoceptive prediction errors can make the world feel unpredictable. One client described her experience as follows: "*I have no idea what to expect. I'm walking around blind. I look to others for guidance.*"
2. Altered interoception influences body distrust and/or body image disturbance.
3. Altered interoception influences anticipatory anxiety and difficulty learning from experience.

   a. For example, one study showed that increased (altered) insula response to touch anticipation was associated with greater harm avoidance and body dissatisfaction. This indicates that individuals with high harm avoidance or body dissatisfaction have more acute altered anticipatory brain responses. This is shown in Figure 11.3

4. Altered interoception impacts avoidance behavior (e.g., avoidance of food or physical changes), intolerance of uncertainty, and a need for structure.
5. Deficits in internal brain signals necessitate reliance on external signals.

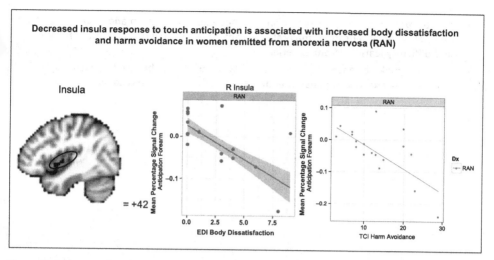

**Figure 11.3** Decreased insula response to touch anticipation is associated with increased body dissatisfaction and harm avoidance in women remitted from anorexia nervosa

## Notes for the Clinician

- It can be helpful to present Figure 11.3.

# Point 6: How Does TBT-S Apply This Information to Treatment?

1. If one cannot rely on internal body-state signals, then it is important for clinicians to use and encourage clients and Supports to
   ○ Rely on a predictable, external structure via meal plan for food and creating specific plans for new events.
   ○ Rely on advanced planning of meals/snacks.
   ○ Increase predictability (reduce anxiety about uncertainty) through routine.

### Summary Key Point

- Eating disorders fundamentally involve disturbances in the experience of the physical sensations in one's body based on internal signals, referred to as interoception.

- Interoceptive prediction errors (mismatch between anticipation and experience of internal physical sensation) may relate to anticipatory anxiety, avoidant behavior, and difficulty learning from experience.
- Deficits in making sense of brain signals related to internal body experience suggest a reliance on external signals is needed as a means to achieve recovery.

# 12 TBT-S Neurobiology Psychoeducation Module
## Reward and Punishment Sensitivity

**Neurobiological and Trait Targets**

- Reward Sensitivity
- Punishment Sensitivity

# Objective

The purpose of the Reward and Punishment Sensitivity Psychoeducation Module is to introduce clients and Supports to the scientific evidence demonstrating the role of altered reward and punishment sensitivity in disordered eating behavior and other symptoms of anorexia nervosa (AN). This module also provides the justification and rationale for temperament based strategies aimed at managing altered sensitivity to reward and punishment. This includes the TBT-S framework for how to use contingency management strategies to motivate behavior change.

## When Is This Module Provided

The module can be provided whenever the clinician wishes to introduce this topic. In the studied 5-day format, it was provided on the third day in one program and the second day in another program.

## Who Is Involved

This module can be offered to clients only and/or Supports only, individually or in a group. It was tested in a 5-day, 40-hour format with a group of clients and their Supports to foster discussion and sharing of experiences among the group.

## What Is Needed

It is helpful to provide visual aids, either via handouts or a formal presentation (e.g., PowerPoint presentation), that may necessitate a computer, monitor, screen, and/or projector. Some visual aids are provided in this chapter and in the Appendices.

# Content

The following six talking points and additional evidence are offered for clinicians to share with clients and Supports. Clinician *scripts* (which can be said verbatim) and notes are provided to help guide discussion.

## Point 1: Individuals with AN Report Reduced Reward Sensitivity and Increased Punishment Sensitivity, Implicating Altered Brain Reward Circuit Function

1. On self-report measures, individuals with AN tend to report experiencing decreased sensitivity to reward and increased sensitivity to punishment. Behaviorally, this may manifest as anhedonia and increased sensitivity to perceived mistakes or criticism.
2. The reward circuit in the brain includes the ventral striatum (which includes the nucleus accumbens, ventral putamen, and ventral caudate nucleus). See Figure 12.1.
3. It identifies and determines the value of rewarding/punishing or emotionally significant stimuli to generate an emotional or behavioral response.
4. It is a target of dopamine transmission, a brain chemical that signals reward to inform learning and the motivation to approach or avoid an environmental stimulus (like food or a predator).
5. Research studies suggest that dopamine signaling may be altered in AN, and this contributes to decreased motivation to eat and increased anxiety.
   a. The release of dopamine tends to cause pleasure or euphoria. For example, food and some drugs of abuse, such as amphetamines cause dopamine release and feelings of pleasure, making eating rewarding for those without AN.
   b. Notably, a few small studies[121, 122] suggest individuals with AN have decreased dopamine (i.e., elevated dopamine D2/3 receptor binding) in the ventral striatum (reward circuit), suggesting this might translate to reduced reward sensitivity.
   c. In addition, reduced dopamine binding in the dorsal caudate (cognitive circuit) is associated with increased anxiety and harm avoidance in AN, suggesting a brain basis for elevated anxiety surrounding rewarding stimuli.
   d. A separate small study[184] found a paradoxical effect of dopamine release in AN; as expected, amphetamine-induced dopamine release in the ventral striatum (reward circuit) increased euphoria in healthy controls; paradoxically, amphetamine-induced dopamine release in the caudate (cognitive circuit) increased anxiety in women with a history of AN. This may help explain why eating tends not to be rewarding and induces anxiety in AN. *Caveat: these are small studies and need replication.*

### Notes for the Clinician
• It can be helpful to present Figure 12.1.

## Point 2: Food–Reward Circuit Dysfunction in AN[35, 46, 47, 106]

1. Brain imaging studies have examined the brain reward response to pictures of food and tastes of food in AN.
2. These studies have found decreased brain response in the ventral striatum (reward circuit) and insula (interoceptive circuit, taste center) for both pictures of foods and tastes of highly palatable food. This suggests decreased reward signaling for food in AN. See Figure 12.2

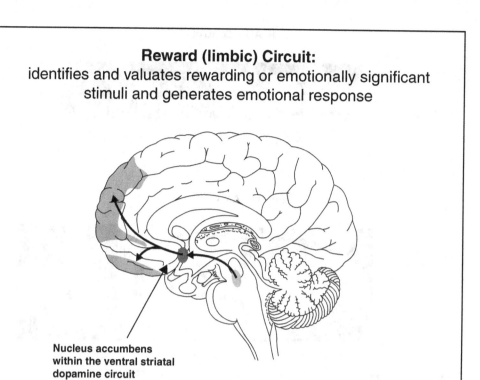

**Figure 12.1** Reward circuit

3. Notably, decreased response to pleasant taste in the dorsal caudate (cognitive circuit) was associated with increased harm avoidance in AN, suggesting there is a biological basis for coding food as risky. In other words, individuals with high harm avoidance experience decreased reward response. See Figure 12.3.

### Notes for the Clinician

- It is important to acknowledge that correlation does not indicate causation; thus, it is unknown whether reduced brain reward response causes anxiety, or whether anxiety hijacks the reward system, resulting in decreased reward sensitivity.
- It can be helpful to present Figures 12.2 and 12.3.

## Point 3: Brain Reward and Cognitive Centers Show Exaggerated Responses to Losses in AN

1. During a guessing game that examined brain response when winning and losing money,

   a. Adolescents with active AN showed an exaggerated response to losses compared with wins in the dorsal caudate (cognitive circuit). This suggests increased sensitivity to punishment in AN.[108] See Figure 12.4.

## III AN < Controls

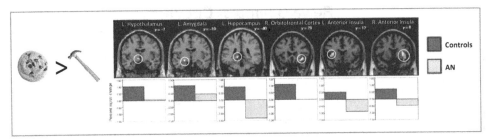

## Remitted AN < Controls

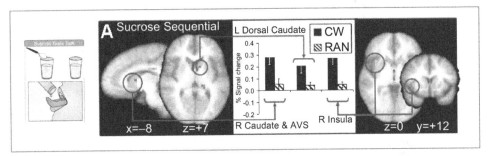

**Figure 12.2** Decreased reward circuit response to food pictures and pleasant taste in anorexia nervosa
From Holsen LM, Lawson EA, Blum J, et al. Food motivation circuitry hypoactivation related to hedonic and nonhedonic aspects of hunger and satiety in women with active anorexia nervosa and weight-restored women with anorexia nervosa. J Psychiatr Neurosci. 2012;37(5):322–32.

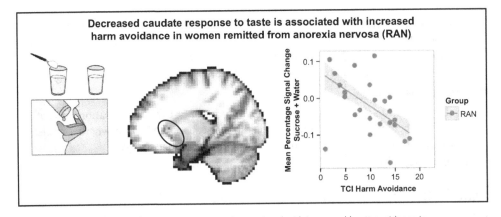

**Figure 12.3** Decreased caudate response to taste is associated with increased harm avoidance in women remitted from anorexia nervosa
From Kaye WH, Wierenga CE, Bischoff-Grethe A et al. Neural insensitivity to the effects of hunger in women remitted from anorexia nervosa. Am J Psychiatr. 2020;177(7):601–10.

b. Adult women with a history of AN had similarly increased ventral striatum (reward circuit) brain response to wins and losses, suggesting they failed to differentiate rewarding and aversive outcomes (which could contribute to difficulties learning from experience if the value of outcome is confusing).[123]

2. Evidence of altered brain reward response to both eating disorder specific stimuli (e.g., food) and general stimuli (e.g., money) suggests that eating disorders involve a broader dysfunction of the reward or motivational circuit that extends beyond food and is seen in trait expressions that do not manifest just around food.

3. This may contribute to a lack of motivation or ambivalence for treatment and recovery often observed in individuals with AN. Treatment "resistance" may actually reflect a biological disturbance of valuating outcomes.

**Notes for the Clinician**

• It can be helpful to present Figure 12.4.

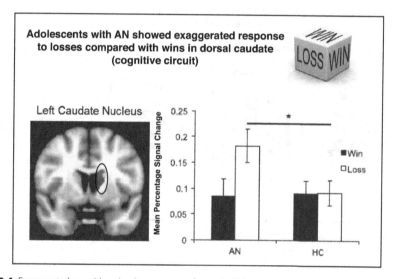

**Figure 12.4** Exaggerated cognitive circuit response to losses in AN
From Bischoff-Grethe A, McCurdy D, Grenesko-Stevens E et al. Altered brain response to reward and punishment in adolescents with anorexia nervosa. Psychiatr Res. 2013;214(3):331–40.

# Point 4: Influence of Hunger and Satiety on Taste Reward Processing in AN

1. One puzzling aspect of AN is the ability to restrict food even when hungry. For people without AN, hunger is a biologically based motivational signal related to energy stores that drives the consumption of food. How are individuals

with AN able to avoid the desire for food despite strong biological signals to eat?

2. Healthy individuals show increased brain response to rewarding stimuli when hungry compared with after a meal. This serves to motivate eating by increasing the rewarding sensation/pleasure from food.

3. Interestingly, individuals with AN show greater reductions in brain reward response to taste when hungry in the ventral putamen (reward circuit) and insula (interoceptive circuit, gustatory cortex) compared with healthy controls, suggesting that hunger may not motivate eating.[107] See Figure 12.5.

4. This is also consistent with altered interoception (e.g., altered sensitivity to the physiological state of hunger) in AN.

### Notes for the Clinician

- It can be helpful to present Figure 12.5.

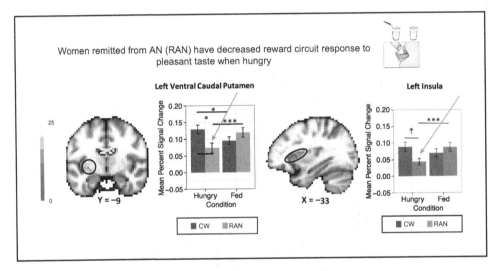

**Figure 12.5** Influence of hunger/satiety on taste reward processing in AN
From Kaye WH, Wierenga CE, Bischoff-Grethe A, et al. Neural insensitivity to the effects of hunger in women remitted from anorexia nervosa. Am J Psychiatr. 2020;177(7):601–10.

# Point 5: What Does Reduced Reward Signaling Feel Like to Someone with AN?

1. It is not a "natural" or dominant brain response to
   a. Eat like those without AN.
   b. Easily trust what and when to eat.
   c. Find pleasure in eating and variety of foods.

2. Eating may cause anxiety, not pleasure (and not eating may reduce anxiety).

3. Altered reward processing may translate to low motivation for recovery and anhedonia.

**Key Points**

For those with anorexia nervosa,

- It is not a "natural" or dominant brain response to eat like those without AN.
- It is difficult to trust what and when to eat.
- It is common not to experience pleasure in eating a variety of foods.
- Eating is anxiety provoking. Not eating may reduce anxiety.

# Point 6: How Does TBT-S Apply This Information to Treatment?

1. Clinicians educate Supports and clients that there is a biological basis for why eating may not be intrinsically rewarding and easy but instead is anxiety provoking.
2. Clinicians encourage Supports and clients to recognize that lack of motivation for treatment may reflect a deficient biologically based reward/motivation system rather than willfulness.
3. Clinicians work with clients and Supports to identify and implement external motivators for recovery-related behavior (aka, contingency management) based on an individual's sensitivity to reward and punishment. External motivators are important for people with AN who often lack intrinsic motivation. By matching external motivators to one's temperament, they can be more effective. For example, for individuals with high punishment sensitivity, avoiding a potential negative consequence might be more motivating that earning a reward.
4. Clinicians work with Supports and clients to provide structure around meals, because it is unlikely that individuals with active AN can eat intuitively given altered brain reward signaling to hunger.

**Summary Key Points**

- Individuals with AN tend to experience reduced sensitivity to reward and increased sensitivity to punishment.
- Altered sensitivity to reward and punishment is observed for both food and general rewards/losses and thus suggests a broader deficit in reward processing.
- Hunger does not increase reward sensitivity in AN, suggesting a deficit in translating physiological signals to motivated behavior, and explaining why individuals with AN can restrict food despite starvation.
- Altered reward processing may be why we see low motivation for recovery and anhedonia.
- Decreased brain response to reward in cognitive circuitry in AN is associated with elevated anxiety, suggesting a brain basis for coding food as risky.

# TBT-S Neurobiology Psychoeducation Module
## Decision-Making and Inhibitory Control

**Neurobiological and Trait Targets**

- Decision-Making
- Inhibitory Control

## Objective

The purpose of the Decision-Making and Inhibitory Control Psychoeducation Module is to introduce clients and Supports to the scientific evidence demonstrating the role of altered decision-making and inhibition in disordered eating behavior and other symptoms of anorexia nervosa (AN). This module also provides the basis for strategies aimed at managing difficulties in decision-making and emphasizing that cognitive control can be redirected to promote healthy eating behavior.

### When Is This Module Provided

The module can be provided whenever the clinician wishes to introduce this topic. In the studied 5-day format, it was provided on the third day in one program and the second day in another program.

### Who Is Involved

This module can be offered to clients only and/or Supports only, individually or in a group. It was tested in a 5-day, 40-hour format with a group of clients and their Supports to foster discussion and sharing of experiences among the group.

### What Is Needed

It is helpful to provide visual aids, either via handouts or a formal presentation (e.g., PowerPoint presentation), that may necessitate a computer, monitor, screen, and/or projector. Some visual aids are provided in this chapter and in the Appendices.

### Content

The following six talking points and additional evidence are offered for clinicians to share with clients and Supports. Clinician *scripts* (which can be said verbatim) and notes are provided to help guide discussion.

# Point 1: Executive Functioning Is Often Altered in AN[110–113]

1.  Performance on cognitive tasks suggests AN is characterized by
    - Cognitive inflexibility
    - Poor set shifting (e.g., stuck in set, perseveration, repetition of previous behavior even if maladaptive)
    - Difficulty task switching (e.g., switching rules)
    - Low central coherence (e.g., greater attention to detail, poor global processing, lose the forest for the trees)
    - Increased inhibitory control
    - Altered decision-making (e.g., less risk taking, less flexibility in adapting to task demands)

# Point 2: The Cognitive Control Circuit Is Responsible for Executive Function

1.  The cognitive or inhibitory control circuit includes the prefrontal cortex (PFC) and the dorsal (upper) part of the striatum, including the caudate nucleus. See Figure 13.1
2.  It is involved in executive functioning, including cognitive control, inhibition, planning and decision-making (sometimes referred to as the CEO of the brain, since it manages complex behavior).[101, 103]

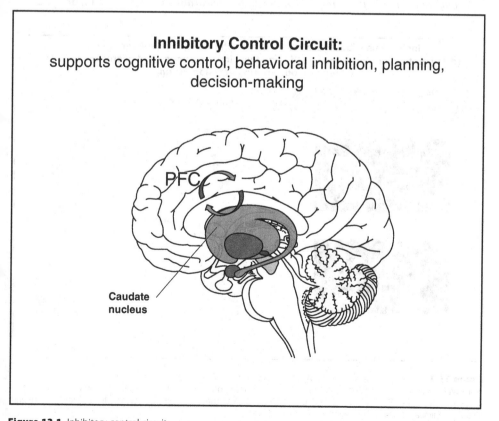

**Figure 13.1** Inhibitory control circuit

**Notes for the Clinician**

- It can be helpful to present Figure 13.1.

# Point 3: Decision-Making Is Sometimes Altered in AN[47, 114, 115]

1. Individuals with AN tend to be willing to wait longer for a bigger reward. For example, studies using "delay discounting" decision-making tasks in the lab show that individuals with AN tend to choose larger-later rewards (like $20 in 4 weeks vs. $15 now) over smaller-sooner rewards (like $15 now vs. $20 in 4 weeks).

2. In contrast, individuals with bulimia nervosa and impulse control disorders like ADHD and substance use disorders tend to prefer smaller-sooner rewards.

3. This suggests individuals with AN are able to delay gratification and inhibit impulses/desires for immediate rewards in favor of perceived better long-term outcomes (this may help to explain the ability to avoid immediately available food in favor of long-term outcome of weight loss).

4. Brain imaging studies show increased frontal brain response during delay discounting decision-making in individuals with a history of AN, suggesting greater recruitment of cognitive control resources. In contrast, individuals with AN show reduced brain reward response (in the ventral striatum) to immediately available monetary reward, *suggesting that AN may be characterized by an imbalance between greater cognitive control/inhibition and reduced reward sensitivity that facilitates the ability to delay gratification or avoid the temptation of something immediately rewarding, like food.* See Figure 13.2.

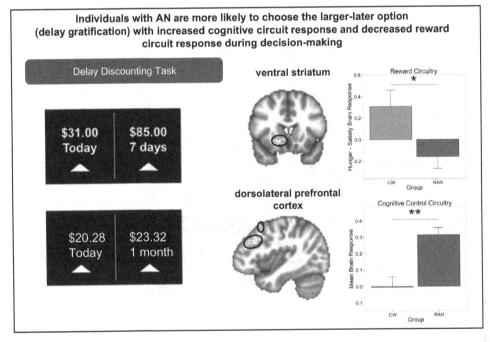

**Figure 13.2** Altered brain response during decision-making in AN: Money
From Wierenga CE, Bischoff-Grethe A, Melrose AJ et al. Hunger does not motivate reward in women remitted from anorexia nervosa. Biol Psychiatr. 2015;77(7):642–52; and Ely A, Berner LA, Wierenga CE, et al. Neurobiology of eating disorders: Clinical implications. Psychiatr Times. 2016;33(4).

## Notes for the Clinician

- It can be helpful to present Figure 13.2.
- "Delay discounting" is a neuroeconomics term that refers to the fact that humans tend to devalue money as time passes, so as the delay in receiving money increases, its value is discounted. Delay discounting tasks are often used to assess impulsivity. The preference of individuals with AN who have restrictive traits to delay monetary rewards indicates that they do not discount its value as much after a delay. In other words, they are not impulsive; rather, they show great ability to inhibit immediate impulses.
- To engage clients and Supports, it can be fun to demonstrate the task and have participants share their decision-making styles. If clinicians opt to do this, it is recommended that this *script* be provided prior to presenting the material in Point 3: *(Script) Delay discounting tasks are commonly used to assess someone's decision-making style and whether they tend to be more impulsive or more inhibited/restrained. In this task, individuals must choose between two options of monetary rewards: a smaller-sooner reward or a larger-later reward. For instance, would you rather receive $31 today or $85 dollars in 4 weeks? Raise your hand if you would choose $31 today. Okay, now raise your hand if you would choose $85 in 4 weeks. Those of you who chose $31, what motivated that decision? Those of you who chose $85, what motivated that decision? What decision-making style do you think individuals with AN who are more restrictive tend to use?*
- To make these finding more relatable, the clinician can ask the clients and Supports for real-life examples of this tendency to delay gratification. Some examples include rationing Halloween candy, saving vacation days for a large trip in the future rather than using them on more frequent (sooner) smaller trips, or saving up for a larger purchase in the future.
- Ask clients if they tend to inhibit an immediate impulse and choose something that is considered of more value down the road, or vice versa. This helps indicate whether their inhibition trait or impulsive trait is stronger.

# Point 4: Individuals with AN Tend to Have Altered Decision-Making Regarding Food

1. Not surprisingly, individuals with AN are more likely to choose low- versus high-calorie food.[102]
2. One study suggests low-calorie food choices may be habit driven. However, there is still debate in the field regarding the degree to which disordered eating behaviors are habit based (automatic) or goal directed (planned). This may depend on individual factors and length of illness (e.g., goal-directed behaviors can become habits over time). See Figure 13.3.

## Notes for the Clinician

- It can be helpful to present Figure 13.3.

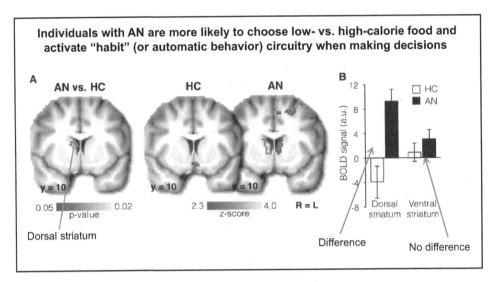

**Figure 13.3** Altered brain response during decision-making in AN: Food
From Foerde K, Steinglass JE, Shohamy D, et al. Neural mechanisms supporting maladaptive food choices in anorexia nervosa. Nat Neurosci. 2015;18(11):1571–3.

# Point 5: What Do Altered Decision-Making and Greater Inhibition Feel Like to Someone with AN?

1. One client described her experience as follows: *"I get overwhelmed by the decision of what to eat. When there are too many choices I don't know what is the right one, so I choose not to eat because it's easier than making the wrong choice."*

2. Increased cognitive control and behavioral inhibition may facilitate food avoidance and dietary restriction.

## Notes for the Clinician

- It can be useful to recite the patient quote and ask the client or group what traits they recognize in the quote.

- The clinician can point out traits such as *anxiety* ("overwhelmed"), *perfectionism* ("the right one," "easier than making the wrong choice"), *interoceptive dysfunction* ("I don't know" suggests no physiological signaling of hunger or reward to inform decision), *inhibition* ("choose not to eat"), and general *difficulty in trusting a decision* ("too many choices").

- In the SE-AN version, the clinician can refer clients to the Trait Profile Checklist to identify other traits that impact their decision-making (see Appendix 2).

# Point 6: How Does TBT-S Apply This Information to Treatment?

1. Clinicians help Supports and clients set clear rules and expectations for recovery-related behaviors (e.g., meal plan, types of movement congruent with current body strength) to capitalize on the ability to follow rules (e.g., rule-bound behavior).
2. Clinicians offer clients options to help them identify motivating pro-recovery *long-term* rewards to take advantage of the ability to delay gratification.
3. Clinicians and Supports offer multiple choices instead of open-ended questions to facilitate decision-making.
4. Clinicians help clients and Supports plan ahead and avoid having to make new decisions on the spot.
5. Clinicians use session time to practice new mealtime routines to re-wire destructive habit circuitry. Supports help clients practice these routines at home.

## Summary Key Points

- Individuals with AN tend to
  - Be able to inhibit impulses and delay gratification, which impacts their decision-making.
  - Have increased brain cognitive control response during decision-making, suggesting they "overthink" to make up for what they "under" sense internally. This response encourages the need for rules to guide behavior.
- Restricted eating may be related to an altered balance between decreased reward sensitivity and increased inhibition.

# Introduction to TBT-S for Young Adults (YA TBT-S)

## Rationale for a TBT-S Model for Young Adults with Anorexia Nervosa

Young Adult Temperament Based Therapy with Support (YA TBT-S) is one of two versions of TBT-S. It has been designed for adults within the age range of 17–27 years. It was developed at the University of California San Diego by Stephanie Knatz Peck to fill a gap in treatment between adolescent family-based therapy (FBT) and adult individual therapy, and as a way to further refine TBT-S by incorporating a YA developmental framework. Despite the fact that eating disorders (EDs) commonly occur in young adulthood, there continue to be few ED treatments that integrate this developmental framework into treatment. The YA version of TBT-S evolved to integrate important developmental concerns and needs associated with "emerging adulthood" that were not specifically addressed in other approaches. It consists primarily of YAs and their parents. Key objectives of YA TBT-S include a model of assistance that is specifically tailored for emerging adults and their parents and addresses temperament and neurobiology within the framework of a continuously developing brain.

"Emerging adulthood" and "transition-aged youth" are developmental terms that have been used to describe the unique life stage of adults between the ages of 17 and 27. Importantly, this life stage has been studied and described extensively and is characterized by distinct developmental milestones and life experiences that differ from those of older adults and younger adolescents. YA clients with anorexia nervosa (AN) are often launching to full independence and living through significant life transitions that characterize these years and challenge the evolving relationship with their parents. Parental encouragement and assistance toward recovery, while necessary, differ from what they once offered during adolescence and what they will offer for future adulthood needs. These key features inform YA TBT-S. The treatment endorses a continuous acknowledgment of what it means to be a YA and encourages the developmental temperament landscape to be woven into all aspects of YA TBT-S treatment. The YA TBT-S model acknowledges that YAs are in a transitional phase, emerging from dependence and entering into independence via interdependence, which necessitates a transition in the assistance offered by parents centered on increasing levels of collaboration. YA TBT-S focuses on fostering a collaborative relationship between YAs and their parents within a temperament framework.

> Key Point: The YA TBT-S model is for emerging adults and their parents. It offers a unique model of assistance tailored for this developmental stage. The model targets temperament and neurobiology in a way that is congruent with YA's developing brain.

# Young Adult Developmental Milestones

Young adults between the ages of 17 and 27 are considered transition-aged youth and/or emerging adults. This life stage is associated with unique developmental needs and milestones that characterize YAs. Assisting healthy growth through this stage, including recovery from AN, requires an understanding of what YAs are oriented toward, and their interdependence on their family of origin, including parents. Clinicians and parents can benefit by knowing common YA developmental milestones. The goal for parents is to assist recovery in a way that converges with this developmental stage.

## Common YA Developmental Features

Young adulthood is often characterized by the following:

- **Identity exploration.** YAs are deciding who they are and what they want from life, such as from work, school, and love.
- **Instability.** YAs are frequently uprooted by residence changes, which can cause changes in social, religious, and other groups or beliefs.
- **Self-focus.** YAs may be stepping away from parents and society-directed school routines. They are deciding who they want to be and where they want to go and are making other life choices. This can be exciting *and* anxiety provoking.
- **Feeling "in-between."** YAs desire to take responsibility for themselves but are still dependent on family and do not "feel" like adults.
- **New possibilities.** This can be a time filled with new adventures and transitions, either for the good or at the expense of their well-being. This can be a time of new self-fulfilling life opportunities.

> Key Point: It is common for YAs to experience a sense of being uprooted, disconnected, and uncertain as they transition from adolescence into adulthood. How they approach this stage of development depends on their temperaments.

# Mental Health Service Utilization for Young Adults

Mental illness is prevalent during the developmental YA life stage.[124–127] In the United States, YAs between the ages of 18 and 25 have the highest prevalence rates of mental illness, yet they are least likely to access mental health services.[1–3] This issue has led to initiatives to develop YA-specific treatments. While treatment underutilization is not wholly understood, it may be related to problems in health care system age designations. Upon meeting the legal adult age, YAs transition from pediatric services, primarily dependent on parental involvement, to adult services with an individual therapeutic approach. YAs do not fit discretely into either of these treatment categories due to transitional development needs. A treatment approach that involves family and focuses on the emergence from dependence toward independence is needed. YA TBT-S focuses on interdependence and an age-appropriate model of parental involvement.

Over the past two decades, YAs have increasingly needed familial financial, interpersonal, and living assistance, compared with past generations. A significant portion of YAs continue to live at home past the age of 18 (or move home upon graduation from college) and receive financial assistance from their families. Currently, many YAs are still embedded in their family systems in ways that have not been accounted for in traditional adult mental health services. Conversely, child/adolescent services and the traditional models of family involvement are not developmentally suitable for YAs who exhibit more readiness for autonomy. These systems' lack of ability to account for these developmental needs is compounded when AN is involved.

Eating disorders are commonly diagnosed and treated in young adulthood.[128] Despite this, few adult eating disorder treatments are tailored for the unique needs of YAs and family to include a developmentally suitable model of parental involvement that matches typical level of YA familial assistance.[129–131] Even fewer adult treatments work within the YA client's temperament framework. YA TBT-S is a treatment for YAs with AN that is developmentally tailored, involves family in YA-specific ways, and targets core temperament and neurobiology.

> Key Point: Mental health services are not designed for YA's developmental needs. YA TBT-S for AN incorporates client developmental needs within a client-parent framework fostering systemic interdependence and integrating temperament.

# What Is the Conceptual Framework of YA TBT-S?

YA TBT-S is rooted in general principles of systemic therapy adapted to account for YA developmental needs and parental collaboration. It is framed within the TBT-S neurobiological model of AN to account for AN temperament within YAs.

## Systemic Principles Integrated into YA TBT-S

YA TBT-S takes a systemic approach to treatment by involving parents in the treatment of YAs with AN. General principles of family therapy for AN are adapted into the YA TBT-S model. Therapy for YAs with AN involves clients and their parents as primary Supports. The following principles, drawn from family therapy for AN (FT-AN) applied to adolescents, are integrated into a YA TBT-S version:

- Explain to the family the seriousness of AN, that it is a potentially life-threatening illness that creates a sense of helplessness and failure in their loved one (See Chapters 6 and 10–13). In the YA TBT-S model, parents are also taught that AN is a brain illness and learn about their YA's strengths and limitations based on temperament traits.
- Utilize results from ED multidimensional assessments and psychoeducation as a foundation for treatment. This includes how YAs are identifying with key AN temperament traits presented within the TBT-S framework. This is key to building awareness and to adapting the treatment accordingly (See Trait Profile Checklist in Appendix 2).
- Emphasize working *with* parents in designated sessions as resources to help their YA recover.
- Accentuate that the family is not the cause of AN, but rather that parents can be a key source of assistance (See Chapter 7).
- Develop a therapeutic alliance that is congruent with key aspects of family organization around the illness, such as client symptoms with a focus on here and now.

- Utilize the family as an agent of change around food and eating, early in the treatment process.

> Key Point: YA TBT-S involves parents as primary Supports who can serve as agents of change collaboratively with their loved one outside the treatment setting.

# How Is Temperament Targeted in YA TBT-S?

The structure inherent in TBT-S directly addresses the common AN temperament profile so that treatment is structured in a way that is congruent with typical innate tendencies. All aspects of treatment are presented in a highly structured format; mealtime rules are established and practiced; and detailed, recovery-oriented rules are established, learned, practiced, and linked to life reinforcers and consequences by both YAs and parents. YA TBT-S addresses key neurobiological targets (anxiety, inhibition, interoception, and altered reward sensitivity) in a sequenced manner where YAs and parents receive psychoeducation → experiential activities → skills training for each TBT-S target. Psychoeducation focuses on providing an interactive, didactic explanation and overview of temperament and neurobiology, and its interplay with AN. From there, experiential activities are used to deepen learning, build parent empathy, and provide opportunities for problem solving in constructive ways for YAs to cope with AN alterations, and for parents to provide assistance in temperament-congruent ways. These coping skills are then reinforced in YA and parent skills training groups, and additional skills targeting temperament and neurobiology are taught and practiced.

YAs and parents alike are provided with opportunities to engage in self-assessment and identify their traits. Importantly, these traits are presented as a "menu," and clinicians should not make any assumptions that YAs identify with all of these traits and be careful to avoid generalizing or assuming that all clients with AN possess them. Instead, YA TBT-S clinicians should provide this information and allow YA clients and their parents to self-determine what is applicable (See Trait Profile Checklist in Appendix 2).

> Key Point: Clinicians should choose skills and interventions that address the traits/neurobiology that YAs self-identify, to provide a more personalized approach.

# How Does YA TBT-S Account for the Developing Brain?

While temperament and personality are relatively stable over the lifetime, it is also important to educate and emphasize that YAs possess continuously developing brains. Clinicians should inform YAs and their parents that the brain does not reach full maturation until individuals reach their mid-20s. This is critical neurodevelopmental information to impart because it encourages YAs and their parents to view the brain as plastic and change as attainable. Indeed, YA TBT-S clinicians should emphasize these implications to instill hope and empower YAs and their parents to strive for full recovery.

Similarly, temperament traits are on a spectrum versus being binary – that is, to what degree do you have the trait, versus you either have the trait or you don't. Presenting information about temperament in this manner encourages individuals to both recognize their innate tendencies as strengths *and to* practice and develop new ways of approaching life. This is particularly important for YA clients who may continue to have considerable capacity to develop new skills and re-wire their brains. This assures that this information does not enable a fatalistic approach, where YAs are discouraged from trying new things – particularly those that may enable recovery.

> **Key Point:** YAs possess continuously developing brains making their brains plastic and more capable of change.

## Disentangling Temperament and Anorexia Nervosa

In YA TBT-S, it is important to distinguish persistent, lifelong traits from eating disorder behaviors and rituals that are enabling illness. This can be difficult because often eating disorder behaviors can be rationalized by temperament. ("I like rules, and that's why I have all these eating disorder rules"). YA TBT-S aims for individuals to recover rather than just restore weight. This means that eating disorder pathology needs to be identified and targeted. Individuals with AN often find their temperament traits playing out in their eating disorder in exaggerated forms. This is an example of destructive trait expression. While these expressions may be guided by temperament, traits are often exaggerated by acute illness and an underweight state.

Furthermore, eating disorder behaviors may be driven by avoiding a feared outcome (such as weight gain) above and beyond just temperament expression ("I like rules"). It is important that this distinction is recognized and addressed in treatment. In general, while traits are stable across the lifetime and present in early childhood, they have increasing impact on eating patterns at the onset of the ED. For example, the YA TBT-S approach will honor a YA for a preference for exactness and precision, *while also* recognizing that the YA's need to simulate exactness and precision in food – for example, by counting an exact amount of calories and eating the same foods – may be a behavior guided by the eating disorder and avoidance of a feared outcome.

In YA TBT-S, the approach would be to encourage the YA and their Supports to use this as a strength. Simultaneously, this would be identified as a potential treatment target to shape and shift trait expressions toward productive expressions. The treatment team would openly discuss this with the YA and parents and develop a collaborative plan to target these temperament traits toward productive outcomes. This provides YAs with the opportunity for full recovery, instead of inadvertently sending the message that this behavior is unchangeable because it is congruent with temperament. That said, if a YA is simply unwavering in their unwillingness to change destructively oriented traits toward productive expressions, YA TBT-S would continue to work with the YA to ensure ED symptom goals (such as weight restoration/weight maintenance) are met. The important aspect of this approach is to avoid sending a message that eating disorder behaviors are acceptable because they appear to be congruent with temperament.

> **Key Point:** YA TBT-S emphasizes that YAs have the potential to develop new skills and learn new behaviors because of their continuously developing brain. It targets changes in eating disorder behaviors using productive trait expressions and shifting destructive trait expressions.

# Rationale for Including Parents as Supports in YA TBT-S

The TBT-S approach views Supports as a necessary part of the AN treatment process for all ages. Chapter 7 describes why and how to include Supports in treatment. The YA version, described in this segment, identifies parents as primary Supports. The YA model of Support involvement is specifically designed to address the unique nature of the relationship between parents and YAs with AN. A YA TBT-S model focusing on parental involvement was developed because parents are most frequently identified as the Supports for YA enrolling in treatment. Additionally, parents are often providing key aspects of assistance (financial, instrumental, emotional) and therefore can make a significant impact in YA recovery.

It is necessary to include Supports in the treatment of AN for persons of all ages, as described in Chapter 7. The YA TBT-S version defaults to using the word "parent" to describe a Support, which most often includes parents or another primary caretaker. "Young adults" (YA) is the term used to describe clients in this age range, and "family" to describe the systemic units presenting for TBT-S treatment. YA TBT-S recognizes a systemic unit as a family regardless of whether or not the parents are part of the family of origin.

> Key Point: Young Adult TBT-S endorses the need for Supports in the treatment process for AN and identifies parents as the primary Supports.

# YA TBT-S Session Format

YA TBT-S was developed and has been studied in a multi-family group format. The concepts and information provided in this chapter can be applied in a wide range of treatment settings including individual YA with parent(s), YA and parents in group therapy settings ranging from outpatient weekly sessions to partial hospital day treatment. Some sessions may involve either the YA only or the parent(s) only, while other specified sessions may combine the YA with parents. Treatment can be virtual or face-to-face. Clinicians may choose to apply YA developmental concepts in this chapter to young adults in the SE-AN TBT-S version of care.

## Aims for Parental Assistance in YA TBT-S

When clinicians begin treatment with YAs who have AN, the initial sessions should facilitate a therapeutic and collaborative relationship between the YA and their parents as primary Supports. The purpose of having parents and/or other family members present is to establish a collaborative relationship working toward recovery that is based on both parent and YA feedback. The clinician can accomplish this goal by establishing designated therapeutic sessions with the client/parents and additional sessions that incorporate input from the dietitian and the medical professional. Clinicians enlist parental assistance to achieve the following aims:

- Include family in designated sessions while respecting the YA's need for autonomy.
- Explore parental beliefs/expectations about the life cycle transition to adulthood.
- Identify barriers to involving parents in treatment.
- Explain the neurobiological bases of AN to both parties simultaneously to establish a common understanding of the illness (See Chapters 6 and 10–13).

- Explain the need for skill development to foster a collaborative relationship and to decrease parental burnout.
- Educate parents on treatment recommendations and progress.
- Recognize and modify parental feelings of guilt and blame.

---

### Summary Key Points

- Parents are primary Supports, or part of the "S" in TBT-S.
- Including parents as Supports is essential.
- YA TBT-S recognizes unique YA developmental needs, and that parental involvement is needed
- Health and maturation are achieved through interdependence among the YA client, parents as primary Supports, and the clinician.

# Chapter 5

# Young Adult TBT-S Multi-Family Group Format

## TBT-S Group Therapy for Parents and Young Adults with AN

Young Adult (YA) TBT-S has been developed and studied in a multi-family group therapy format by Stephanie Knatz Peck at the University of California San Diego. It consists of multiple young adults (YAs) with anorexia nervosa (AN) and their parents as primary Supports. Multiple YAs and their parents are treated together over 5 days and 40 hours, in a 1-week program. When possible, this context allows for a rich therapeutic experience where parents and YA clients can learn from one another. Clinicians provide time for YA clients and parents to connect, observe, relate, validate, and advise one another on issues important to their recovery. This chapter describes the multi-family group process within a 1-week TBT-S format. Qualitative feedback from the YA TBT-S groups suggests that the multi-family milieu is a powerful experience.

> **Key Point:** The young adult version of TBT-S has been studied in a multi-family 5-day, 1-week format that provides opportunities to learn together and from one another.

## Multi-Family Therapy Techniques

The YA TBT-S version derives some of its practices from multi-family therapy techniques that facilitate connection and cross-communication. Examples of multi-family therapy activities used in YA TBT-S are described in Chapters 16 and 17.[71, 132, 133]

## Mixed Parents Groups: Encouraging Cross-Fostering for YA Clients

### What is cross-fostering:

Cross-fostering is a format that encourages family members to connect with YAs and parents of other families. The YA TBT-S program does this in a variety of ways such as mixing group members into smaller "mini-groups" where subgroup members have the opportunity to speak to group members outside of their family. (For example, client from Family A talks with parent from Family B.)

### Why do we recommend cross-fostering:

Bringing YA clients and their parents together for treatment provides the opportunity to foster new connections with others who have similar lived experiences, and to create a recovery network. Receiving treatment with others with similar concerns and developmental needs stimulates ideas for recovery by learning from one another. In a multi-family context, clinicians can utilize a variety of techniques to facilitate cross-fostering of learning among group members (For example, see Appendix 22). Doing so can amplify important recovery messages and provide additional assistance and validation from peers, which facilitates motivation and change that can facilitate recovery.

Significant outcomes from TBT-S open trials may be in part related to the multi-family milieu. A group format allows participants to share ideas and learn from one another just as they learn from the clinicians and dietitians. Group members interact, model, and stimulate new ideas when they have the opportunity to engage in interventions and interactions together. When group members have the opportunity to hear others' experiences, they tend to adjust their perspectives of AN, expanding empathy and understanding. This can generate new perspectives and awareness of effective ways for parents to assist and communicate with their loved ones.

Inter-parent cohorts (pairing participants with clients and parents outside of their families) provide a useful format when skill building together. Learning and practicing skills together allows participants to practice new tools and to learn from different vantage points. Relevant information and actions are then practiced among YAs and their parents. Dividing the group of parents and YAs into smaller mini-groups allows for personalized feedback among group members. Participants have the opportunity to ask for and receive more feedback, and it engages group members who may be less comfortable to share in the larger group.

> Key Point: The multi-family group format is a natural therapeutic setting for participants to learn from one another in ways that could not be achieved in an individual client and clinician therapy session. This may enhance motivation and strengthen outcomes.

## How to Facilitate Cross-Group Interactions

To facilitate cross-group interactions, the clinician assigns group members to mini-groups that consist of parents and clients from different families. *It is important for the clinician to make assignments deliberately and strategically.* For example, pairing a person who is inhibited and reserved with someone who is more extroverted and talkative allows traits to be complemented. Furthermore, a smaller cohort (grouping) can draw out more discussion and sharing than a larger group setting because it enables active participation by all members.

In this format, the cohorts are given a prompt by the clinician and instructed to engage in a discussion on that topic. It is important to provide time for members in the cohorts to connect. This usually takes 20 to 25 minutes. Mini-group interactions increase connections and opportunities for members to ask questions relevant to recovery, even if they stray from the group prompts.

If a clinician is facilitating a series of the group sessions with the same clients and parents, the clinician could reassign group members to different cohorts each time or continue with the same cohort for a designated number of sessions. Although there are benefits to both ways, it is recommended that the same cohort is repeated at least once. This allows each cohort to increase familiarity and comfort in discussions enhancing content and feedback. The mini-groups are given a therapeutic prompt to discuss with time to engage in responses. The clinician then brings the entire group back together to share.

> **Key Point:** Mixing client and parents with other families expands understanding, empathy, and perspectives.

> **Therapeutic Sequencing of Multiple Parent and YA Client Groups**
> 1. **Clinician assigns mini-groups** by mixing family members.
> 2. **Clinician provides a brief introduction** and discussion prompt (see Discussion Prompts).
> 3. **Mixed mini-groups discuss answers to prompts.** Clinician may periodically (and briefly) join the mini-groups to amplify a topic or conversation or provide an additional prompt.
> 4. **Larger group sharing.** Mini-groups return to the larger group to discuss answers shared in the mini-groups. This can be done in two ways.
>     a. The clinician facilitates each group member to share information.
>     b. The clinician assigns clients and parents as a mini-group to provide relevant feedback together to other group members.

# Cross-Group Prompts and *Scripts*

(Do not read the scripts. Use them as notes and speak directly to clients and Supports to increase therapeutic impact.)

A list of prompts is provided to facilitate recovery-related discussion in a multi-family context. These prompts are primarily intended for mini-group interactions. Clinicians should use their own judgment and creativity to formulate discussion prompts and activities relevant to group members' concerns. The prompts can be flexible and varied.

### Discussing Meals outside of Treatment

The clinician asks the mini-group how meals, snacks, and specific skills taught in treatment are being applied outside of treatment. Using this prompt reinforces the use of TBT-S tools and guidelines outside of the program and ensures that treatment providers are aware of progress outside of treatment, to assist with problem-solving difficulties.

○ *Discuss how dinner went last night. What went well? What was challenging? What tools did you practice? What tools did your family members practice? What is important for you to practice today? What would you like your family members to practice today?*

### Ask the Expert

This prompt is less structured and allows mini-group members to get feedback on their actions. Clients are introduced as eating disorder (ED) "experts." This empowers them to share their stories and provide feedback on effective methods of assistance. This approach engages clients to help others by offering feedback on what parents do that works and what does not work. Clients are asked to provide advice and feedback to parents regarding questions or struggles that they have in working with their loved one. It allows parents to hear first-hand accounts of AN experience from someone other than their family member, which is often a powerful way to learn about the illness and see the general commonalities across family experiences. This approach reduces blame and the over-personalization of problems with recovery. For more detail, see Appendix 22.

○ *You have the privilege of sitting with a true expert in AN, someone with first-hand experience! Use this time to ask questions about anything you have wanted to know about the illness or seek any feedback you need on being an effective parent. This could include specific struggles you have had in assisting your loved one.*

○ *Similarly, clients, you are sitting with a parent who has lived experience in providing assistance. Reflect on your relationship with your parent and use this time to seek feedback or ask for advice that will help you work more effectively with your parents.*

### Practicing a Skill

Practicing skills (skillful actions) in mini-groups allow for participants to practice skills that include new ways of communicating or receiving assistance. Practicing with persons outside of one's family neutralizes the experience by eliminating past emotionally charged, family patterns. Clients and parents are often more motivated to practice with neutral participants. The process often triggers new ideas and responses.

### Discussions after TBT-S Neurobiological Experiential Activities

Mini-groups can be assigned after TBT-S experiential activities. This is an efficient method that allows each group participant to share their experiences, identify constructive coping skills, and learn "take-home messages" from each exercise. Mini-group participants are prompted to discuss their experience and which aspects of the activity apply to their experience. Mini-group members are encouraged to apply what they experienced in the activity to what they can do outside of treatment. Clients can offer feedback to parents on effective ways to help them practice the solutions that they explored in the activity.

○ *Talk about the aspects of the exercise that struck you the most. What traits and responses did you and your parents use to complete the activity? These same traits and responses hold solutions for your recovery.*

### Appointing an Advocate

A parent in a mini-group is instructed to be an advocate for the client to the client's family. The parent in the mini-group is responsible for providing feedback to the client's family based upon what they discussed. The client is assigned to report what assistance their parents are offering that helps and to describe an example of what does not help. The parent advocate then meets with the parents of the client and shares the feedback. Hearing input nonjudgmentally from someone outside the family has the potential to decrease defensive responses.

It can be helpful to assign mini-groups of parents to summarize information learned from the parent advocate instead of facilitating all group members together. This increases communication. This method is applied less in the beginning of treatment when it is more effective to have mixed mini-groups practice skills or advocate for a client to enhance understanding of the illness and build empathy.

### Large Group Discussions

Once mini-group interactions occur, it can be helpful to share the new ideas with the large group. This can be done at the clinician's discretion. It allows for clients and parents to hear information from different perspectives. This approach broadens understanding for recovery. Clinicians facilitate sharing in the large group by using "circular questioning." A group member is asked to discuss what another person in the mini-group said or discussed instead of sharing what they said. The clinician asks questions like, "*What did you hear XX say?*" or "*What was XX's perspective on this?*"

Using the circular method allows YA clients and parents to hear one another's stories and perspectives from different points of view. It can be a powerful way to deepen understanding and increase empathy. Sharing on behalf of someone else also creates a natural advocacy role for a group member. Common themes shared in mini-groups can be identified and amplified within the group. The clinician may then ask other group members to share or relate: "*Does anyone have a similar experience?*"

**Summary Key Points**

- Open trials suggest that the multi-family context in YA TBT-S may play an important role in positive outcomes.
- The multi-family milieu improves participants' understanding of the illness as participants hear multiple perspectives that broaden their viewpoints on effective ways to manage recovery and to generate new ideas.
- This method of treatment can assist in identifying and practicing productive actions in a safe environment.

# Young Adult TBT-S Parent Skills Training

## Purpose and Description of the Parent Skills Training Module

The Parent Skills Training Module provides parents with information about young adult (YA) development and the opportunity to learn and practice skills to improve their ability to facilitate and assist with recovery in a temperament-congruent manner. This module is intended to be delivered in a parent-only format. In the multi-family YA TBT-S model studied, parent-only skills training groups occur on a daily basis. The activities presented in this module were developed to be delivered sequentially; however, clinicians can choose any/all activities, and any order of delivery that is relevant or applicable to their setting. The framework and skills applied in this module are flexible and can be applied in any therapeutic setting with parents of YAs in treatment. For example, clinicians can schedule parent-only meeting(s) to augment individual out-patient sessions, or YA parent skills training could be offered for a group in a higher level of care setting (virtually or in-person). The YA parent information and skills are presented in a framework for clinicians to include parents in designated treatment sessions. Parents are oriented to a Model of Parenting that was specifically developed for YAs with anorexia nervosa (AN) (the Dialectical Model of Parenting). They learn specific skills in line with this approach, in addition to parenting skills related to key temperament and neurobiological targets.

> Key Point: Parents attending YA TBT-S are oriented to a Model of Parenting that was specifically developed for YAs with AN. They learn skills to assist their YA, including skills addressing key temperament features.

## Parent Support for Young Adults with AN

As discussed in Chapter 14, parental assistance for a young adult with AN can be significantly different from helping a child or adolescent through AN treatment. The YA TBT-S framework differs from traditional models of family treatment for adolescents with AN in various ways. YA TBT-S was specifically designed for the YA developmental stage and incorporates a model that accounts for developmental milestones associated with this life stage, as described in Chapter 14. When parents of YA clients with AN are invited into treatment, it is important to begin by orienting them to the developmental backdrop of YA TBT-S by providing a brief overview of developmental milestones associated with this life stage. The neurobiological and developmental information shared focuses on parental assistance that is developmentally congruent with YA needs. See Chapter 14 for more background information.

# Parenting a Young Adult Activity

The activity described here orients parents to the broad framework of supporting a young adult and should be conducted at the outset of any skills training conducted with parents to orient them to the structure of support.

## Objectives

- Provide a parent group activity that orients parents of YAs to the importance of the YA developmental stages.
- Lead parents to intuitively access their own experiences and memories of being young adults, their priorities, experiences, and feelings when they were young adults.
- Provide an opportunity for parents to share their experiences.
- Characterize young adulthood as a time of transition and change, the desire for independence and autonomy, as a struggle for identity development outside of the family, and a change in familial relationships.
- Lead parents through the guided imagery exercise to recall their own YA experiences.
- Build empathy and understanding for the YA life stage in preparation for parental assistance in treatment.

## Materials and Time Needed

- Fifteen minutes.
- Clinician guided imagery script.

## Clinician Checklist for YA Parent Skills Training

⇒ Provide an overview of the aims of YA Parent Skills Training as a way for parents to learn and practice effective strategies assisting their YA with AN.
⇒ Prepare and lead the guided visualization and related discussion: "What does it mean to be a YA?"

## Steps

1. Orientation and introduction: The clinician leads parents through a guided imagery exercise to recall what their experiences were during their own YA life stage.
2. Provide a brief introduction on the purpose of the activity: To recall aspects of their own developmental life stage to promote an effective recovery relationship more empathically, and to help parents learn and practice skills to assist their YAs through recovery.
3. Guided imagery exercise: The clinician directs parents to assume a comfortable position (seated comfortably, eyes closed or focused on one point). The clinician then directs parents to recall being in the life stage that the young adult is currently in by directing them to remember details of this time including internal and external experiences.

## Clinician *Script*

1. *We will start this group by taking some time to reflect on what it means to be a young adult. I would like for you to recall your own experiences as a YA.*
2. *I will be leading you through a guided visualization to do this.*
3. *Take a moment to get comfortable in your chair. Find a position you can stay in for a few minutes. Once you are settled, direct your attention inward.*
4. *Be aware of your breathing. (Pause) The pace of your breaths as they go in and out.*
5. *If your attention wanders, gently bring yourself back to the topic.*
6. *Take yourself back to the age your son/daughter is now. (Pause)*
7. *What was happening in your life at this point? (Pause)*
8. *Where did you live? (Pause)*
9. *Who were you surrounded by? (Pause)*
10. *Who was most important to you at this time? (Pause)*
11. *What were you dedicated to? (Pause)*
12. *What were your interests? (Pause)*
13. *As you are the age of your daughter/son, overall did you feel more stable or more stressed? (Pause)*
14. *What were the challenges you faced? (Pause)*
15. *How did you manage them? (Pause)*
16. *What help did you want from your parents? (Pause)*
17. *What help did YOU need? (PAUSE)*
18. *Now bring yourself back to the present day, to this session where you are sitting and slowly open your eyes.*

## Discussion Points

- Ask parents to share their experiences during the exercise.
- What stood out to them as important memories during this life stage?
- Highlight common developmental milestones (see Chapter 14).

**Key Points**
- Parents and other Supports can be more empathic when they are aware of unique YA developmental needs and conflicts and offer appropriate assistance toward AN recovery.
- An experiential activity on guided reflections can enhance empathy for YA development *and orient parents to developmentally appropriate support.*

# Dialectical Parental Support Module

## Objectives

- Help parents learn and practice skills that can assist their YAs through recovery.

# Who Is Involved
- Parents of YAs with AN.

# Materials and Time Needed
- Thirty minutes.
- Dialectical circles, blank and filled in examples of dialectical dilemmas.

# Clinician Checklist for YA Parent Skills Training
⇒ Introduce the general concept of a dialectic first by drawing the research from dialectical behavioral therapy (DBT).
⇒ Review the dialectical parent model including the primary domains of (a) emotional assistance and (b) instrumental assistance.
⇒ Highlight dialectical skills: Parents are to fill in the model by reflecting on skills that fall under each domain.
⇒ Parents' Self-Assessment: Parents conduct an assessment of their strengths and weaknesses (See Appendix 2).
⇒ Skills Training: Parents identify skills that they would like to improve upon and practice. Skills training is conducted using the method: identify → teach → learn → practice. (After the dialectical model is reviewed and completed, subsequent parent skills training sessions are spent teaching and practicing skills identified in the self-assessment.)
⇒ Facilitate sharing and connection (for group formats): Provide time for parents to connect and share.

Note that a set of steps and instructions is presented for each point in the clinician checklist.

# Introduce a Dialectical Parental Model

**Steps**

1. The philosophical concept of a dialectic is explained in relation to providing YA parental assistance that can be divided into two broad domains: emotional assistance and instrumental assistance. <u>Emotional assistance</u> refers to the skillset and ability to be understanding and provide encouragement and validation. <u>Instrumental assistance</u> refers to the skillset and ability to ensure that YAs are progressing in recovery via structure and accountability.
2. Figure 16.3 represents a completed Dialectical Parent Model. This is not presented until all of the activities outlined in this section have been completed. This allows parents to build their own model with personalized skills and strategies. This completed model is intended to be an example to augment the personalized dialectical parental models outlined here.
3. Describe what a dialectic is.

   - A dialectic is the synthesis of two perspectives, depicted by two overlapping circles.
   - Explain that a dialectic means holding opposite truths simultaneously. It is being willing to hear or discuss opposing points of view. The synthesis of the opposing parts is greater than either singular viewpoint or approach.

- An example of a dialectical theme is to allow for both acceptance and change simultaneously instead of defending one perspective or the other.
- When two perspectives are held simultaneously, parents can benefit from both viewpoints. For example, a dialectic reality includes both contentment with the situation (acceptance), *and* commitment to change.
- Highlight that two seemingly opposite perspectives can be synthesized by using the words "both/and," instead of keeping the perspectives separate and opposing with the words "or/but."
- Practicing dialectical responses is an effective way to underscore the idea of synthesis or integration that underlies the dialectal philosophy.
- TBT-S participants are encouraged to practice using "and" statements throughout treatment, as is practiced in dialectical behavior therapy (DBT). An example may be one's attitude toward smart phones. Smart phones are essential and make life easier AND are problematic for a variety of reasons.

4. Present the dialectic blank diagram, Figure 16.1, or ask parents to draw the dialectical circle image shown in Figure 16.1.

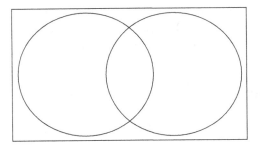

**Figure 16.1** Blank dialectical model of parent support

5. The blank dialectical model is presented as the framework for learning effective methods of assistance that frame parent skills.
6. The primary dialectical dilemma in providing assistance for YAs with anorexia nervosa is transforming the conflict of (a) emotional assistance using validation and understanding, and simultaneously offering (b) instrumental assistance using firmness and accountability.
7. Clinicians present parental assistance within two primary spheres consisting of emotional assistance (validation) and instrumental assistance (firmness, accountability), with a brief explanation of each.
8. Emotional assistance is the ability to communicate understanding and validation of the YA's experiences surrounding anorexia nervosa and recovery. See Figure 16.2.

- The left circle the empathic (validation) sphere.
- It is referred to as the "soft skills" sphere.

9. The complementary (versus opposing) sphere of assistance is instrumental (firmness) responses is on the right.

- This sphere sets healthy boundaries to facilitate recovery.

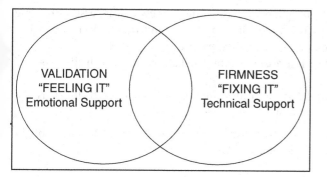

**Figure 16.2** Dialectical model of parent support, overview

10. Parents are asked to reflect on accommodating or enabling behaviors that have inadvertently enabled their loved ones with AN to continue their eating disorder (ED) symptoms. Have they made it easier in any way for their loved ones to do ED behaviors?
11. Clinicians highlight that both domains of assistance and expression are necessary and equal.

    • Neither one is sufficient alone.

12. The dialectical parent model for YAs allows parents to achieve a balance by practicing skills from both domains to simultaneously provide both aspects of assistance.
13. This overarching model contains the big picture view from which specific skills are practiced to assist in recovery.

    • It allows parents to reflect in more general ways on their capacity and effectiveness in being encouraging in both "soft" and "hard" ways. See Figure 16.2.

**Key Points**
• Parents, as Supports, are taught that a dialect is the synthesis of two simultaneous opposing points of view or approaches.
• The dialect serves as the framework for parental skills to be applied in varying situations based on the dilemma at hand.

# Highlight Dialectical Skills and Parent Self-Assessment

## Steps

1. Give each parent a handout of the dialectical model with empty spheres or have them draw the spheres on a piece of paper (See Figure 16.1).
2. Ask parents to reflect on and list skills and actions that fall under each sphere.
3. Once each parent completes the skills list, the clinician facilitates sharing within the group and completes a full model including all participant ideas. If key skills are missing, then the clinician can add those in.

- It is more effective to have group members generate their own ideas versus providing a dialectical model that is already filled in. It allows for individual specificity and variations of ideas that are particular to each parent.
- Parents are able to generate impressively complete lists without much clinician involvement.
- Parents come up with novel and clever ideas that often serve to teach clinicians and other parents about important aspects of providing assistance.

4. Actions that are key aspects of parental assistance are bolded. It is important to highlight these actions to parents if they are not generated.

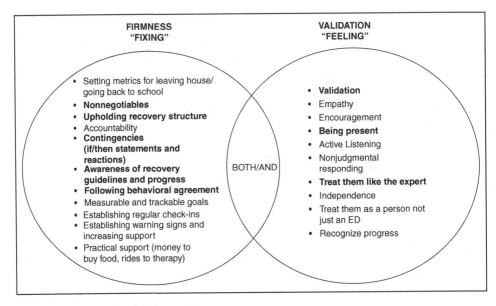

**Figure 16.3** Dialectical model of parent support

5. <u>Self-Assessment</u>: Parents are asked to identify and circle
   a. Three skills that they identify as their strengths.
   b. Three skills that they would like to improve upon because they would positively impact recovery.
6. The clinician leads a discussion and informs parent(s) that these skills will be reviewed and practiced in subsequent parent skills training sessions.

**Key Points**
- **Parents are directed to think of assistance as dialectically multi-faceted and are oriented to various ways to provide assistance to YAs.**
- **Parents self-asses their strengths and weaknesses and choose skills to improve their ability to assist.**

# Parent Skills Training

## Steps

1. Clinicians share a rationale for skill use (**teach-learn**).
2. Clinicians choose a skill from the following list to highlight during any given session based on the needs of parent(s) present.
3. Clinicians provide a brief explanation and example of the skill. (A relevant example is a poignant way to highlight the way a skill can be used.)
4. Invite parents to "try it on" (**practice**) with other parents/Supports.
5. Seek parent feedback of their experiences.
6. Provide time for parents to apply the skills with their YA loved ones or as homework.
7. Seek feedback from parents at the next session on how the skills were applied. Use the "Self-Critique Tool," in the Toolbox in Appendix 9.

## Parent/Supports Skills

Following are brief definitions of key strategic skills, or methods, that clinicians can teach parents and help them practice during treatment sessions and at home. Their order below is not prioritized. Skills address the need for emotional and technical assistance and effective parental responses to key neurobiological alterations. Skills should be chosen based on the Parent Self-Assessment (see Steps 3 and 4). The purpose of outlining the skills in one chapter is to provide a holistic picture of the expectations of parents based on the YA-TBT-S model. It raises awareness and enables parents to internalize their diverse roles when offering assistance to their YA. Some of the strategies, particularly those included under the "Instrumental" domain, are covered in the YA Behavioral Agreement.

### Nonnegotiables

#### Neurobiological and Trait Targets

- Rule oriented
- Harm avoidant
- High need for structure and certainty

Nonnegotiables are boundaries that parents and YA clients identify for recovery. Each parent is encouraged and prompted to develop and articulate their own nonnegotiables based upon both their needs and their own tolerance. Clients identify and articulate their own nonnegotiables. Clarifying the "line in the sand" means that it is the place beyond which different actions are required to move toward recovery. If the YA steps outside the nonnegotiable, parents and their YA agree upon critical actions that are necessary to take to ensure recovery and/or prevent relapse. Critical actions are planned contingencies for progress and relapse that promote compliance with identified goals and enhance motivation to recover. Nonnegotiables define situations or actions that are critical or unacceptable for recovery to occur. This appeals to the tendency of those with AN to need structure and certainty.

Establishing nonnegotiables enables parents and clients to clarify actions that they are committed to change. Nonnegotiables can change over time based on various situations. Clinicians could explain nonnegotiables as "fires" in recovery, signs or actions that would be highly alarming or signals of an emergent situation. Common examples of parent nonnegotiables for YAs include establishing a minimum weight requirement and clarifying a minimum amount of contact with treatment providers. If the client is unable to meet the nonnegotiable, then consequences can be identified, such as the need for a higher level of care.

Common examples of YA nonnegotiables include boundaries for parental involvement such as *"It is non-negotiable for me that I prepare my own breakfast."* Nonnegotiables/parent commitments are established by YAs during YA sessions individually or in groups. See YA Behavioral Agreement in Appendix 27 and SE-AN Behavioral Agreement in Appendix 28.

## Upholding a Recovery Structure

### Neurobiological and Trait Targets

- Rule oriented
- High need for structure and certainty

Upholding a recovery structure is another method for parents to assist in structure and certainty. This refers to parents' involvement and ability to uphold the prescribed structures, including mealtime rules and other specific recovery recommendations surrounding meals and snacks and activities amid other treatment, work, and school activities. This addresses the need for structure for many with AN. For example, TBT-S and most ED treatments approach meal plans with three meals and three snacks, and individual movement/activity plans for each client. At a minimum, parents should be aware of meal plans and identify ways that they can assist in upholding this structure.

## Contingencies: If/Then Statements with Planned Responses to ED Behaviors

### Neurobiological and Trait Targets

- Sensitive to punishment
- Harm avoidant
- Altered reward sensitivity (motivational deficits related to recovery)

Contingencies are defined as planned responses to particular behaviors. Assisting parents with developing planned responses to ED behaviors, as well as progress in recovery, is an important aspect of parent involvement in AN treatment. This strategy relates to altered reward sensitivity in AN, which may affect motivation. Contingencies provide alternative means for motivation; when parents establish "bottom-line" contingencies or nonnegotiables, they are appealing to the common AN temperament trait of being sensitive to punishment/harm avoidant. Contingencies are also addressed in the Behavioral Agreement (see Appendix 27). Parents are encouraged to think through appropriate responses to improvements and relapses in their loved one's ED symptoms. They also need to practice articulating these conditions to their YA in neutral, nonjudgmental ways using if/then statements. For YAs who continue to receive various types of assistance from their parents, this may also include guiding parents to consider how financial and instrumental assistance may change based upon progress with recovery. (See YA Behavioral Agreement, Types of Support in Appendix 27.)

## Knowledge and Continued Awareness of Recovery Guidelines and Progress

### Neurobiological and Trait Targets

- Driven by external structure
- Sensitivity to social criticism

TBT-S places a strong emphasis on parents being involved in identified segments of treatment. This is important because those with AN may benefit from external accountability due to lack of internal motivational drives to recover. An important aspect of this includes being knowledgeable about recovery guidelines and progress so that parents have the information needed to provide effective assistance and can adjust their methods based on progress. Examples include being knowledgeable and aware of the prescribed meal plan, established body composition goals, and weekly physical strength progress. Parents of YAs are encouraged to attend dietary sessions in TBT-S. See Chapter 20 on dietary strategies to ensure continuity of dietary recommendations including body strength expectations and movement guidelines.

## Validation

### Neurobiological and Trait Target
• Sensitivity to social criticism

Validation is an important skill for parents to learn in their communication with their YA loved ones with AN.[134, 135] Validation by parents demonstrates their affirmation of YA experiences, even when they are painful and hard to hear. Individuals with AN are often sensitive to criticism and concerned about negative evaluation by others. Teaching parents skills for verbal validation may improve their YA's resolve and provide affirming feedback if and when a YA feels uncertain or worried. Dialectically, a parent can validate what their YA shared about an ED behavior *and* simultaneously move forward to the agreed plan of action.

## Being Present

TBT-S focuses on the present, recognizing it is the time when a person holds control to take action or not. It also means that parents agree to designate when they can be available to offer assistance. This skill also extends to more specific circumstances, such as being present during particular mealtimes or difficult times of the day, and/or being engaged in an interaction.

## Appointing the Client as the Expert

As adults, clients with AN understand their experience better than others, even clinicians in many cases. Parents are encouraged to ask and learn from their YA regarding puzzling or confusing behaviors, instead of assuming their own cause or reason. When parents observe or identify a problem, parents are taught to ask observational questions that will facilitate their YA to participate in problem-solving. Seeking understanding through specified questions helps the YA explore options, instead of making unsolicited suggestions or criticisms. Parents are taught to encourage problem-solving, and then ask what type of assistance their YA needs versus providing solutions or engaging in unnecessary "rescuing." This approach allows clients to be respected as autonomous individuals in their recovery and emphasizes a collaborative working relationship between clients and parents. For example, a parent may ask, *"Help me understand what it is like when you arrive at a meal? Do you do the same thing each time? How do you feel before? How do you feel afterward?. That is helpful for me to know."*

## Understanding and Viewing AN as a Biological Illness

Many, if not all of the neurobiology exercises applied in TBT-S share the objective of building empathy and understanding of the AN experience. There are biological reasons that individuals with AN engage in destructive behaviors such as restriction, that are both damaging AND have a purpose and explanation from a biological perspective. Clinicians can help parents develop a knowledgeable skill-base by educating them on the neurobiological and temperament bases of AN (see Chapters 9–13). This establishes a deeper empathy when parents offer other skills.

## Constructing and Forming a Behavioral Agreement (BA)

### Neurobiological and Trait Targets

- Rule oriented
- Highly structured
- Achievement oriented

The YA BA, explained in detail in Chapter 22, is an explicit agreement between the YA client and parents/Support(s). It provides the framework to integrate and outline the skills presented in this chapter that are practiced in parent skills group. Outlining a specific plan between YA clients and their parents or other Supports in detail includes establishing recovery guidelines and outlining treatment recommendations and a contingency plan for parental involvement. Creating the YA BA is a skill in and of itself. The BA provides a structure that summarizes concepts in a detailed plan and identifies useful and needed rules for YA clients with AN. The BA establishes consistency and clarity between the YA client and parents, as well as with the clinician, dietitian, and medical professional involved in treatment.

## Redirection/Distraction

### Neurobiological and Trait Targets

- Anxiety
- Obsessionality
- Rumination

Redirection refers to the ability to assist and facilitate with moving away from obsessive eating disorder thoughts and negative rumination. Parents learn effective ways to assist with redirecting their YA's attention by using directive prompts (for example: *Let's take a walk to the other room*) and assisting with distraction activities such as facilitating a conversation about a non-eating disorder–related topic during meals or when doing an activity together. Clinicians teach parents to avoid rationalizing or providing facts to reduce anxiety because facts cannot fight fear (i.e., anxiety). Clinicians also teach parents to avoid asking open-ended questions, which can be overwhelming for an emotionally aroused brain. (For example: in response to a statement about being fat "*Why do you think you are fat?*" would be discouraged.)

## Prompting

### Neurobiological and Trait Targets

- Anxiety
- Excessive inhibition

Clinicians teach parents to provide clear, concise prompts to assist their YA with initiating a desired behavior or to provide direction when a YA is anxious and unable to make a clear decision. Clinicians teach parents to break down questions into steps, and to prompt for the next step needed, if the YA is unable to act on the next needed step. For example, if a YA is staring at a plate of food and feels unable to get started, a parent could provide a prompt such as, "*Pick up your fork and take a bite of your fish*." Prompts can also be used in response to anxiety and a negative repetitive thought or behavior to facilitate redirection. (For example, "*Let's play* Uno, *please deal the cards.*"

## Consistent and Predictable Response-Sets

### Neurobiological and Trait Targets

- Highly structured
- Intolerant of uncertainty

Clinicians direct parents to identify commonly occurring eating disorder behaviors and developed planned responses, referred to as "parent protocols" that they can deliver consistently in response to eating disorder behaviors. Parents are taught to inform their YAs of these responses and then encouraged to follow through consistently. This ensures that YAs know what to expect, which reduces uncertainty and anxiety and can help promote compliance with recovery.

# Forming a Network of Supports

In addition to skills training, parent groups could be resources of encouragement and assistance for one another. TBT-S advocates from the very beginning to involve Supports, resulting in a high level of parental involvement in treatment of YAs with AN. In group settings, ongoing Support networks are easily and naturally established. Supports will likely experience distress and potential burnout. This illness is best assisted with a team of Supports, including peers and other important relationships where possible. When TBT-S is offered in a 5-day group format, and parents have spent 40 hours together in 1 week discussing extended histories of illness, Support networks are naturally formed. Parents realize their needs are shared by an entire system of Supports who hold a wide range of stressors and solutions. Supports may benefit by meeting outside of treatment to share with other Supports. A network may occur for a period of time.

Supports are encouraged to connect with national and international nonprofit organizations whose missions are to offer a network of assistance to other parents. Examples are the National Association for Eating Disorders, F.E.A.S.T., and Eating Disorders Families of Australia.

---

**Key Point**
- Clinicians teach parents a broad range of skills to effectively assist their YA to reduce symptoms of AN.

---

**Summary Key Points**

- The dialectical model of parent support is a unique framework for parenting YAs with AN
- Parents need a portfolio of skills to help their YA loved one toward recovery.
- Skills are actions taken that improve recovery.
- Different skills are needed for different situations.

# Young Adult TBT-S Client Skills Training

## Purpose and Description of the Young Adult Client Skills Training Module

TBT-S teaches and practices temperament based skills that young adult (YA) clients with anorexia nervosa (AN) can use to cope with the challenges of long-term recovery. The YA TBT-S skills modules augment eating disorder (ED) therapies. They are aligned with clients' temperaments. Each individual has different traits and needs. Determining which skills apply is based on client temperament and a needs assessment. Clinicians administer the Trait Profile Checklist (see Appendix 2) and assess aspects of the clients' ED that need to be addressed. Clinicians work with YA clients to explore their destructive traits that are contributing to their ED symptoms to identify what skills could help reshape trait and symptom expressions. This information serves to determine a focused plan for skills training. Identified skills can be trained and practiced in individual or group settings at all levels of care. TBT-S draws from other skills-based treatments, such as dialectical behavioral therapy (DBT) and encourages clinicians to conduct a needs assessment and draw from other skills-based treatments that are applicable. Clinicians weave TBT-S and other ED skills together that are congruent with client(s) temperaments to maximize motivation.

YAs are taught how skills address traits and underlying brain responses, drawing from information presented in the Psychoeducation Modules. Clinicians can augment the skills outlined in this chapter with the Neurobiological Psychoeducation Modules to explain underlying causes of ED symptoms and why specified skills are needed for recovery (see Chapters 9–13). Specifically, YA TBT-S focuses on skills that address key aspects of the neurobiological model of TBT-S treatment, which include **anxiety**, altered **interoception**, motivational deficits via altered **reward sensitivity**, and **inhibition** (see YA Skills Worksheets in Appendices 4 and 5).

TBT-S emphasizes skills *practice*. Skills learned can be practiced during YA skills training sessions and assigned to continue to be practiced during therapeutic mealtimes and outside of treatment.

> Key Point: YA skills training is based on a needs assessment of YAs using the Trait Profile Checklist. YA TBT-S skills reflect the TBT-S neurobiological model of AN and target: anxiety, altered interoception, motivational deficits (via altered reward sensitivity), and inhibition.

# Clinician Checklist for YA Skills

⇒ Assess client ED symptoms that need management or reduction.
⇒ Administer the Trait Profile Checklist to assess client productive traits (internal resources for motivation and action) and destructive traits that contribute to and/or cause ED symptoms.
⇒ Learn and practice skills in treatment sessions.
⇒ Assign skills for practice outside of treatment sessions.

Table 17.1 summarizes YA skills training modules. It matches common AN treatment targets with client productive traits (internal strengths and resources). It then shows corresponding TBT-S skills (clients and Supports) and experiential activities. Clinicians are encouraged to include skills from other treatment modalities that address the clients' needs and traits, with an emphasis on in-treatment practice.

# Targeting Anxiety Module

## Neurobiological and Trait Targets

- Anxiety
- Inhibition
- Avoidance
- Obsessiveness
- Difficulty Set Shifting

# Objectives

Clinicians provide clients who have AN with methods that

- Decrease anxiety before, during and after meals.
- Clarify actions that refocus or distract attention away from ED thoughts to another topic or activity.
- Redirect fears of weight gain and intense feelings of fullness to intense productive actions.
- Identify client traits that productively help manage ED symptoms and motivate forward action.
- Explore underlying causes that trigger mealtime anxiety (see Chapter 11).
- Identify ways that AN miscodes food signals as dangerous (see Chapter 11).
- Match low intensity with a verbal activity and high intensity with physical activity.
- Are simple and practical.
- Can be practiced during treatment first and repeated at home.
- Introduce skills as actions to be practiced and mastered.

# What Does the Research Say?

- An eating disorder study comparing the use of distraction strategies with mindfulness strategies applied before mealtimes found that distraction resulted in a greater caloric intake for those with AN.[185]
- See Chapter 11 for neurobiological research addressing anxiety and interoception.

**Table 17.1** YA TBT-S treatment targets matched with skills

| Trait treatment targets | Potential productive AN traits (motivate and activate) | Skill module | Description/instructions | Support skill reinforcement | Related TBT-S activities modules |
|---|---|---|---|---|---|
| Anxiety Inhibition | Determined<br>Cautious<br>Routine<br>High achievement<br>Perfectionism<br>Optimism<br>Extroversion<br>Novelty seeking<br>Cooperative<br>Active<br>Conscientious<br>Sociable<br>Attentive | Distraction Redirect Attention | • Clients identify times when anxiety is greatest (pre, during, post meals)<br>• Clients practice re-directing attention to another simple activity or task to manage intrusive internal experiences related to AN<br>• Clients choose distraction activities<br>• Clients construct a distraction routine to be used surrounding meals | • Effective re-direction<br>• Support and participation with distraction activities<br>• Effective Prompting | • Experiential Activity: Anxiety Brain Sculpt (Appendix 16)<br>• Experiential Activity: Anxiety Wave Handouts (Appendix 15)<br>• Psychoeducation: Anxiety<br>• Psychoeducation: Inhibition |
| | Assertive<br>Curious<br>Imaginative<br>Altruistic<br>Dutiful<br>Disciplined | Mealtime Rules and Structure | • Clients formulate rules and habits to follow around meals<br>• Practice repetition (to reinforce habit and reduce anxiety) | • Upholding structure<br>• Consistency and predictability in responses and behavior | • YA Behavioral Agreement |
| | Detailed<br>Committed<br>Persistent | **RAD:** Recognize | • Describe hunger and fullness signals in AN as a faulty gas gauge | • Consistency and predictability in | • Psychoeducation: Altered Interoception |

| | | | | | |
|---|---|---|---|---|---|
| Interoception | Competitive Diligent Empathic Reliable Hard-working | Acknowledge Distract/De-Identify | • Identify discrepancy between prescribed meal plan and what "feels" like the right amount<br>• Review/practice ways to acknowledge and tolerate discomfort<br>• Practice following prescription (meal plan)<br>* See Rules and Framework for Meals and Snacks Handout (Appendix 6) | responses and behavior<br>• Uphold meal plan structure | • Psychoeducation: Alterations in Reward Processing<br>• Experiential Activity: YES/NO Game<br>• YA Behavioral Agreement SE-AN Worksheet 1- Red Flags |
| Motivation Deficits | | External Reinforcers and Consequences | • Identify reinforcers and natural consequences of recovery | • Supports enable external reinforcers and consequences | |

> **Neurobiological Key Points**
> - Anxiety is distressing and can lead to restriction around mealtimes.
> - Learning to redirect attention and action to other skillful actions (skills) can reduce distress and be an effective anxiety management tool.

# Practicing Distraction and Redirecting Attention

## Steps and *Scripts*

(Do not read the scripts. Use them as notes and speak directly to YAs and parents to increase therapeutic impact.)

Clinicians are encouraged to learn (not read) the scripts and express them in their own voices, so that they can look clients in the eyes (virtually or face-to-face) to provide the information and to lead discussions.

1. Provide an introduction to anxiety and a rationale for distraction/redirection, using information from the Neurobiology of Anxiety Module in Chapter 11.
2. The clinician leads a discussion about the anxiety and distress experienced during recovery or around mealtime.
3. Once the clinician thinks that the interaction has reached a serious tone, the clinician abruptly shifts to a distraction activity without warning and without explanation.

   o *Take out a pen and paper and write the word NEUROBIOLOGY on the top of the paper.*
   o *You have two minutes to write down as many words as possible by using combinations of letters from the word.*
   o After two minutes ask, *Are you still thinking about ED mealtime anxiety?*

4. Discuss how the activity forced thoughts to be distracted from the discussion to a mental game. Action forces thoughts to shift.

   o *Identify times when ED thoughts and other related experiences are intense for you.*
   o *Please look over the List of Distraction Activities Handout and choose actions you are willing to practice before, during, and after meals (Appendix 7).*
   o *The more you practice an action, the more it becomes a routine, and habitual, for your thoughts to turn to a different focus from the anxious thoughts.*
   o *Your mind is already practicing habitual thoughts. They are simple but anxious, frustrating, and distressful thoughts. You are forcing your mind to shift topics and to establish a less distressing habit.*

5. See Table 17.1.

**Homework**

- Practice a distraction activity before each meal, a distraction activity during each meal, and a distraction activity after each meal every day. Practice the same distraction routine daily to establish a pre-meal and post-meal routine (to reduce anxiety).

# Mealtime Rules and Structure

### Steps and *Scripts*

(Do not read the *scripts*. Use them as notes and speak directly to clients and Supports to increase therapeutic impact.)

1. TBT-S dietitians and/or clinicians identify sessions to eat with clients and Supports multiple times during the therapeutic process (virtually or face-to-face). (During the studied TBT-S model, YAs and parents prepare and partake in 20 therapeutic meals and snacks over 1 week at structured times each day.)
2. Instruct parents and YA clients to identify rules and a meal structure at the outset, both of which are methods to provide safety from fearful mealtime experiences.
3. Although the mealtime rules may initially add to the distress, once clients with AN practice the rules and structure repeatedly, they establish predictability and comfort.

   ○ Ask: *Do you use rules to guide the small amounts of food you have been eating?* (Clients with AN often have a tendency toward rule making and routine.)

4. Since clients with AN tend to be rule bound and to prefer structure, TBT-S uses those same traits by working *with* the client to adjust the rules and structure to move toward recovery, using Figures 17.1–17.2.
5. After practicing the new rules and structure in sessions, developing an imprint on the change process, assign clients and Supports to use the same rules and structure outside the treatment sessions for every meal.
6. This structure is the first phase of preparation for the YA Behavioral Agreement. Information identified for the worksheet is refined after testing it out and before writing the YA BA.
7. This information is then included in the Behavioral Agreement.
8. Use the handout pictured in 17.1 for a brainstorming session; the handout is in Appendix 6.

**Homework**

- Practice new rules and structure at all meals outside of therapy.

## Young Adult Behavioral Agreement Template: Meals and Snacks, by Stephanie Knatz Peck

☐ Eat 3 meals and____snacks every day following the schedule below:

    ☐ Breakfast at____AM
    ☐ AM Snack at____AM
    ☐ Lunch at____PM
    ☐ PM Snack at____PM
    ☐ Dinner at____PM
    ☐ Evening Snack at____PM

☐ Complete 100% of meals and snacks
☐ SUPPLEMENTING: Supplement drinks (or bars) will be used if meal/snack is not completed.
    ☐ If more than 50% but less than 100%, 1 supplement will be consumed.
    ☐ If less than 50%, 2 supplements will be consumed.

☐ Meals follow the USDA plate model. Examples that could be default meals:

| BREAKFAST EXAMPLES | | |
|---|---|---|
|  |  |  |

| LUNCH EXAMPLES | | |
|---|---|---|
|  |  |  |

| DINNER EXAMPLES | | |
|---|---|---|
|  |  |  |

1

**Figure 17.1** Young adult client rules and framework for meals and snacks

☐   Snacks will be based on approved snack list. Default snacks include:

_____          _____

_____          _____

_____          _____

☐   Meals will be eaten in____minutes and snacks will be eaten in____minutes.

☐   I will remain in the presence of a Support for 60 minutes following meals and snacks to avoid purging.

☐   Bathroom visits will be supervised by a Support.

☐   Support persons,_____and_____,will remain informed of meal plan and any changes.

☐   Supports will attend the following regular appointments:_____

_____

☐   Supports will be present for the following meals and snacks regularly:

　　☐   Breakfast at____AM
　　☐   AM Snack at____AM
　　☐   Lunch at____PM
　　☐   PM Snack at____PM
　　☐   Dinner at____PM
　　☐   Evening Snack at____PM

☐   When Supports are not present, I commit to:

　　☐   Having meals with others who can assist me (Name:_____)
　　☐   Reporting back to Supports by: (describe how you will keep them updated).
　　☐   Video chatting during meals and snacks (list which ones).
　　☐   _____
　　☐   _____

☐   When Supports are present, I will:

　　☐   "Check off" that my meals/snacks meet dietary requirements.
　　☐   Assist with distractions.
　　☐   Provide the following feedback if I am having difficulty initiating/completing my meal:
　　　　Discuss and write strategies you would like your Support to use:

　　　　_____
　　　　_____
　　　　_____

　　☐   Provide the following feedback if I am engaging in any ED behaviors during meals/snacks:

　　　　_____
　　　　_____
　　　　_____

2

**Figure 17.1** (cont.)

# Targeting Interoception Module

## Objectives

- Explain the impact of altered interoception in those with AN.
- Provide actions and a RAD skill (**RAD: Recognize, Acknowledge, Distract/De-Identify**) that clients can take to respond to altered interoceptive experiences.

## What Does the Research Say?

- AN fundamentally involves disturbances in the experience of physical sensations in one's body, referred to as *interoception* (see Chapter 11).
- Interoception includes internal physical body-state experiences, such as hunger and fullness, taste, pain, touch, heartbeat, breathing, and gastrointestinal sensations.
- Many AN symptoms relate to altered interoceptive experiences such as increased gastrointestinal discomfort/distress and an inability to sense hunger and/or fullness and/or pain from excessive exercise.

> **Neurobiological Key Point:** Altered interoception, inability to sense hunger and/or fullness and/or pain from excessive exercise, is related to more acute eating disorder symptoms.

## Steps and *Scripts*

(Do not read the scripts. Use them as notes and speak directly to clients and Supports to increase therapeutic impact.)

1. Review the neurobiological research information presented in Chapter 11 with the clients and/or Supports.

   - Ask clients with AN, *Can you sense when you are hungry?*
   - *Can you sense when you are full? How do you experience pain?*
   - *Some clients with AN are not able to experience some or all of these sensations.*
   - *If you are not able to internally experience body signals that tell you what to do about eating or not eating, it is understandable that you would be anxious to eat, because you don't know if you should eat now if you can't sense hunger. If you can't sense fullness, it makes sense you won't know when to stop eating. You are in essence eating blind.*
   - *Research tells us that the more severe your inability to experience your body sensations, the more severe your eating disorder symptoms are.*
   - *What about that is true or not true for you? Listen to how clients apply this to their experiences.*
   - *If you are less able to experience necessary internal sensations to guide your decisions, then you need to rely to external signals to indicate what to do. How does this fit with your experience?*
   - *If you are unable to sense hunger, then rules can help you determine what to do each time you eat.*
   - *You have naturally used and practiced ED rules that structure how to eat or how to eat less.*

2. Action: Emphasize the importance of using rules when a person has altered interoception. Use rules. Replace ED rules with healthy rules related to eating or other areas of life.

   ○ *If you are able to experience fullness, it can be extremely uncomfortable when you are expected to eat more energy than your stomach is used to taking in. That is why it is important that you work with your dietitian to identify energy needs that take up less volume as you are getting stronger.*

3. Offer metaphors that could represent this physical response. For example, faulty interoception is like a faulty gas gauge in a car.

4. When a "gauge of hunger or fullness" is faulty, external requirements are needed to compensate, such as adjusting the prescribed "fuel" plan.

5. Action: Instruct clients to work with the dietitian to shift fuels to a "higher octane" that offers more energy and less volume if they experience pain when eating high-volume foods.

6. Share with the clients that being aware of their discomfort is necessary for them to identify what to do.

7. **RAD** is a skill that provides a way to manage uncomfortable body states that are at odds with a prescribed meal plan.

8. Review the client handout titled "Young Adult RAD Skills Training Handout for Clients with Anorexia Nervosa" in Appendix 8.

9. Practice RAD skills in session. Provide non-ED examples of practice responding to an uncomfortable body state using RAD. Clinicians pass out small feathers to each client and have each client lightly rub the feather over a sensitive area of skin to provoke a tickle. YAs practice experiencing the tickle without reacting to it by using the RAD skill.

## Homework

• Practice RAD at home.

# Targeting Altered Reward Sensitivity/Motivational Deficits Module

**Neurobiological and Trait Targets**

• Harm avoidance
• Punishment sensitivity
• High achievement

## Objectives

• Describe neurobiological reasons why persons with AN may not be intrinsically (self) motivated.
• Parents are identified as a source to whom clients can turn to uphold structure.
• Encourage consistency in established structures creating safety and impacting motivation.

## What Does the Research Say?

- Brain imaging studies have examined the brain reward response to pictures of food and tastes of food in AN, finding decreased brain responses in the reward circuit (ventral striatum) and the interoceptive circuit that signal hunger, fullness, and taste (insula) for both pictures of foods and tastes of highly palatable foods.
- This finding suggests decreased reward signaling occurs for foods among persons with AN.
- Notably, decreased response to pleasant taste in the cognitive circuit (the dorsal caudate) is associated with increased harm avoidance in AN, suggesting a biological basis for coding food as harmful.
- For people without AN, hunger is a biologically based, motivational signal related to energy stores that drives the consumption of food.
- Healthy individuals show increased brain response to rewarding stimuli when hungry compared with after a meal. This response serves to motivate eating by increasing the rewarding sensation/pleasure from food.
- Individuals with AN show greater *reductions in brain reward response to taste when hungry* in the reward circuit (ventral putamen) and interoceptive circuit (insula) compared with healthy controls.
- This result suggests that hunger may not motivate eating.

> **Key Points**
> - There is a biological basis for why eating is not easy in that food is not intrinsically rewarding, contributing to why the brain may code food as harmful.
> - Lack of motivation for treatment may reflect a deficit in biologically induced reward/motivation system rather than willfulness.

## Steps and *Scripts*

(Do not read the scripts. Use them as notes and speak directly to clients and Supports to increase therapeutic impact.)

1. Describe and discuss the key neurobiological points presented about motivation in those with AN.
   - *Do you feel motivated to eat most foods?*
   - *Do you experience distress and dysphoria versus an internal sense of pleasure and satisfaction?*
   - *Eating and the consequences from eating can be punishing instead of rewarding for those with AN. How does that fit with your experience?*

2. Identify valued reinforcers. Since the intrinsic value of recovery can be low for clients with AN, YA TBT-S focuses on linking recovery to other activities and objects of value to the YA, such as maintaining a job, independence, or the ability to attend college.

3. Set recovery metrics with treatment team and parents. Lead YA clients to collaborate with parents to set clear recovery metrics.

4. These recovery metrics are then attached to each of these valued outcomes/reinforcers. Encourage YA clients to tell their parents, who are willing to offer assistance in meeting those goals, what they need from them to move forward.

5. In YA TBT-S, parents and other Supports are important stakeholders as external agents who help compensate for the YA client's inability to be internally motivated.

6. This process becomes preparation for the YA Behavioral Agreement to be filled out by the YA and parents and/or other Supports.

7. Work with YA clients and their parents or other Supports to identify backup contingencies if they go off course. This is a management skill. The ideas are refined in the YA Behavioral Agreement Module.

8. Direct clients to think through the following prompts and to provide answers via self-reflection and group discussion. Answers serve as preparation for the YA Behavioral Agreement. They are discussed with Supports to include in the YA Behavioral Agreement.

---

**Motivators:**

- List life goals that you would like to achieve within the next year that will motivate you to recover (Ex. leaving home, attending college)
- List things you want to earn that are tangible (Ex. a desired object or trip).

**Parent reinforcements:** What can your parents do/provide, or what goals can they support that will motivate you to progress?

- Extra privileges and reinforcements. (List things you want to earn. They can be tangible (a desired object or trip) or privileges like independence).
- Nonnegotiables. Discuss with your parents what would cause them to increase their involvement or reduce their assistance of your goals.

**Self-identifled consequences if I begin to relapse:**

**Red Flags\*** What are indicators that I am not doing well?

- What do I expect I should do about them?

**What would lack of progress look like?**

- o Ex. Failure to restore at recommended pace.
- o Weight drops below xx.

**How will parent involvement change if I am slipping?**

\*If clients have trouble generating their own ideas, see SE-AN Worksheet 1 (Appendix 28), which provides a list of red flags from which clients can choose.

---

**Figure 17.2** Young adult prompts to identify healthy external motivational sources

**Summary Key Points**

- Clinicians can help clients turn to Supports to identify external motivators since they may not experience intrinsic motivation.
- Provide structure around meals because it is unlikely that individuals with active AN can eat intuitively given altered brain reward signaling to hunger.

# TBT-S Tools to Manage and Reduce ED Symptoms

## Tools for Severe-and-Enduring Anorexia Nervosa (SE-AN) and Young Adult (YA) Clients

### What Are the Tools?

TBT-S provides a wide range of tools, that are simple steps (sometimes one-word responses) and when practiced become skillful verbal responses and actions to shape patterns of recovery. The TBT-S toolbox has been developed with SE-AN clients' input, see Figure 18.1. The TBT-S Toolbox handout is in Appendix 9. The toolbox is a rectangle with a border, representing a toolbox. The border lists the client's productive traits. This reflects that one's actions, thoughts, and feelings are framed and impacted by one's temperament traits. Traits contribute to why one tool may be chosen over another.

The tools are a list of possible actions that clients and Supports could choose to manage eating disorder (ED) symptoms. Any tool may seem like a good idea to use, but if it is not aligned with the client's and Support's traits, it would not be a "good fit" for the person. To endorse trait-aligned tools, clients and Supports identify six of their productive traits from the Trait Profile Checklist (see Appendix 2) and write their productive traits in the borders of the toolbox. This strategically aligns traits with tools to develop long-term productive habits.

> **Key Point: Tools that are a "good fit" align with the client's and Support's productive traits.**

## The Difference between Symptoms and Traits

As shared in Chapter 1, drawing on Cloninger's model, traits are biological (nature) influences of one's personality. Character is one's outward expressions, the socialized, environmentally shaped side of one's personality (nurture).[136]

TBT-S tools come in all shapes and sizes. They can be a person's productive traits as well as verbal statements, objects and actions that one can use to manage ED symptoms. As explained in Chapter 1, the difference between symptoms and traits are outlined next.

### Symptoms

- Are outward behavioral expressions, such as self-induced vomiting or binge eating.
- Are reactions to one's illnesses.
- Have the potential to be reduced and eliminated.

## Traits

- Are inherited, innate features in one's personality that guide one's thoughts, feelings, and behaviors.
- Can be altered by *intentionally* shifting their expressions.
- Cannot be eliminated. They are with one throughout life.

## TBT-S Toolbox

**List 4 traits that I express productively** (from Trait Profile Checklist)

*My Trait:*

Say, **"Give me two/three options"** when others ask me open questions, e.g., "What do you want to do?"

**Delay** ED behaviors by doing: _____

**Give a compliment** to another person via text: ID one _____

**Walk** ____ minutes.

**Actively listen and participate in a conversation**

**Do one hour of a project that takes my concentration**_____

**Deep breathe** – inhale 4 seconds, exhale 4 seconds.

**Distract** by: Fill in two actions:_____   _____

**Ground myself** to this moment. ID: 2 things I see; 2 things I hear; 2 things I can touch; 2 things I smell.

**Walk Tall** (Stretch up as much as possible as walk).

**Hold myself accountable** by telling (ID the person) ____ if I act on a destructive behavior.

**Stop, reboot, reroute:** If waking toward destructive action, "Stop," turn 180° Walk in new route.

**WW** ____ **D?** Ask self, "What would ____ Do? ID person I admire _____, Then do it.

**WWID4** ____? "What would I do for_____?) ID the person_____, Then do it.

**Ask for help** ID 2 people _____

**Use my wise mind** using the dialectic "I think/or feel_____ AND I think/feel:_____."

**Earphones with music** of my playlists

**Food is my medicine:** I will eat my planned breakfast, lunch, dinner, snacks.

**Take my prescribed medication: food, pills/supplements**

**Restorative Yoga** with ID person _____ when, ID days _____.

**Self-Critique** an action/interaction/event: In this order: What would I do the same? What would I do differently? How would I do it differently?

**Use a premeal routine.**_____

**Help another person by doing** _____

**Accept myself for who I am** and use my traits in the current situation.

Instead of **walking toward** a destructive action, I will **walk to** _____.

Instead of **counting** _____ to restrict, I **will count** _____

Instead of holding back on (food or interactions), I will hold back on _____ to focus on _____.

*My Trait:* *My Trait:* *My Trait:*

**Choose three tools/skills that work WITH my traits.**

**Figure 18.1** TBT-S Toolbox

TBT-S approaches temperament traits on a continuum ranging from destructive to productive. Any single action is an expression of one's state. Trait expressions establish cognitive, emotional, and behavioral tendencies over time. Trait expressions begin at birth and are genetically determined. A trait could be dormant through much of a person's life and then genetically shift and become dominant as specific developmental stages or environmental pressures (such as trauma or high-stress life experiences) shape trait expressions. It is traits that trigger thoughts, feelings, and actions internally, while environment shapes trait expressions externally. TBT-S tools are used to help shape or chisel away at destructive traits and ED symptoms to form productive expressions.

Key Point: The TBT-S Toolbox contains simple and practical tools to reduce and manage ED symptoms encased by one's productive traits that are inner resources to reduce symptoms and live life more fully.

## Who Are the Tools For?

The TBT-S Toolbox is for ED clients and Supports. They are encouraged to "try on" tools to experimentally discover which tools are congruent with their own temperaments. The more aligned each tool is with a client's traits, the more likely they will use the tools to interrupt and manage their ED symptoms. The more adept one becomes at using a tool, the sooner it becomes a skill. Repetitive practice develops habits to replace the destructive ED habitual behaviors.

Supports need tools too. If Supports are left out of treatment sessions, they do not know what to do to help their loved ones. This causes Supports to experience repeated failure and exhaustion. It is common for young adult (YA) and SE-AN clients to push Supports away, feeling they should be able to manage the illness on their own. Regardless, Supports need tools that are helpful to the clients.

Selecting tools is part of the SE-AN Behavioral Agreement (see Appendix 28). It provides a means for clients and Supports to structure and coordinate their tools to work toward their goals.

Key Point: The TBT-S Toolbox is for clients and Supports.

## When to Use the Tools

The TBT-S Toolbox can be in introduced into treatment settings at any time. The earlier tools are introduced into treatment, the sooner clients can "try on" new actions to interrupt and counter ED behaviors.

Clinicians can practice tools while entering, during, and at the end of treatment sessions to initiate their use outside of therapy. For example, a clinician asks a client to "walk tall" as they enter or leave the therapy room before or after a treatment session or at the beginning and end of virtual sessions. To stretch up and walk tall allows a client to slow their pace and breathe more deeply. This action biologically forces a client's heart to slow down, which in turn slows thoughts and lowers anxiety. Clients have reported that it takes two or three tools to interrupt any one ED symptom.

> **Key Point:** Tools are an active means to change and shape traits and behaviors. The sooner clients identify and practice using tools, the better.

## Where to Use the Tools

The Toolbox can be used in all levels of care, individual or group settings, virtually or face-to-face.

## Why

TBT-S tools are verbal statements, objects or uncomplicated practical actions that can be applied in most places to distract, replace, manage, and reshape ED destructive behaviors into more productive expressions. They should be as simple and easy to use as ED behaviors are simple and easy. From a temperament approach, tools should be congruent actions with client's traits. This increases the potential for a "good fit" that could be sustained over time. The toolbox holds tools that are helpful to the client. This could include tools from other therapeutic approaches.

## How Can Clients Work toward Eliminating ED Symptoms Using Tools?

Clinicians enable clients to use their temperaments to reduce, manage, and eliminate ED symptoms by
- Identifying their productive traits, which are natural tendencies and internal resources.
- Practicing identified tools more frequently than ED symptoms are expressed.
- Asking for assistance from Supports.
- Working with the clinical team.
- Taking medications if needed.

## TBT-S Toolbox Instructions

The border or "container" of the toolbox represents each client's productive temperament traits. To know what traits each client has, client and Supports need to identify their traits so that traits and tools can work hand-in-hand.
1. Administer the Trait Profile Checklist handout, in Appendix 2. Instructions are included in the form.
   a. After clients score their checklist, they are asked to identify four current productive and three destructive traits.
   b. Identifying their productive and destructive traits allows them to acknowledge their innate strengths and weaknesses.
2. Give the TBT-S Toolbox Handout to clients and their Supports.
3. Ask the client(s) to choose four productive traits and write them in the border of the toolbox. Just as a toolbox contains or holds tools, clients contain traits that hold the capacity for what they can do most naturally.

4. Discuss each of the tools in the toolbox with the client(s).

5. Have each client fill in the blanks and actively "try on" each tool.

   a. A tool may look interesting or seem relevant, but test this by having the client try it on to determine if it is a good fit.

6. Optional: Have clients practice the tools with other clients by playing the TBT-S experiential activity, "Charades" (see Appendix 21).

7. Have clients circle the tools that reflect or fit with their productive traits. This increases the potential for them to use the tools.

8. Have each client choose three tools.

   a. These tools should be actions that are congruent with their traits, not incompatible with their temperament.

   b. Tools that work *with* their traits are easier to become habit.

9. Point out that it may take two or three tools to manage one ED symptom.

   a. One tool may not interrupt an ED behavior.

   b. Some tools may work better as a set when interrupting an ED symptom.

10. Ask Supports to identify tools for themselves. Then have Supports share with the client:

    a. Which tools they chose to assist in helping their loved one.

    b. To affirm if the client would find those tools helpful or unhelpful.

    c. That Supports may use tools that the client identifies or different ones.

    d. The tools used by Supports that are congruent with the Supports' temperaments.

# Tool Descriptions

- Ask: *"Give me two/three options"* when others ask open questions (e.g., *"What do you want to do?"*)

  o This addresses clients' inability to trust their decisions due to reward circuit abnormalities (see Chapter 12). Adult clients report that having two to three options (versus an infinite number when asked open ended questions) allows them to think through specific options and trust their decisions.

- **Delay** ED behaviors by doing: _____

  o ID a productive and distractive actions.

- **Give a compliment** to another person via text: ID one person _____

  o For example, by text, face-to-face, written note, emoji, Instagram image.

- Walk ____ **minutes.**

  o Based on the medical/dietary recommendations for movement.

- Actively **listen** to and participate in a conversation.

  o Practice repeating back what was heard without judgment.

- Do one hour of **a project** that takes intense concentration:_____

- ○ Intense focus distracts from ED "noise" or continual body shape and calorie thoughts.

- **Deep breathe** – slowly inhale four seconds and exhale four seconds.
  - ○ To slow the heart, which slows thoughts, which creates a temporary calmer state.

- **Distract** by doing two actions:_____ _____
  - ○ Editing a paper, rearranging a closet, a yoga pose, punching a pillow, stepping high 10 times.

- **Ground myself** to this moment. ID: two things I see; two things I hear; two things I can touch, two things I smell.
  - ○ Self-orchestrated distractions that stimulate all five senses.

- **Walk Tall** (Stretch up as much as possible as you walk.)
  - ○ Encourages deep breathing and staying in the present moment and strengthens muscles.

- **Hold myself accountable** by telling (ID the person) ____ if I act on a destructive behavior.
  - ○ Practices humility and honesty and decreases potential of repeating negative action.

- **Stop, reboot, reroute.**
  - ○ When heading toward a destructive object or location, say out loud "stop," turn around 180° and walk in that direction, regardless of where it goes. It is away from the place of self-harm.

- **WW** _____ **D?** (Ask self, "What would ____ Do?") ID person I admire ID what they would do_____. Then do it.
- **WWID4** _____? "What would I do for_____?" ID a person you want to help. Then do it.
  - ○ Transforms advice projected onto another person (I know what you could do) and reflects it back to self (I will do that myself).

- **Ask for help:** ID two people _____ _____
  - ○ Usually this needs to be planned ahead. A person can ask for help when anxiety is low. When anxiety is high, the person needs help but is unable to ask for it (see Anxiety Wave Handouts, Appendix 15). Schedule vulnerable times for a Support to text, FaceTime, visit.

- **Use my wise mind,**[134, 135] using the dialectic, "I think or feel both _____ AND:_____ "
  - ○ See Chapter 16 on dialectical responses. Relevant for clients and Supports.

- **Earphones with music** of my playlists.
  - Play music with a volume that interrupts intrusive ED thoughts.

- **Food is my medicine:** I will eat my planned breakfast, lunch, dinner, snacks.
  - Refer to default meal plan in the Behavioral Agreement.

- **Take my prescribed medication:** Food, vitamins, medications/liquid supplements.
  - Food, vitamins, and medications provide chemical, nutrient, and mineral requirements for body strength and stability.

- **Restorative Yoga** with _____ (ID person) when _____(ID days).
  - Engages the body to physically align in the moment with emotional and physical experiences.

- **Self-Critique a specific action/interaction/event:** in this order: What would I do the same? What would I do differently? How would I do it differently?
  - Use after any action, interaction, work or school assignment to affirm what the body/mind did well, acknowledge it to more confidently repeat it, and to reshape what was not helpful into a productive action.

- **Use a pre-meal routine:**_____.
  - The same one before each meal *if* it decreases anxiety.

- **Help another person by doing:** _____.
- **Accept myself for who I am by using my traits** in the current situation.
  - Acknowledging what traits one has and working within one's temperament.

- **Instead of walking toward a destructive action,** I will **walk toward** _____(name object/place) to do _____(productive action).
  - This is a variation of stop/reboot/reroute.

- **Instead of counting** _____ to restrict, I **will count** _____ _____ (topic).
  - For example, Sudoku.

- **Structure my plans clearly** describing what I will do and when.
  - Such as, when I get out of the car, I am going to go in the house and do XX and then do YY.
  - A healthy enjoyable default action to slip in whenever unsure of what do to and to prevent an ED behavior, e.g., slowly get out a stick of gum, slowly take off the wrapper and chew it for a minute.

## Summary Key Points

- The TBT-S Toolbox provides a variety of tools for adult clients to choose to use that are practical and easy to practice.
- Tools are used to reshape and re-wire ED symptoms and destructive trait expressions.
- Clinicians need to provide time for clients to practice tools in the toolbox during sessions to initiate practice at home/work/school.
- Tools should be congruent with a client's temperament.

# Chapter 19

# TBT-S Experiential Activities

## What Are TBT-S Experiential Activities?

TBT-S activities are structured, playful activities that provide opportunities to learn experientially. Some of the TBT-S activities reflect eating disorder (ED) brain processes, and others provide metaphoric scenarios for each client to discover solutions to ED problems by exploring options and realizing firsthand what worked.

Client traits are identified and owned as internal resources that either help the client through the activity or block the client's ability to complete the activity alone. Owning and utilizing all that one is and acknowledging all that one is not (is *not able* to do) sharpens the client's ability to move forward by drawing upon internal and external resources as needed.

> Key Point: TBT-S activities are structured playful experiences that metaphorically enact complex ED brain responses and empower clients to explore how to overcome ED symptoms by utilizing their traits.

## Where to Use the Activities?

Many of the TBT-S activities can be accomplished virtually. All of the TBT-S activities can be experienced in face-to-face groups. A few can be done in one-on-one therapeutic interactions, for example, "Nondominant hand" and "Wire–re-wire". See Table 19.1.

## Who Are Participants of TBT-S Activities?

- Young adult ED clients (YAs).
- Severe-and-enduring clients with AN (SE-AN).
- Supports of those with ED.
- Students and professionals in classrooms and trainings.

## When Are TBT-S Experiential Activities Implemented?

TBT-S experiential activities can be implemented at any time during the treatment process. Clinicians typically identify an activity that plays out current issues being addressed in ongoing treatment sessions whether in outpatient or higher levels of care.

---

There are videos of some of the TBT-S experiential activities in the electronic text titled *A Brain-Based Approach to Eating Disorder Treatment*, by L. Hill, 2017 www.BrainBasedEatingDisorders.org/.

**Table 19.1** TBT-S experiential activities

| Setting | | | | | |
|---|---|---|---|---|---|
| Activity name | Group classroom | One-on-one | Virtual | Face-to-face | Appendix |
| **Activities associated with AN brain responses** | | | | | |
| Yes/no activity | ✓ | | | ✓ | 10 |
| Nondominant hand | ✓ | ✓ | ✓ | ✓ | 11 |
| Telephone | ✓ | | | ✓ | 12 |
| Neuron activity | ✓ | | | ✓ | 13 |
| Brain Wave | ✓ | | | ✓ | 14 |
| **Problem-solving activities** | | | | | |
| Nondominant hand | ✓ | ✓ | ✓ | ✓ | 11 |
| Anxiety wave activity | ✓ | | | ✓ | 15 |
| Anxiety brain sculpt | ✓ | | | ✓ | 16 |
| Wire–re-wire | ✓ | ✓ | ✓ | ✓ | 17 |
| Stop, reboot, reroute | ✓ | ✓ | ✓ | ✓ | 18 |
| Landmine | ✓ | | | ✓ | 19 |
| Social gauntlet | ✓ | | | ✓ | 20 |
| Charades | ✓ | ✓ | ✓ | ✓ | 21 |
| What will you do? | ✓ | | ✓ | ✓ | 22 |
| Expert client advice | ✓ | ✓ | ✓ | ✓ | 23 |
| Communicating and listening | ✓ | ✓ | | ✓ | 24 |
| Family circuits | ✓ | | ✓ | ✓ | 25 |
| Family wise mind | ✓ | | ✓ | ✓ | 26 |

The TBT-S studied program offered one to two experiential activities daily over 5-days in 1 week to facilitate a better understanding of neurobiological influences on ED and to explore problem solving. A clinician could augment ongoing therapy by inserting a TBT-S experiential activity.

## TBT-S Neurobiological Experiential Activities

The brain-based, experiential activities were developed by applying ED neurobiological research findings to metaphoric scenarios to help clients with ED understand how their brains appeared to be responding, triggering, and contributing to ED symptoms. Clients were asked to give their input on how the activities represented their experiences. The activities were continually refined until most clients reported the experiences to be true for them, *and* the activity reflected research findings.[137]

# TBT-S Problem-Solving Experiential Activities

The TBT-S problem-solving experiential activities model what the brain does, which is solve problems by using an active process. While the brain process is quite complex, essentially resolution occurs through trial and error: trying on options and finding which fits best for each person. TBT-S sets up game-like activities, such as "The Landmine," with conditions placed on each client that symbolize anorexia nervosa (AN) or other ED brain responses, requiring each client to figure out how to move through and around "land mines" to solve the problem and get to the other side.

# How to Apply TBT-S Activities

Playfully. That is how to apply TBT-S activities. If they are read and administered in a serious linear manner, the energy and purpose are removed. Complex brain responses, complex problem-solving processes, can be "played out" and solutions discovered within the game in one session that may otherwise have taken months to solve. The clinician takes the client's own "played out solutions" and helps the client integrate them into experiences at home, work and interpersonal interactions. These actions are client identified productive responses that can become new habits. Newly forming habits take encouragement from Supports and clinicians to develop. The client tends to discover that their own motivation may be heighted to repeat their playfully discovered solutions because each client utilizes their own traits in their solutions. It is the clients' traits that carry them forward into new habits. The habits fit well and are more comfortable than externally recommended actions that may look right but not fit as well.

# How Experiential Activities Are Organized

The TBT-S experiential activities are described in detail in Appendices 10–26. Each experiential activity is structured by using the following format:

➤ Neurobiological and trait targets.
➤ Objectives.
➤ Who is involved?
➤ Materials and time needed.
➤ What does the research say?
➤ Neurobiological key point.
➤ Clinician checklist.
➤ Experiential activity instructions.
➤ Activity rules.
➤ Steps and *scripts*.
➤ Group discussion prompts.
➤ How to treat to these traits.
➤ Homework.
➤ Clinician notes.

---

**Summary Key Point**

Clinicians can augment their ongoing therapies with TBT-S experiential activities to actively explore and "play out" new behaviors based on the client's own exploratory and temperament based responses that reshape destructive ED traits and symptoms.

# Chapter 20

# TBT-S Strategic Dietary Approach

## Purpose and Description of the Dietary Approach

This chapter provides dietitians with strategies on how to apply meal plans with young adult (YA) and severe-and-enduring clients with anorexia nervosa (SE-AN) within a temperament based approach. TBT-S promotes a dietary approach similar to many eating disorder (ED) dietary approaches. Where it differs is that it involves the dietitian in a larger more active role through the treatment process. In addition to meal planning, TBT-S dietitians are involved in dietary food preparation and encourage food intake in outpatient sessions as well as higher levels of care. Dietitians include Supports in designated dietary sessions and during meals with adults who have anorexia nervosa (AN) to ensure everyone is aware and is practicing portion sizes and prescribed food combinations for balanced meals and snacks. TBT-S dietitians also use more structure in response to temperament needs for those with AN.

Dietary structure is established through the TBT-S Behavioral Agreement (BA). There are two versions of the BA, one for YA and the other for SE-AN clients. They are described in Chapter 21, under "Framework for Action via the Behavioral Agreement" and detailed in Chapters 22 and 23. The BA includes Supports in the meal-related process because they are critical agents of assistance outside of treatment for adults with AN and a critical part of the treatment team for adults with AN. The BA also provides dietitians with a means to individualize meal planning by integrating client traits into the meal plan process. The TBT-S approach provides the dietitian with multiple opportunities to apply neurobiological nomenclature and acknowledgment of temperament during meal planning and coaching with both adult clients and their Supports.

Working with ED as a dietitian is difficult. It is hard work that requires determination and recognition that the path forward often has many steps backward. Structure, consistency, small steps, and persistence pay off when adults with AN achieve and maintain a strong and healthy body. Structure and planning are core to that process.

> Key Point: TBT-S dietitians extend their ongoing ED dietary approach of meal planning to also include (a) the practice of food preparation and food intake at all levels of care with Supports, and (b) the use of increased structure via the Behavioral Agreement for adult clients with AN.

# Temperament Based Role of the Dietitian

## Establishing a Meal Plan That Meets Healthy Targets *with* Clients Is the Primary Role for ED Dietitians

It is necessary to assess food intake relevant to the client's resting metabolism, body composition, physical activity, and work/mental activities to determine a healthy nutrient balance. Dietitians should have accurate biological information to develop accurate meal plans. This includes working with medical professionals, seeking feedback from blood tests that clarify client physical stability and possible food allergies, and using information on the client's body composition (see "Meal Plan Revisions and Body Composition" later in this chapter). Dietitians identify and recommend food portions based on underlying biological factors just as physicians assess medical problems before identifying and dosing medications.

Eating disorders are biologically based illnesses. In light of this, dietitians recommend or "dose" each macronutrient to ensure dietary balance. Macronutrients are categories of foods needed in large portions for health and body strength. They include carbohydrates, proteins, and fats. It is important for dietitians to take time to explain why macronutrients are essential to the body. This reframes food fears into food functions. This brings the biologically based purpose of food into meal planning and opens the opportunity for dietitians to provide concrete facts about why, when, and how much food is needed to establish a biological balance.

Key Point: Dietitians develop meal plans by drawing upon clients' biological information from labs and physicals by medical professionals, and providing biologically based purposes of macronutrients to reframe food fears to food functions.

## Use the TBT-S Behavioral Agreement to Structure the Meal Plan Application

As stated earlier, there are two BAs, the young adult and the severe-and-enduring anorexia nervosa Behavioral Agreements (see Appendices 27 and 28). Both are structured handouts that help clients develop and carry out their personal meal plans. The agreement addresses pre-meal, post-meal, and mealtime rules with adult client Supports. The BA provides the structure for who does what, when, and how.

The SE-AN Behavioral Agreement has a section for the dietitian to place the newly developed meal plan into the BA, and provides a framework for the client to decide *how* to complete the meal plan throughout the week (see Appendix 28). For example, the SE-AN BA comes in three parts. The second worksheet (Appendix 28), provides a list of options to help adult clients decide what to do, when and how for "Goal 2: Commit to my meal and movement plan."

Once the dietitian has developed a meal plan with the client, either the dietitian or the clinician could work with the client and Supports to review the detailed choices on the handout, asking the client to choose which options work best for them to establish a practical weekly meal structure. The worksheet includes options for the client to identify who purchases the food and who prepares identified meals. The treatment team, including Supports, is given a copy of the BA (with written authorization if needed) to increase strategic reliability among the treatment team.

Creating a meal plan structure is central to helping reduce food avoidance, binging or purging. Supports need to be an active part of the BA process. SE-AN clients choose which actions they want their Support(s) to do. Supports share whether or not they can assist in the identified ways. If they cannot, then another Support is identified. Clients and Supports may decide how to eat specified meals together via, for example, Zoom, Skype, FaceTime, or phone time. Eating together tends to reduce meal resistance, increase meal assistance, and provide opportunities for Supports to contribute.

> Key Point: The TBT-S Behavioral Agreement is the structure within which the adult client and their Support(s) develop clear strategies on how to carry out the meal plan.

## Provide Dietary Psychoeducation

Dietitians have the unique opportunity to provide nutritional information that addresses each client's biological needs at all levels of care. Shifting food myths into biological nutrient-based facts changes cognitive paradigms. Dietitians explain why, how much, and how often a client's body needs proteins, carbohydrates, and endurance fuels (fats) to establish physical strength. Educating clients on the importance of fueling their metabolic "fire" each morning and keeping it burning with snacks and meals throughout the day is critical for brain and body function.[186]

It is cognitively distressful to eat more and different foods for many persons with AN. As explained in Chapter 11, a client with AN feels less anxiety and is calmer when not eating. To restore physical strength requires clients to eat more and to feel worse. It is helpful for the dietitian to acknowledge that there are cognitive "side effects" when eating. Eating creates more distress due to altered neurocircuits.[187] If SE-AN clients do not know this, they may continue to avoid foods due to the struggle provoked, instead of realizing that distress is an inevitable biological process when moving forward. It is recommended that the dietitian discuss cognitive distress with each client. The medical professional may choose to recommend medication while anxiety is acute. If a client declines medication, the dietitian informs the adult client and Supports that even more structure for meals may be necessary to provide increased assistance as clients move through cognitive, and at times physical, discomfort.

> Key Point: Dietitians educate clients and their Supports about the neurobiological bases of increased distress from changes in food intake.

## Include Supports in the Implementation of Meal Planning

Supports need to be involved in the implementation of meal planning with adult clients who have AN to ensure consistency and stability to help compensate for altered neurobiological brain responses, such as hunger and fullness signaling. Whether the Support person is a spouse or a friend who lives at a distance, or a parent of a YA, their inclusion in the process is critical. The BA provides structured questions that help clients identify and plan what is needed from their Supports, what is nonnegotiable, what to do when stress rises and avoidance increases, and what to do if ED behaviors are triggered. The BA brings the clients and Supports together to confirm meal process strategies. Supports are as central to the team as nurses are to a hospital setting. They need to know what is "prescribed," what recommendations have been identified, and what needs to be done to help carry out the recommendations *with* the adult client. They also need to know what to do when things do not go as planned.

> **Key Point: Supports are a central part of the team that works with adult clients and the dietitian and clinician to help carry out the meal plan in various settings.**

## Integrate Client Traits

AN temperament (the biological underpinnings of personality) needs to be acknowledged and incorporated into dietary planning to assure that the dietitian is working *with* the client, not counter to their temperament. For example, clients with AN tend to be concrete thinkers, focus their attention on details, are sensitive to making errors, and are often avoidant when presented with new foods. These hardwired traits are not symptoms that can be eliminated. Working *with* these traits, instead of ignoring them or trying to remove them, allows clients to feel understood, igniting trait-aligned actions toward healthier eating patterns.

Dietitians are urged to plan meals with adult clients by using multiple-choice options instead of asking open-ended questions to work congruently with AN traits. For example, it is less helpful to ask an adult with AN, "*What dairy would you like to eat or drink?*" It is more trait aligned to ask, "*Would you prefer three slices of Colby cheese, a yogurt (giving specified brand and amount), or 3 oz. of chicken for your lunch protein?*" This level of specificity is counter to the way many dietitians are trained. However, research has increasingly found that persons with AN temperaments need more specificity and detail to lower anxiety and utilize their traits productively. These traits are hardwired. Adults with AN report that multiple choice options minimize new food avoidance, increase relief, and decrease fear of making an erroneous choice.

> **Key Point: Dietitians work *with* AN traits by asking detailed questions and offering multiple-choice options instead of asking open-ended questions for meal planning.**

## Dietary Nomenclature

The dietitian is a key member of the ED treatment team. TBT-S expands the treatment team to include the adult client (as the expert) and Support(s) in addition to the clinician, dietitian, and medical professionals. Since clients with AN often face food with marked resistance, the dietitian often has a particularly difficult role on the team. Patience and endurance are required.

Because EDs are biological and brain based, the treatment team may benefit by approaching food biologically, recognizing that it is the substance that fuels the body. This helps clients see the biological role of food. All members of the treatment team are encouraged to use the same vocabulary to describe the biological purpose of food and its impact on the body. Table 20.1 explains the TBT-S nomenclature.

The TBT-S vocabulary substitutes "food" with "fuel." This term speaks to the medicinal source of energy that restores and retains body strength. For many adult SE-AN clients who also have obsessive and/or compulsive traits, dietitians may refer to "dosing" foods, shifting food portions to medication-like doses. This provides a medicinal association with food quantity necessary for health. "Fats" are called "endurance fuels," addressing the biological, long-burning nature of fats in the body.

**Table 20.1** TBT-S dietary nomenclature

| "Loaded" words | TBT-S word replacement | TBT-S rationale |
|---|---|---|
| Behaviors | ED Behaviors<br>*Healthy* Behaviors<br>*Purge* Behaviors<br>*Interactive* Behaviors<br>*Restricting* Behaviors<br>*Productive* Behaviors<br>*Destructive* Behaviors | Clinically, "behavior" needs a specifier. Behavior is the central word for both symptoms and solutions. Each type of behavior needs to be stipulated. If it is not specified, by default the clinician is implying unhealthy behaviors and removing the opportunity for the client to realize their behaviors are the means for their solutions. |
| Food | Fuel or medicine | The source of energy and healing. |
| Fat | Endurance Fuels or (EFs) | Fats have a social connotation of globules of lipid stores, instead of the biological reality that fats have multiple crucial body functions, e.g., brain axon coating allowing neurons to fire. Fats burn longer than proteins and carbohydrates allowing them to provide complex body services. Small amounts of fat fuel enduring tasks in the body. Lipid stores are but one. |
| Weight gain | Strength gain | Weight is associated with fear for those with AN. Strength is a goal. The more body composition shifts to healthy levels, the stronger the brain and body becomes. |
| Calories | Energy | Biologically, calories are energy units. Heating the body and maintaining equilibrium transform the fearful word "calories" to its scientific function, energy. |
| Exercise | Movement/actions | All movement ranging from verbally speaking words, body posture, walking, running, yoga uses energy to express cognitive, emotional and behavioral responses. |

*Source:* Hill (1993); Hodgekiss (2014).

---

**Key Point: A biologically based nomenclature unites the organic function of food with body needs, confronting food-related fears.**

## Meal-Planning Strategies

Developing a default meal and snack plan is helpful and at times necessary for many ED clients. Default plans need to be practical, easy meals and snacks that meet required macronutrient doses in response to the client's current metabolic and activity needs that can be eaten anywhere at any time. It is appropriate for persons with SE-AN who are extremely uncomfortable to eat new macronutrients recommended to restore body strength. If one meal and snack plan is established *with* the client that meets all nutritional requirements, then it could be the "fall back" meal for the client to eat when overwhelmed, stressed at work, or too tired to make a different meal.

Research finds that eating a variety of food predicts better outcomes.[189,190] When establishing meal plans at the outpatient level of care for SE-AN clients, who have comorbid obsessive and compulsive traits, introducing new foods in smaller steps and at a slower pace may be necessary to prevent food avoidance. This is in contrast to YA clients with AN who should be pressed to eat new foods more frequently while brain circuits are still growing. SE-AN clients re-wire their brain faster when repetitively eating the same new food within a routine (see Trait Profile Checklist in Appendix 2). For example, the dietitian may recommend a new food once a week instead of once a day for those with SE-AN. Healthy habits form for both YA and SE-AN; it takes longer and more practice for the latter.

Key Point: Developing a default meal and snack plan *with* an SE-AN client aligns AN traits such as the need for sameness, structure, and detailed planning to work toward sustained health and strength over time.

## Who Should Know the Meal Plan?

The dietitian establishes rules with the adult client about who receives the meal plan during the first session. The whole team should receive a copy of the meal plan, which includes the client, the Supports, the clinician, and medical professionals. Release of authorization may be required. Resistance to sharing information tends to increase with each subsequent session if rules are not created from the beginning. TBT-S works from a collaborative, interdependent approach, ensuring that the treatment team is regularly updated and informed. The dietitian may emphasize different aspects of the meal plan with different treatment team members. For example, the dietitian provides the clinician and Supports with the meal plan and answers clinician and Support questions while discussing nutrient deficiency concerns with the medical professional. This ensures the meal plan meets dietary recommendations when eaten in therapy sessions with the clinician as well as at home/work settings with Supports.

Key Point: The dietitian ensures that the whole treatment team has the client meal plan and subsequent updates.

## Meal Plan Revisions and Body Composition

The meal plan is continually revised as YA and SE-AN clients' body compositions change regularly when restoring body strength. The level of care often determines how often the plan changes. It may be weekly in higher levels of care, monthly as they transition to outpatient care, and extends to quarterly to maintain client strength. Regardless of level of care, regular body composition assessments need to be completed and meal plans updated to maintain strength.

Traditionally meal plans are developed using the client's weight. Technological advancements now offer practical, affordable devices that measure multiple physiological dimensions of body composition, such as water weight and fat mass, instead of simply weight. Weight is a single number that includes unaccounted water retention, dehydration, constipation, or diarrhea, if a meal was just eaten or a large amount of water was drunk. Weight alone does not provide measurements of lean mass, fat mass, and water weight that are important when determining if the client's body composition has changed and biologically warrants meal adjustments. Since eating disorders are a biologically based illness, they need comprehensive biological measures of body composition to inform meal planning.

A wide variety of body composition analyzers range in accuracy, number of body composition dimensions measured, and price. In general, body composition analyzers measure the rate at which an electrical current travels through the body. This is as physically painless as stepping on a traditional scale. They can be as simple as a scale-like device that measures low weight to extremely high weight, with percentage of fat mass and water mass. The more advanced devices are walk-on body composition analyzers that measure total body water, extra- and intracellular water, quality of somatic cells, fat mass, fat-free mass, and resting energy expenditure. If the client has too little muscle and lean and fat mass, recommended adjustments to macronutrients and movement can be recommended to rebuild body mass.

> Key Point: Meal adjustments need biologically based resources, such as body composition analyzers or feedback from medical professionals to accurately determine what macronutrient adjustments need to be made.

## Role of Dietitian during Meal Sessions

### Use Practical Methods for Dosing Fuel

Food visuals (pictures) and food replicas help adult clients and Supports understand how much food and in what combinations are needed. Replicas are three-dimensional imitations of foods and drinks that look realistic. Dietitians can use visuals to demonstrate appropriate portion sizes and to teach combinations that maximize metabolic and physiological balance for each client. Adults with AN may be unable to estimate portions intuitively. For example, using a practical food visual, the dietitian might say, "*Let's see if the cooked chicken is equal to the size of the palm of your hand*" or "*Your portion of rice is equal to two handfuls of cooked rice. Your hand, not your child's hand.*" Use concrete and practical suggestions to increase accuracy. Figure 20.1 is a visual example that uses one's hand to determine normal food portion sizes.

If the client reports gastric pain from increased fuel volume, the dietitian can suggest alternatives that have less volume with the same macronutrients, such as a tablespoon of olive oil instead of a piece of cake to meet one's endurance fuel need. This is similar to a physician offering a client options to take a medication in either pill or liquid form. Work *with* the client and Supports to ensure that foods are easily accessible. Clarify who buys the foods. This helps reduce food avoidance.

Many eating disorder dietitians use grams instead of calories to dose food portions. Dietitians should use a method that most accurately allows them to assess and ensure (a) macro- and micronutrient balance, (b) energy sufficiency, and (c) body composition restoration and maintenance.

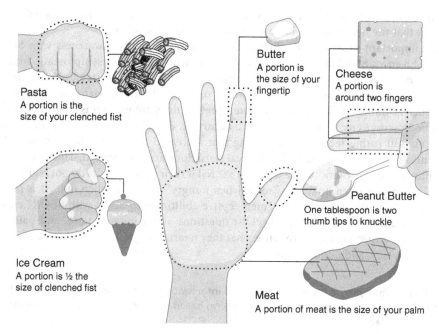

**Figure 20.1** Practical food portions

Key Point: Dietitians offer clients who have AN and their Supports clear practical ways to dose fuel, such as food visuals and replicas, to ensure nutrient balance is understood.

# Provide a Range of Structure Based on AN Symptom Severity

Clients with AN temperaments tend to need structure. Forms of structure can change as the client stabilizes and maintains body strength. A tighter temporary structure is required when new and different meals and foods are introduced. A looser structure could be planned when a client is in outpatient care and maintaining a meal plan. The more severe the ED symptoms, the more structure needed on a daily basis, even if the client is in outpatient treatment. Structure empowers AN treatment providers and clients by offering consistency and mutually agreed limits to address the high need for certainty, fear of error, need for repetition, and attention to details. These trait tendencies are genetically and biologically ingrained and shaped by environmental influences. Working with them by planning structure through the day to integrate meals allows clients to work with their traits productively, not against them.

Dietitians can establish a clear and dependable meal structure through the BA. The BA structures the details needed when faced with eating in various settings each day. For example, it is easy for dietitians to get pulled into SE-AN resistance and rationalizations for not eating a new food during that week. Hearing the concern is important *but* moving forward by eating the new food together is necessary. New foods cannot become habitual until they are practiced. Practicing them first with the dietitian and Supports and clinician solidifies that the new food can be eaten again in different settings.

It is important to address the limitations of "mindful eating" awareness with SE-AN clients who encounter daily stressors. Many persons who are actively symptomatic with AN have a reduced ability to sense hunger/fullness cues due to brain circuit alterations that decrease interoceptive ability. Interoception is one's ability to experience physical sensations, such as hunger, fullness, or pain. Interoception does not mean it is how one "thinks" about body sensations. It is one's ability to accurately sense body signals. Dietitians could teach mindful eating techniques assuming that increased awareness increases sensation. Awareness does not ensure that the physical sensations are experienced. This is similar to color blindness. One cannot make a person see red if their brain circuits do not register red. SE-AN clients are often unable to "sense when hungry" or "sense when full." It is recommended that dietitians assess what interoceptive abilities each client with SE-AN experiences by using the Trait Profile Checklist questions about hunger, taste, and pain (see Appendix 2). Expecting clients to sense what they neurobiologically cannot sense increases guilt, inadequacy, and noncompliance.

> **Key Point: Dietary structure is a fundamental intervention that aligns *with* AN traits and can range from high to low, temporary, or long-term based on client traits, dietary changes, and ED symptom acuity.**

## Meal Coaching

The dietary meal session is the time for clients to practice planned fuel intake in different settings. The dietitian is the coach in TBT-S meal sessions. Virtual technology is ideal for meal-coaching sessions, allowing fuel intake to be practiced in home/work/school settings. With virtual treatment, the dietitian has greater opportunities to answer questions and observe how adult clients prepare, eat, and cleanup after meals. This allows dietitians to offer input that sharpens procedures for healthier habits to be practiced in different environments. The dietitian acknowledges the difficulty for those with restricting-type AN to begin eating and recognizes those who binge eat may have difficulty stopping. The TBT-S Toolbox (described in Chapter 18 and found in Appendix 9) offers tools to manage anxiety for each phase of the meal.

> **Key Point: Virtual coaching during meals with YA and SE-AN clients and their Supports ensures accurate fuel intake and promotes healthy habit formation over time.**

## Pre-Meal and Post-Meal Exercises

Beginning a meal and ending a meal are often difficult and vulnerable times for persons with ED. It can be helpful to train clients and Supports to identify and use specific tools that can become ritualized at the beginning and end of meals, especially for those with SE-AN. For example, one tool is the $4 \times 4$ deep-breathing activity (in the TBT-S Toolbox) that could be used before meals. The dietitian teaches the tool the first time and has the client or the Support lead the activity in subsequent scheduled meals together. Post-meal exercises could include the client clearing the table and putting the dishes in the dishwasher or sink after each meal. Depending on the client's level of severity, the meal could be followed by X minutes of the TBT-S tool, "walking tall." This is easily accomplished virtually by adult clients and Supports walking tall at their own locations.

The TBT-S Toolbox provides many tools for clients to use during pre- and post-meal phases to manage ED symptoms. Practicing them during dietary sessions demonstrates the importance of the pre-meal and post-meal rituals and establishes healthier habits. The tools also help reduce anticipatory anxiety and replace post-meal destructive ED behaviors. This does not mean the exercise takes away the anxiety or temptation, but it does divert attention and promotes positive action.

> Key Point: Repeatedly practicing pre-and post-meal activities creates healthy rituals to lower anxiety and replace ED behaviors.

## Distraction Tools

Distraction is a targeted tool that can break through AN obsessions and temporarily lower anxiety. Thought-provoking interactions force thoughts to shift from obsessive food fears and body image disturbances to different cognitive challenges. Distraction tools can range from a discussion on a topic that requires the client to actively participate to mind games that require the client to solve problems. Many phone apps have mind games to draw clients into fun and challenging interactions while preparing and eating and then use during post-mealtimes. These are helpful when clients are alone and need to interrupt ED tendencies such as compulsive calorie counting during meal preparation.

A simple meal distraction tool for clients to use when with Supports is to choose a topic and then go back and forth identifying a word that corresponds with each letter of the alphabet. For example, the topic is animals. One client has "A" and says antelope. The Support has "B" and says bear. Adult clients tend to like complex topics that require more mental demand, such as sports or music, to divert attention away from obsessive food fears. SE-AN clients report that wearing headphones or earbuds and listening to music is a helpful distraction in all three meal phases.

> Key Point: Dietitians coach clients and their Supports to identity and practice distraction tools that can be used in various situations to lower anxiety triggered by food and body-image obsessions.

## When Meals Fall Apart

Meals often fall apart. For example, when new foods and expanded portions are introduced to a SE-AN client who has practiced and refined ways to restrict, avoid, inhibit, and circumvent foods for years, emotional outbursts rise up. Meals tend to fall apart on holidays when more people gather to eat together. They can fall apart because the effort needed to eat the whole meal is more than the client can muster after a long day of work or school.

The dietitian works with SE-AN clients, and their Supports, to explore solutions that are congruent *with* their temperaments to work through meals that are particularly stressful. A common scenario of a meal that "goes bad" for an adult client with SE-AN could be a holiday-planned group meal. The client may become overwhelmed and upset and has left the table in the past. There are some clients with SE-AN who have never eaten with their children or other family members during holidays. An avoidance trait tendency dominates to diminish and cope with food fears and distress. A structured plan is needed that addresses what the client wants to do in these circumstances, and what the client needs from Supports when this happens.

SE-AN clients report that when they become overwhelmed, they tend to need time out. Acknowledge that. Time out is valid to take when distress is high. Establish *with* the client a designated amount of time that is typically needed when they feel like "erupting" and their anxiety is high. If the client wants to be with family members and return to the table, a step-by-step plan developed ahead of time, could help the client return to the table. In some cases, eating the "default meal" (describe earlier in this chapter), endorsing the need for sameness could bring the client back to the table, eat with others, and perhaps participate in conversations. The plan could include that the client warns Supports that they may need to leave the table but to continue eating and they will return. The client may walk around in the kitchen, allowing movement and distraction to lower the distress and then walk back to the table. The client's meal may need to be an adjusted meal instead of the meal others are eating if it helps the client feel less overwhelmed when eating and being with others. The bottom line is that the client eats foods that meets the meal plan whether alone or with others. The best-laid plans can fall apart when anxiety becomes overwhelming for the SE-AN client. When, not if, that happens, step back and refine the plan, then move forward and practice it. And then practice the plan again.

> Key Point: When meals go awry, the dietitian steps back with the client, refines the plan, and moves forward to practice different tools and responses with structure to contain anxiety.

### Summary Key Points

- Structure is strategically central for dietary interventions for AN.
- Dietitians enhance empathy when aligning meal planning with client AN traits.
- Meal planning for adults with AN needs to be practical, consistent, and structured regarding how to obtain and prepare foods.
- Supports are treatment team members who need to learn the meal plan and strategies to provide assistance at home or work/school.
- After the meal plan is identified, the dietitian is a central agent in coaching and practicing pre-, post-, and mealtime fuel intake with both the client and their Support(s) virtually or face-to-face.

# Framework for Action via TBT-S Behavioral Agreement

TBT-S Behavioral Agreements (BAs) are like treatment plans and more. They provide a structure for goals and concrete strategies that are actively developed by the adult clients and their Supports, with the clinician coaching the process. The clients and Supports lead the activity, not the clinician, as they work through the worksheets and BA forms. The BAs become the working plan that adult clients and Supports identify, and mutually agree to, regarding what needs to be done to achieve the stated goals. The BAs are ideal for electronic medical records (EMRs) treatment plans. If an EMR has its own treatment plan, the BAs can be attached to the client's session notes.

The BA incorporates clients' temperaments into their treatment goals and strategic plan. Clients identify their productive traits that can help them achieve their goals and carry out their identified strategies. This allows the client to work with their own strengths to manage and reduce their eating disorder (ED) symptoms. Recognizing and utilizing a client's traits increases self-worth and affirms the client's unique temperament to carry out the intended goals.

In intensive TBT-S programs, the BAs take two to three hours to complete. In outpatient settings, some of the worksheets could be completed as homework by the adult client and Supports, leaving two hours of clinical sessions for both the client and Supports to develop and refine the BA together. The clinician schedules these sessions, ensuring that the agreement is completed, and everyone involved is onboard to carry out their identified roles.

There are two forms of BAs. One is for young adult (YA) clients with anorexia nervosa (AN), and one is for severe-and-enduring clients with anorexia nervosa (SE-AN).

---

**Summary Key Point**

TBT-S Behavioral Agreement is a framework for action that incorporates client-identified strategies (actions that detail how) to reach their intended goals with their Supports.

---

# 22

# Young Adult TBT-S Behavioral Agreement (YA BA)

## What Is the YA BA?

The young adult (YA) Behavioral Agreement (BA) is a written document that represents an agreement between the YA and parents. It is a summary of agreements and actions to achieve recovery based on the skills and activities learned and practiced throughout TBT-S treatment. The YA BA is a document that outlines the client's primary plans for recovery, including activities, nutrition, and weight recommendations by the professional treatment team. The YA BA also outlines how YA and their parent(s) will collaborate during recovery. This includes both YA and parent commitments related to their responsibilities and roles in recovery and indices that describe what recovery looks like for the YA clients and parents.

The purpose of the YA BA is to ensure consistency in the way in which clients and their parents are approaching recovery based on agreements made during TBT-S treatment sessions. Additionally, the YA BA provides a way to track progress in recovery based on indicators determined and outlined in the document, determined by the professional treatment team and the YA and parents. Lastly, the YA BA is a motivational tool. YAs identify valued reinforcers that are tied to recovery metrics based on YA and parent input and, conversely, define planned consequences for not meeting recovery metrics. For YA clients, this may include additional directives on what is needed to gain more independence, and for parents to facilitate autonomous and independent client goals such as living transitions, higher education goals, and/or to provide continued financial assistance.

> Key Point: The YA BA is a written agreement between the YA client and their parents that addresses plans and actions toward recovery based on the skills and activities learned and practiced throughout TBT-S treatment.

## How to Use the YA BA

The construction and development of the YA BA is completed in two stages. First, clients and parents work separately to formulate their ideas. This can be done during YA Skills Training and Parent Skills Training groups based on prompts provided in Chapters 16 and 17. Stage 1 (see *Stages* in later sections of this chapter) could be completed during two scheduled individual therapy sessions with the YA client and their parents virtually or face-to-face. After the ideas are worked through in Stage 1, clients and parents begin Stage 2 by working together to construct the final YA BA document. In the 5-day, 40-hour TBT-S program, this occurs over two to three hours on the fourth day.

The YA BA is developed after TBT-S skills training sessions, where YA and parents are formulating their own goals and commitments for the YA BA. Additionally, some of the TBT-S experiential activities emphasizing communication and relationships are helpful to position YA and parents to work together to formulate this collaborative plan. Developing the YA BA after participation in these TBT-S activities allows ideas to formulate and a summary plan to be developed on what the client and their parents want and need from one another. *The YA BA is the end product* to serve as the strategic plan for future actions and interactions. Developing the YA BA after TBT-S modules have been implemented, such as the neurobiological psychoeducation and skills trainings, ensures that both parties have practiced effective communication, which helps diminish ineffective styles of relating. For clinicians orchestrating the YA BA during outpatient sessions, the client-parent interpersonal relationship should be assessed first to ensure that the relationship structure is intact to be able to work collaboratively. If warranted, the clinician offers a TBT-S experiential activity focused on communication and family structure to prepare for the development of the YA BA. See Chapters 16 and 17.

> Key Point: The YA BA is completed in two stages: (1) preparation (where YA and parents work separately) and (2) construction of the final document prepared by the YA client with AN and their parents with input from the professional treatment team *after* TBT-S skills have been practiced.

# Time Requirement and Clinician Involvement in YA BA Development

Ample time is needed to engage in each of the two stages. Stage 1 of the YA BA requires up to two hours for preparation with clients and parents working separately with a clinician leading the sessions. Once both parties have had time and clinician assistance to reflect on their expectations and commitments, the second stage (Stage 2) involves the YA client and their parent(s) working together to construct the written agreement collaboratively. This could be accomplished in individual outpatient sessions or in a group of clients and parents with subunits of client and parents working simultaneously, virtually or face-to-face. The writing of the final YA BA takes up to three hours to complete.

Stage 2 of the YA BA generally requires clinician oversight. It is not necessary, however, for the clinician to be present for all of the work being discussed between clients and parents. In the 5-day, 1-week studied TBT-S format, YA BA writing is conducted in a multi-family group format. One to two clinicians provide group time with multiple sets of clients and their parents working together while clinicians oversee and step in only when necessary or requested. Between two and three hours is a feasible amount of time for clients and parents to spend working through the YA BA (see Chapters 16 and 17).

> Key Points
> - **YA BA Preparation:** 1.5–2 hours (in group format)
> - **Support BA Preparation:** 1.5–2 hours (in group format)
> - **Constructing the BA Collaboratively:** 2–3 hours (in group format)

## YA BA Clinician Checklist

⇒ Introduce the YA BA

⇒ Conduct YA BA preparation sessions with clients and parents (separately).

⇒ Facilitate session for client(s) and parents to collaboratively write the YA BA.

## Stage 1: Behavioral Agreement Preparation

In this one- to two-hour session, the clinician introduces and addresses the importance of developing a YA BA that unites both YA's and their parents' intentions regarding various concerns, such as ED symptoms, trait expression, meal plan, and nonnegotiables. The YA BA becomes the client's and parents' mutually agreed script and strategy to achieve treatment goals, effective interactions, and social expectations.

The clinician should emphasize the purpose of the YA BA as a structured format that ensures clients have a roadmap and parents provide assistance in effective ways based on the clients' feedback and input. Additionally, the YA BA serves as an important motivational tool for clients because it is their structured plan of action. Often times overall recovery in and of itself is not intrinsically motivating. Through the BA, YA clients are directed to think of recovery as a means of actualizing their productive traits to attain important life goals, for which a strong body and health are necessary. This may include attending or staying in a university, pursuing travel desires, and anything else that is salient and important for the YA client. Developmentally, YAs are poised to focus on increased autonomy and larger life goals.

> Key Point: The YA BA is a comprehensive structure connecting YA clients with their life goals in concrete and measurable ways.

## YA Prompts to Prepare the BA

The following prompts in Figure 22.1 are used to direct YA clients with AN to reflect on needed aspects of the YA BA. Clients review the prompts with time to reflect on each and write down information that they would like to include in their BAs.

When engaging in Stage 1 YA BA preparation, YAs are encouraged to include treatment recommendations and their commitments to fundamental aspects of recovery, including nutrition, movement plan, and weight recommendations. Outlining this in the YA BA ensures that parents are aware of recovery recommendations and that professional treatment team members are explicit with recommendations to the YA client with AN.

YAs should also include their parents' involvement, including needed check-ins on progress, and the level of involvement the client needs for nutrition monitoring. In this way, they are actively determining the parents' level of involvement and role in meal preparation and eating.

The 5-day, 40-hour TBT-S program has parents learning the dietitian-recommended meal plan with the client on the first day and practicing providing feedback to their YA related to nutrition on the following 4 days. In this 5-day model, parents practice 20 therapeutic meals and snacks and attend dietitian sessions together with their YA during

> - My plans and commitments based on treatment recommendations
>   - Outline Meal Plan
>   - Outline Physical Activity
>   - Outline Weight Recommendations
> - Parent commitments
>   - What would be helpful for my parents to do to help me?
>   - What is unhelpful and I do NOT want them to do?
> - How often will I meet with my parents for a recovery check-in and what will be discussed?
> - Parent reinforcements: What will motivate you to progress?
>   - Extra privileges and reinforcements
>   - Consequences
> - Red Flags
>   - What are they (be specific)? For the client? For the parents?
>   - What do I commit to doing about them?
> - How will parent involvement change if I am slipping?
> - How do we define lack of progress or lapse?
>   - Ex. Failure to restore at recommended pace
>   - Weight drops below xx

**Figure 22.1** Young adult prompts to prepare for the Behavioral Agreement

the week. This allows time for YAs and parents to determine and practice how parents will provide assistance surrounding mealtimes.

In the YA Behavioral Agreement section titled "Parent Reinforcements and Consequences," YAs and parents clarify YA goals (set by the YA) and how parents will assist those goals based on recovery progress or decline. This can include financial assistance and other tangible methods of needed assistance using contingency management.

**TBT-S Sessions Completed Prior to Parents and YA Preparing the BA**

- Mealtime/coaching
- Communication
- Skill development
- Experiential activities

## Defining the Roles of Parents

Parents are directed to consider a multi-faceted way of providing assistance and encouragement to their loved ones. Broadening the definition of assistance and what it entails allows parents to explore various levels of involvement. This increases parent efficacy even though their roles as "primary caretakers" have shifted to broader roles of assistance. This is important given the age and developmental needs of YAs. The YA BA integrates a wide range of assistance techniques in a diverse array of family presentations and levels of acuity, with flexibility based on YA and parent needs. Offering assistance in a multidimensional approach encourages parents to consider and adopt other ways of providing assistance that may be distinctive and complementary to their former ways of engaging with their YA.

A spectrum of forms of assistance is listed next that parents can draw upon and "try on." Once these are reviewed, parents are encouraged to reflect on how they can broaden their assistance for their YA in ways suitable for their situations and roles. Doing this prior to engaging with Stage 2 of the YA BA allows parents to maintain a flexible and adaptive attitude toward assisting their loved ones.

# Types of Parental Assistance

**Emotional Support:** The ability to be accepting, understanding, and validating. In this realm of assistance, one can practice empathy and offer words of encouragement and affirmation. This also includes simply being present to listen and comfort during times of challenge.

Emotional Support Skills: Parents are taught and provided time to practice

- Validation
- Empathy and understanding
- Being present and available
- Offering words of affirmation and encouragement

**Informational Support:** This involves providing information that fosters intellectual growth. Information can (sometimes) assist recovery, create certainty, and be helpful and make someone feel safe. Generally YAs will request this type of assistance when it is needed or helpful. As such, it is important to avoid providing unsolicited facts and information, repeating recovery facts that are already known, *or* responding to emotional concerns with facts and logic (which can be perceived as invalidating).

ED Information Skills: Parents are taught to:

- Be willing to research or search of more information for the loved one when asked.
- Ask questions that clarify the "what, when, where, when, why and how" to help guide/lead YAs to consider facts and information. (For example, *"You plan to pack your snacks. Do you have what you need to ensure there is enough energy for the day?"*)
- Provide options when a YA is unable to make decisions independently.

**Instrumental (Tangible) Assistance:** Provide concrete services or resources for the YA. This can include assistance with making meals, financial assistance, and/or help with making appointments. Tangible assistance demonstrates parental willingness to offer needed structure for YAs who are not yet fully autonomous.

Instrumental skills: Parents can offer

- Financial assistance that could be on a contingency basis, meaning that parents determine recovery criteria with their YA to merit the financial assistance.
- Assistance with living arrangements.
- Meal and snack assistance, being present and helping to prepare.
- Additional favors and assistance to decrease stress.

**Belonging Skills:** Assist by encouraging a sense of belonging, for the YA in the family and/or community. Parents are taught to:

- See the YA as a person versus an ED.
- Engage in non-ED, non-recovery–related dialogue.

- Invite and help the YA prepare to participate in specified activities and events.
- Express gratitude and appreciation for the YA's role in family/community.

## Parent Behavioral Agreement Preparation

Clinicians are encouraged to invite parents or other Supports into designated treatment sessions without YA clients present to clarify their perspectives of levels of involvement and monitoring necessary to facilitate their YA's recovery. To do this, clinicians offer parent prompts listed in Figure 22.2. The parent session(s) could be virtual or face-to-face, individual or group discussions.

## Stage 2: Constructing the Final Behavioral Agreement

Clinicians facilitate a collaborative 2- to 3-hour meeting with the client and parents to share ideas based on their separate behavioral agreement preparation handouts and sessions. This could be accomplished in an outpatient session with one YA and parents, or in a group setting, or part of a group series. The clinician provides time for the YA and parents to meet to review their work and to construct the final, written YA Behavioral Agreement jointly.

During group sessions, a clinician remains present while units of YA and their parents work together. It is not necessary, however, for clinicians to be actively involved in every minute of the group session with each of the family units. Clinicians should be attentive and offer assistance if/when requested by the YA or parents. This allows families to practice working collaboratively without the need for a clinician-mediator. Once the family (YA and parents) has completed their draft, the clinician reviews it with them to ensure that it addresses the client's recovery needs based on the clinician's expertise and working knowledge of the family and the client. In the 5-day, 40-hour TBT-S program

---

- Be aware of the professional treatment recommendations that include meal plan, body composition changes, and movement.
- Identify how you will know whether or not your loved one is progressing?
- Clarify how often you should check in to know the status of progress.
- Identify and communicate your nonnegotiables:
    What would it take to be critical enough to intervene? (Define this as specifically as possible.)
    What are you unwilling or unable to cope with from your YA?
    What are your requirements for treatment?
- Parent contingencies:
    What are your YA's primary life goals?
    What are the minimal requirements that you need to continue to offer to reach these life goals?
- What assistance/reinforcement will you offer if your YA is progressing in recovery?
- What will be your measures if your YA is not progressing in recovery?
- What is your definition of "progress" in one week? In one month? In one year?

**Figure 22.2** Parent prompts to prepare for the Behavioral Agreement

studied, one to two clinicians oversee families as they work together in a shared group room space.

A YA Behavioral Agreement template is provided in Appendix 27. It provides a structure for YA and parents to use in creating the agreement together if requested. Every family has a unique set of circumstances and requires a different plan to suit their needs, and therefore agreements that are highly tailored and family-specific end up being the most useful. The template is available for those who seek out additional structure, but families are encouraged to come up with their own document so that it is more personal. The YA BA prompts are intended to provide a broad structure to allow for focus and diversity, so that YA and parents tailor their needs to their own situations. When using the template, clinicians emphasize using the YA BA sections that are relevant and remove what is not relevant. Similarly, YAs and parents can add in additional concerns as needed. It is most useful if the YA BA is edited, before completed, to remove extraneous wording and sections, and includes only the aspects that are relevant. This will ensure that the document is usable, practical, and applicable.

---

**Summary Key Point**

The YA Behavioral Agreement is collaboratively written by the YA and parents addressing criteria that meet their unique concerns.

# 23 Severe-and-Enduring Anorexia Nervosa Behavioral Agreement (SE-AN BA)

## What Is the SE-AN BA?

The SE-AN Behavioral Agreement (BA) is a structured TBT-S document that is central in addressing details regarding who is going to do what, when, and where in relation to managing food intake and eating disorder (ED) symptoms. It is a detailed plan for collaborative action led by the adult client that incorporates input from Support(s), clinicians, and dietitians who are involved in developing it. The document format was constructed to maximize and utilize AN temperaments. For example, it is usual for persons with AN to be uncertain and lack confidence in trusting decisions (see Chapter 13). As a result, the BA is designed with lists, multiple-choice options, and narrowly focused fill-in-the-blanks. This format of questioning facilitates cognitive reasoning, a strong trait in many adults with AN. The BA minimizes open-ended questions, which persons with AN tend to respond to with doubt. The BA provides a structured format that fosters safety, containment for uncertainty, and direction. Persons with SE-AN tend to be highly detailed, and the BA matches trait expression with strategic plans for health and strength.

> **Key Point:** The SE-AN BA is a structured document developed to utilize AN traits and includes Supports, clinicians, and dietitians.

## Stage 1: Behavioral Agreement Preparation

The SE-AN BA consists of three worksheets that the client and Support(s) complete sequentially.

First, the **Trait Profile Checklist,** shown in Figure 23.1 is to be completed. The complete handout is in Appendix 2. Temperament is one's internal resources that fundamentally influence who one is, one's strengths and weaknesses. Temperament consists of trait tendencies. The Trait Profile Checklist is completed by the client and Support(s) to clarify what strengths (productive traits) and weaknesses (destructive traits) each person brings to the table. It is a list of fifty-four traits identified compiled from personality models and eating disorder research. It is transdiagnostic and includes a wide range of traits that impact various diagnoses. Persons identify the traits they have and how they are currently expressing each trait on a continuum from productive to destructive. The client scores the checklist by adding the number of traits identified and counting the number of productive and destructively expressed traits to clarify the proportion of traits that are working for or against the client currently.

## Trait Profile Checklist

**1st:** Check the traits that characterize me.
**2nd:** Circle how I have expressed those traits <u>on average</u> over the past few months, on the continuum:

"I have <u>tendency</u> to ..."

<u>How I am currently expressing this trait</u>

| Trait | More productive | | | | More destructive |
|---|---|---|---|---|---|
| ☐ Be perfectionistic | 5 | 4 | 3 | 2 | 1 |
| ☐ Be determined | 5 | 4 | 3 | 2 | 1 |
| ☐ Be anxious, worry | 5 | 4 | 3 | 2 | 1 |
| ☐ Be cautious | 5 | 4 | 3 | 2 | 1 |
| ☐ Have low self-esteem, see what's wrong in me | 5 | 4 | 3 | 2 | 1 |
| ☐ Want similarity and routine | 5 | 4 | 3 | 2 | 1 |
| ☐ Be Introverted, energized when alone/few people | 5 | 4 | 3 | 2 | 1 |
| ☐ Be high-achieving | 5 | 4 | 3 | 2 | 1 |
| ☐ Think the same thoughts repeatedly (obsessive) | 5 | 4 | 3 | 2 | 1 |
| ☐ Do the same things repeatedly (compulsive) | 5 | 4 | 3 | 2 | 1 |
| ☐ Be extroverted, energized being with others | 5 | 4 | 3 | 2 | 1 |
| ☐ Be optimistic, tend to see the best in things | 5 | 4 | 3 | 2 | 1 |
| ☐ Be pessimistic, tend to see negative in things | 5 | 4 | 3 | 2 | 1 |
| ☐ Avoid what seems harmful or uncomfortable | 5 | 4 | 3 | 2 | 1 |
| ☐ Prefer novelty, new or different | 5 | 4 | 3 | 2 | 1 |
| ☐ Be agreeable, cooperative, or kind | 5 | 4 | 3 | 2 | 1 |
| ☐ Be aggressive, antagonistic, or hostile | 5 | 4 | 3 | 2 | 1 |
| ☐ Be physically active | 5 | 4 | 3 | 2 | 1 |
| ☐ Be conscientiousness, dutiful, or deliberate | 5 | 4 | 3 | 2 | 1 |
| ☐ Be stubborn | 5 | 4 | 3 | 2 | 1 |
| ☐ Be shy, timid | 5 | 4 | 3 | 2 | 1 |
| ☐ Be attentive, focused | 5 | 4 | 3 | 2 | 1 |
| ☐ Pursue pleasure or rewards | 5 | 4 | 3 | 2 | 1 |
| ☐ Be adaptable or flexible | 5 | 4 | 3 | 2 | 1 |
| ☐ Be reactive | 5 | 4 | 3 | 2 | 1 |
| ☐ Be assertive, speak out for self | 5 | 4 | 3 | 2 | 1 |

1

**Figure 23.1** Trait Profile Checklist

Clinicians are encouraged to help clients focus on applying their productive traits in as many ways as possible, focusing on the client's temperaments, not the clinician's traits, for problem solving. Clinicians address how destructive traits can and do shift toward productive expressions as recovery improves. Clinicians can encourage clients to use their productive trait expression to manage symptom change.

| "I have _tendency_ to …" | How I am currently expressing this trait | | | | |
|---|---|---|---|---|---|
| | More productive | | | More destructive | |
| ☐ Be curious | 5 | 4 | 3 | 2 | 1 |
| ☐ Be imaginative, creative, esthetic | 5 | 4 | 3 | 2 | 1 |
| ☐ Be altruistic or concerned for others' well-being | 5 | 4 | 3 | 2 | 1 |
| ☐ Be dutiful, following rules or principles | 5 | 4 | 3 | 2 | 1 |
| ☐ Be disciplined | 5 | 4 | 3 | 2 | 1 |
| ☐ Be impulsive, act on urges in the moment | 5 | 4 | 3 | 2 | 1 |
| ☐ Be detailed | 5 | 4 | 3 | 2 | 1 |
| ☐ Be committed | 5 | 4 | 3 | 2 | 1 |
| ☐ Be independent or self-directed | 5 | 4 | 3 | 2 | 1 |
| ☐ Be uncertain or not trust my decisions | 5 | 4 | 3 | 2 | 1 |
| ☐ Be persistent | 5 | 4 | 3 | 2 | 1 |
| ☐ Be competitive | 5 | 4 | 3 | 2 | 1 |
| ☐ See errors over successes | 5 | 4 | 3 | 2 | 1 |
| ☐ Be hesitant, concerned about consequences | 5 | 4 | 3 | 2 | 1 |
| ☐ Be sensitive (emotionally, smells, sounds, etc.) | 5 | 4 | 3 | 2 | 1 |
| ☐ Be diligent or thorough | 5 | 4 | 3 | 2 | 1 |
| ☐ Be inhibited, hold back, or procrastinate | 5 | 4 | 3 | 2 | 1 |
| ☐ Have thoughts get stuck on something | 5 | 4 | 3 | 2 | 1 |
| ☐ Be empathic (aware of the needs of others) | 5 | 4 | 3 | 2 | 1 |
| ☐ Be social, interactive | 5 | 4 | 3 | 2 | 1 |
| ☐ Be uncertain | 5 | 4 | 3 | 2 | 1 |
| ☐ Be reliable or dependable | 5 | 4 | 3 | 2 | 1 |
| ☐ Plan ahead or prefer structure or organization | 5 | 4 | 3 | 2 | 1 |
| ☐ Be addicted to_____ | 5 | 4 | 3 | 2 | 1 |
| ☐ Be hard-working | 5 | 4 | 3 | 2 | 1 |

I tend to sleep less than 6 hrs. a night: ☐ Yes ☐ No

I tend to have difficulty falling asleep: ☐ Yes ☐ No

2

**Figure 23.1** (cont.)

Key Point: The Trait Profile Checklist is administered prior to the behavioral agreement. It is a worksheet that offers clients fifty-four traits, drawn from multiple personality and ED models. Clients are instructed to identify their dominant traits to recognize and utilize how they impact their thoughts, feelings, and behaviors to promote or interrupt recovery.

To what degree do I *sense* (not think about, but internally sense) the following?

**Degree of Average Sensation**

| | Highly Sensitive | | | No sensation | |
|---|---|---|---|---|---|
| Hunger | 5 | 4 | 3 | 2 | 1 |
| Pain | 5 | 4 | 3 | 2 | 1 |
| Physical touch | 5 | 4 | 3 | 2 | 1 |
| Taste | 5 | 4 | 3 | 2 | 1 |
| Fullness | 5 | 4 | 3 | 2 | 1 |
| Need to urinate | 5 | 4 | 3 | 2 | 1 |
| Pleasure | 5 | 4 | 3 | 2 | 1 |

☐ Other trait tendencies: _____

**Scoring:**

1. Count the number of traits I identified _____
2. Count how many traits I have been expressing productively (4 or 5) _____
3. Count how many traits I have been expressing destructively (1 or 2) _____

**Scoring interpretation:**

a) If the productive number is higher, I can use the momentum of these traits to reduce my eating disorder symptoms.

b) If the destructive trait number is higher, I can use tools to assist my productive traits to *shift* my destructive traits toward productive expressions. Practice will hold the productive expressions in place.

c) If the numbers are equal, I can use tools and my productive traits to eliminate my symptoms.

**Four** productive traits I have (scored as 4 or 5) that I can use to help manage my symptoms are:

_____

_____

_____

_____

**Three** destructive traits I have (scored as 1 or 2) and want to shift to be less destructive and more productive are:

_____

_____

_____

3

**Figure 23.1** (cont.)

The **"Preparation for SE-AN Behavioral Agreement"** is the first worksheet. It is a two-page handout that sets the stage for the adult client with AN and their Support(s) to develop a working plan together. It is shown in Figure 23.2 (see Appendix 28 for the handout). It

**Preparation for SE-AN Adult Behavioral Agreement**
for Anorexia Nervosa Ages 18–60+
**Worksheet 1**
**Temperament Based Therapy with Support (TBT-S)**

Written by (Client name): _____

My Diagnoses 1:_____Diagnosis 2:_____
 Diagnosis 3:_____Diagnosis 4:_____

**Support** is critical for my recovery. To make myself stronger and my treatment more successful, I am willing to enter into the following agreement with the following person(s) to be my "Support":

Support person 1: _____

Support person 2: _____

Support person 3: _____

Support person 4: _____

<u>Identify the errors, or what is not true for me in the sentences below.</u>
<u>Change any word(s), phrases, or sentence to make the statements true for me.</u>

I recognize that I can be my own worst enemy. In my desire to become stronger physically, psychologically, and interpersonally, I at times sabotage my own efforts in moving forward. While I may want myself to improve, I at times block myself from progress and push others away who want to help me.

## I agree to be honest (Client)

Truth is essential. If I am not honest with myself and others, trust is lost. If I am to recover, then honesty is the first step.

- [ ] I agree to share the full truth, even if it makes "ED" angry. Honesty keeps me accountable to myself and others.
- [ ] I recognize that honesty is a skill that needs to be practiced. If I am not honest, then I will share the truth with the person via text, email, phone, or face-to-face.
- [ ] I can be honest one day at a time.

## I agree to offer interpersonal respect (Client)

Interpersonal respect can sometimes be difficult to manage while in the midst of eating disorder noise and anxiety. (Check what you are *willing to try* to offer.)

- [ ] I agree to take responsibility for my actions and to act kindly and show respect for others in and outside of treatment.
- [ ] If I am not taking responsibility and/or am not respectful, I agree to apologize to the person(s).

1

**Figure 23.2** Preparation for SE-AN BA Worksheet 1

addresses who the Support(s) is/are, client warning signs, Support(s) strengths, and the client's commitment to be honest and offer interpersonal respect.

If the client cannot commit to honesty, the clinician needs to pause, and directly address this issue before moving forward. Without honesty, the clinician, dietitian, and Support(s)'

## My (Client) Warning Signs or Red Flags Include:

I need to help my Supports know what I do when relapsing into ED thoughts, feelings, and behaviors:

- [ ] Eat longer than others, or delay eating snacks and meals.
- [ ] Change my attire (i.e., wearing baggier clothes).
- [ ] Be more argumentative about food/eating/treatment/recovery.
- [ ] Avoid reaching out for help or to my Support.
- [ ] Direct my anger and negative emotions onto Supports.
- [ ] Increase my social withdrawal and isolation or avoid previously enjoyed activities.
- [ ] Increase my negative body comments.

## Support Person(s) Strengths:

S-1 S-2 S-3 S-4   (Support numbers are names indicated above)

[ ][ ][ ][ ]   Listens: Reflects back what they hear with no judgment
Willing to practice new tools
Models and owns their own emotions
(e.g., this is scary for me, I am exhausted, and I am determined.)

[ ][ ][ ][ ]   Willingness to try/learn
Able to be accountable
Is logical

[ ][ ][ ][ ]   Won't give up
Keeps an open mind
Problem solves
Other_____

## I agree to do/not do the following (Supports):

S1 S2 S3 S4

[ ][ ][ ][ ]   Encourage the balanced meal plan and the Behavioral Agreement. (Do)
Instead of judging, ask questions by starting with, "Can you help me understand ...?"
or "I don't understand ..." (Do)

[ ][ ][ ][ ]   Offer 2–3 options to help my loved one with decisions. (Do)
Active Listening: Rephrase what you heard your loved one say without adding your
own judgment. (Do)

[ ][ ][ ][ ]   Refrain from endorsing "diets." (Not do)
Other things that are *bothersome* to the client: _____

[ ][ ][ ][ ]   Other things that are *helpful* to the client: _____

2

**Figure 23.2** (cont.)

actions would be meaningless. The SE-AN client needs to make a commitment to these fundamental qualities before goals are identified and strategies established. Supports in turn identify what they are able to offer when assisting the adult client.

> Key Point: The "Preparation for SE-AN Behavioral Agreement" is the first worksheet. It establishes SE-AN client commitment to accomplish identified goals.

# Stage 2: Goals and Objectives

The "Goals and Objectives, SE-AN Behavioral Worksheet 2" is a four-page document that provides strategies for how the client wants to accomplish the TBT-S treatment goals. Three goals are listed in order, based on adult client feedback. It is shown in Figure 23.3. The complete handout is in Appendix 28. Goals are the "what" or overall aim of the client. Objectives are the strategies (the how) adult clients plan to accomplish the goals. The SE-AN provides detailed lists that fit AN temperament from which clients choose plans for action. Adult clients pinpoint specifications for change based on their individual temperaments. The strategic options included in the worksheet were developed over a 10-year period by adult clients. The three goals are:

- **Goal 1:** Identify my strengths and weakness: My temperament
- **Goal 2:** Commit to my meal and movement plans.
- **Goal 3:** Reduce my eating disorder symptoms.

Goal 1 addresses the client's trait profile recognizing that the client's temperament is fundamental to how the client can accomplish identified objectives over time. Goal 1 is the stage from which Goals 2 and 3 play out. It consists of filling out the Client Trait Profile Checklist, described above, and then reviewing the TBT-S Toolbox together (See Appendix 9). The SE-AN client tends to want to work on treatment goals autonomously. However, little of significance in life can be accomplished and maintained alone. The clinician orchestrates the adult client to be the leader to ascertain what is needed from the Support(s). The Supports determine if they have the traits, energy, and time to do what is requested from the adult client.

Goal 2 addresses strategies for applying the meal plan day-by-day. The dietitian works with the client to complete the meal plan and the clinician or dietiain helps the client complete the objectives with the Supports. The clinician reviews the strategic options chosen by the client.

Goal 3 identifies ED symptoms and strategies, with repairs, to reduce ED behaviors. The client identifies current ED symptoms and detailed strategies to reduce or eliminate destructive behaviors. The clinician can have the client work through this goal as homework with the client's Support(s) and then review it in the next session, or have it filled out during the treatment session. The complete worksheet is in Appendix 28.

> **Key Point:** The second SE-AN BA worksheet provides a structure for adult clients to identify their meal plan and goals and objectives congruent with AN temperament.

# Goals and Objectives
## SE-AN Behavioral Agreement
### Worksheet 2
### Temperament Based Therapy with Support (TBT-S)

Name _____ Date: _____

**Goal 1:** Identify my strengths and weakness: My temperament
**Goal 2:** Commit to my meal and movement plans.
**Goal 3:** Reduce my eating disorder symptoms.

---

**Goal 1:** Identify my strengths and weakness: My temperament

My temperament is the biological foundation of who I am, my natural tendencies that influence my thoughts, feelings, and behaviors. When I express my traits productively, they are my strengths. When I express them destructively, they are my weaknesses. How I express my traits is up to me and it takes work.

### Be true to who *I am*:

1. Take the "Trait Profile Checklist."

2. Identify and practice tools from the "TBT-S Toolbox" to reshape destructive traits and reduce my ED symptoms.

**Goal 2:** Commit to my meal and movement plans

*Biologically, Food is Medicine.* Food is the fuel or energy fundamental to life. For me, food is medicine with uncomfortable side effects. However, I need to eat prescribed meals and snacks each day as my medication for physical and mental strength. I will probably experience higher anxiety when eating certain foods, increasing irritability and distorted thoughts. My thoughts may become "noisy" and negative, making it harder for me to interact with others. These "side effects of food" can keep me from eating or trigger me to binge eat. In spite of these biological reactions, I can better manage my "medication side effects" by choosing from the options below.

## Check the options I could do to manage my meal and exercise plan:

☐ Develop a meal plan with a dietitian, virtually or face-to-face.

    ☐ a. Due to my temperament, inform the dietitian that the meal plan should

        i. Be practical, with foods easy to buy at my grocery,
        ii. Have clear portion sizes, and
        iii. Allow food combinations that can be easily prepared and repeatedly practiced.

1

**Figure 23.3** Goals and Objectives, SE-AN Behavioral Agreement Worksheet 2

☐ b. Include identified Supports whom I want to eat with at times_____, _____.

☐ c. Supports have a copy of the meal plan.

☐ Identify a strengthening movement plan with my dietitian or my medical professional to develop stronger muscles and body strength.

☐ a. Include identified Supports to do active movement together_____,_____.

☐ b. Supports have a copy of the movement plan.

☐ Due to my temperament, I agree to **not eat "intuitively"** when in new eating situations. at this time.

## Check the options I could use to manage my meal plan

Eat 100% of ☐ Breakfast ☐ AM Snack ☐ Lunch ☐ PM Snack ☐ Dinner ☐ Evening Snack

☐ Create a Plan A or default meal and snack. It becomes the meal /snack to eat when stressed.

☐ Take my default meal and snack with me when I leave home.

☐ Exercise or do my movement plan IF I eat/drink 100% of prescribed foods within the past 24 hours.

☐ Go to the grocery alone to purchase foods/drinks in my meal plan.

☐ Keep accurate food logs via, e.g., app_____or using form_____.

☐ Keep accurate movement logs via e.g., app_____or using form_____.

☐ Drink liquid supplements if I cannot eat the food in the prescribed doses, e.g., Boost, Ensure, electrolyte beverages, milk, juice

☐ Drink_____oz of fluid per day (non-caffeinated).

☐ Eat within 1½ hours of getting up and every 3–4 hours.

☐ Text, Skype, or virtually be with_____following_____meal(s).

☐ Set phone alarms for meals/snacks and other reminders.

☐ Use the tools I identified in my TBT-S Toolbox.

☐ Ask_____to shop for my groceries at this time.

☐ Eat at least 1 protein, 1 carb, 1 EF (fat) per meal/snack.

☐ If there are bowel movement problems, talk with medical clinician about supplemental medication.

☐ **Use my productive traits, from my Trait Profile Checklist,** to help me manage my food and movement plans. List 3 of my productive traits that will help me eat my meal plan.

_____, _____, _____

☐ Ask my Supports to offer a couple of options when discussing what to eat at a restaurant, instead of open-ended questions, e.g., "What do you want to eat?"

☐ Ask my Supports to have foods for my default meal on hand. If I am having a stressful day, that is what I'll eat.

☐ Ask my Supports to buy the foods on my meal plan when they are going to the store, instead of my going to the grocery myself.

☐ Ask a Support to go with me to the grocery to get the foods I need. Identify when I will do this_____.

☐ Ask a Support to eat together in person or via face time (ID when and where)_____.

☐ Ask a Support to text or FaceTime me to offer assistance before or after eating. If so, identify when_____.

☐ Inform my Supports if the dietitian adjusts my food or movement plan.

Other:_____

2

**Figure 23.3** (cont.)

**Repairs:** If I don't meet my Meal and Movement Plans:

☐ Text_____(Support) while eating next meal face-to-face or remotely.

☐ Eat or drink missed servings (carbs, pros, and endurance fuels) within 24 hours of the day they are missed, in the form of smoothie, bar, liquid supplement, etc.

☐ If I delay eating, ask_____to text me at set time and talk while I eat.

☐ Have my dietitian or_____monitor my food logs.

☐ Return to the Plan A default or backup meal plan.

☐ If I am unable to eat all my "medicine" more than 3 times a week, I will seek more structure by either setting up more structure with my Supports_____or enter a higher level of treatment_____

☐ Other:_____

## Goal 3: Reduce my eating disorder symptoms.

### Check all ED symptoms that are true for me:

☐ Fasting or restricting

☐ Binge eating

☐ Self-induced vomiting

☐ Cutting or self-mutilating

☐ Weighing myself more than_____

☐ Body checking to self-monitor

☐ Chewing and spitting

☐ Excessive alcohol, marijuana, or smoking (circle one(s) relevant)

☐ Other_____

☐ Hiding or stealing food

☐ Excessive exercising

☐ Laxative abuse

☐ Abusing alcohol or drugs

☐ Using diet pills

☐ Delaying eating

☐ Isolating > 4 hrs. a day.

### Who: I need to work with the following to help reduce my eating disorder symptoms (virtually or face-to-face)

☐ Myself using my productive traits

☐ Supports to know what is being planned and to learn the tools to apply

☐ My clinician

☐ My medical professional

☐ My dietitian

### Ways I could reduce or eliminate ED symptoms

☐ Use my productive traits (Trait Profile Checklist), to help me manage ED symptoms.

☐ Combine 2–3 tools from the TBT-S Toolbox to divert, interrupt or reshape ED symptoms.

☐ Use my_____ and _____ productive traits to help me push forward.

☐ Have my weight monitored (if relevant) by _____.

☐ Agree to have my vitals monitored (if relevant) by _____.

☐ Not exercise until I have eaten 100% of my meal plan in the last 24 hours with no purging, e.g., vomiting or laxatives.

3

**Figure 23.3** (cont.)

☐ IF I am of legal age and IF it is legal in my state or country, I can use marijuana within the limit identified by my medical professional and IF I have no addiction trait.

☐ I agree to not drink alcohol due to urges it triggers.

☐ Ask my Supports to learn the following tools from my Toolbox to help me practice new skills to shift my destructive traits and reduce my symptoms.

_____, _____, _____

☐ Describe my symptoms to my Supports so they know what to look for.

☐ Clarify when it helps and when it does *not* help for my Supports to offer assistance.

☐ Inform my Supports that it may take multiple tools from the Toolbox to help me manage

_____symptom and_____symptom.

☐ Inform Supports that if they become afraid and uncertain of what to do, they have my permission to request time with my therapist and me to discuss the issue together.

☐ Other_____

## Repair: If I do an ED symptom:

☐ If I self-induce vomit or take more laxatives than recommended, then immediately drink an electrolyte beverage (16 oz minimum).

☐ If I do ED symptoms more than two times a week, I understand more structure is needed. This may mean I need more assistance at work, home, or school to help me or more treatment during the week.

☐ I agree to return to work or school only when the following conditions are met.
1. _____
2. _____
3. _____

☐ If I body check, I will take down the mirror (or cover it) and use a "distract" tool: (see TBT-S Toolbox)_____.

☐ If I use laxatives or self-induce vomiting, I will replace the meal eliminated with an equal amount of liquid supplement or foods.

☐ If I restrict, I agree to refer back to my meal plan and eat the carbs, proteins, or endurance foods (fats) to make up the difference.

☐ If I cannot repair restriction or over-exercise, or other ED behaviors by myself, I agree to a higher level of care.

☐ If I do not follow my meal plan, I will do NO exercise for the following 24 hours.

☐ If I purge in any way, I must eat 100% of my meal plan for 2 days and with no additional movement/exercise, and then I could continue with my movement plan.

☐ Do movement with_____(Supports).

☐ Share the ED symptom with_____Support(s) to hold myself accountable.

☐ Agree to have more assistance during_____(time of day).

☐ Text/zoom/Skype/FaceTime_____(Support) to share time with me during the vulnerable time.

☐ Take three tools (from TBT-S Toolbox) with me to distract or reroute from destructive actions for a specific vulnerable time period.

☐ When I return home, I will enter my home *after* I identify 1–2 tools that can help me reroute from a destructive action.

☐ Other: _____

"Always bear in mind that your own resolution to succeed is more important than any one thing."
—Abraham Lincoln

4

**Figure 23.3** (cont.)

## Stage 3: SE-AN Behavioral Agreement Summary

The "Summary SE-AN Behavioral Agreement, Worksheet 3" is a three-page document that summarizes and prioritizes the strategies identified in worksheets 1 and 2 on commitment, meal planning and ED symptom management drawing on the client's traits and Supports' identified actions. It is completed by the adult client with Support(s) present, facilitated by the clinician. It provides a structure for clients to choose their most important objectives to increase focus, repetition and the potential for new habit formation. It serves as the bottom line guide toward recovery. See Figure 23.4.

> Key Point: The Summary SE-AN Behavioral Agreement, Worksheet 3, allows clients to choose the primary strategies identified in the Preparation and Goals/Objectives Worksheets that address how to follow the meal plan and reduce ED symptoms within one's temperament framework. It is completed with Support(s).

## Who Is Involved in Completing the SE-AN BA?

The clinician facilitates the clients and their Supports in completing the Preparation Worksheet, Goals 1–3 and the Summary SE-AN BA. The dietitian is actively involved in Goal 2, which identifies the meal plan with the clinician or the dietitian assisting the client and Support to develop strategies to carry it out. The dietitian recommends meal planning strategies to ensure the "prescribed medicine" of foods is consumed daily, drawing on the client's temperament to motivate and fulfill the goal.

The adult client is the leader who orchestrates their own BA. The client writes/completes the SE-AN BA with at least one identified Support as homework for session preparation or during the therapy and/or dietitian sessions. One to four Supports can be involved in developing the BA with the adult client. Adult clients with AN often do not want Supports involved in their treatment. Nevertheless, TBT-S advocates that Supports are a necessary part of adult AN treatment. The clinician becomes the agent to incorporate dietitian and Support involvement (see Chapter 7) in virtual sessions or face-to-face discussions during treatment.

> Key Point: The adult client leads the behavioral agreement process by filling out the SE-AN BA Worksheets 1–3 with their Support during treatment sessions or as homework for the dietary and clinical sessions.

## When Should the SE-AN BA Be Completed?

The SE-AN Behavioral Agreement can be administered at any time during the treatment process. It could serve as a treatment plan document in the early stages of ED treatment to structure future sessions, in the middle of care as a working document for change as temperament is being introduced into ongoing therapy, or as a summary document at the end of a series of treatment segments before stepping into another level of care. For example, a clinician in a partial hospital ED program has the client and Support complete the SE-AN BA at the end of care, before the client completes treatment and returns to their outpatient (OP) clinician. The OP clinician "picks up the baton" to use the completed BA as the initial OP treatment plan knowing it is the *client's* goals and keeps the same structure, plans, and Supports in place for outpatient client stability.

# SE-AN Adult Behavioral Agreement Summary
## Worksheet 3
### Temperament Based Therapy with Support (TBT-S)

Name _____ Date: _____

## My Problem:

ED symptoms I express are:

_____

_____

**I agree to commit to:** (draw from my responses in **Worksheet 1**)

**Honesty by doing:** _____

**Interpersonal respect by doing:** _____

## Three of my "Red Flags" are:

    1. _____

    2. _____

    3. _____

## My Supports

### Three things my Supports agree to do are:

    1. _____

    2. _____

    3. _____

### Two things I want my Supports to do to help me to reduce my ED symptoms
**are:** (draw from Worksheets 1 and 2)

    1. _____

    2. _____

### Two **tools** I would like my Supports use are: (draw from TBT-S Toolbox)

    1. _____

    2. _____

1

**Figure 23.4** Summary SE-AN Behavioral Agreement, Worksheet 3

The Trait Profile Checklist takes about 10 minutes to complete. The Preparation Worksheet 1 takes 20 to 30 minutes to complete *with* the Support(s). The Goals/Objectives Worksheet 2 takes 60 to 90 minutes to complete *with* the Support(s). The Summary SE-AN Behavioral Agreement takes 30 minutes to complete by the adult client *with* the Support(s), facilitated by the clinician.

**Goal 1:** (Drawing from **Worksheet 2, my "Trait Profile Checklist and TBT-S Toolbox"**):
<u>Be True to Who I Am: Draw upon my own Temperament or Traits:</u>

Three traits I express productively that I can draw upon to help manage my symptoms are:

    1. _____
    2. _____
    3. _____

Two of my current destructive traits that I express without thinking and want to reshape are:

    1. _____
    2. _____

**Goal 2:** Commit to my meal and movement plans.

I have a meal plan identified with the dietitian_____:

Three ways I plan to complete my meal plan each day are: (from Worksheet 2)

    1. _____
    2. _____
    3. _____

Three of my productive traits that I can draw upon to complete my meal plan are: (Trait Profile Checklist)

    1. _____
    2. _____
    3. _____

Two Supports who can help me carry out my plan to eat are:

    1. _____
    2. _____

Two things I want my Supports to do help me with the meal plan are: (draw from Worksheet 2)

    1. _____
    2. _____

2

**Figure 23.4** (cont.)

Key Point: The SE-AN BA is completed when clients, clinicians, and/or dietitians need to establish new goals and objectives that integrate AN temperament. This could be at the beginning of treatment or at times when new goals or meals plans need to be established.

# Where Is the SE-AN BA Completed?

The 3 SE-AN BA Worksheets and the Trait Profile Checklist could be completed in virtual or face-to-face sessions at all levels of care from outpatient to residential care. They can be implemented in individual or group settings.

The documents could be completed in individual and Support(s) sessions or group sessions where several adult clients are working on their own BAs with their Support(s). The Worksheets and Trait Profile Checklist could be assigned as homework to prepare for the SE-AN Behavioral Agreement Summary during therapy, with the instruction that the client and Support(s) complete both.

**Repairs:** Two things I will do if I do not complete my meal plan: (Worksheet 2)

1. _____
2. _____

What action that I identified in my meal and movement plan is nonnegotiable? (Worksheet 2)

_____

## Goal 3: Reduce my Eating Disorder Symptoms:

I plan to use the following 3 methods to reduce my ED symptoms: (Worksheet 2 and Toolbox)

1. _____
2. _____
3. _____

Three of my productive traits that I can use to reduce my ED symptoms are: (Trait Profile Checklist)

1. _____
2. _____
3. _____

Two Support persons who can help me reduce my ED symptoms are:

1. _____
2. _____

Two things I need my Supports to do to help me reduce my ED symptoms are: (Worksheet 2)

1. _____
2. _____

**Repairs:** When I Do an ED symptoms I will make one of the following two repairs: (Worksheet 2)

1. _____
2. _____

## Living with purpose:

By the time I am_____years old, I will live my life with more purpose by doing
Or, I will be upset with myself if I am not doing_____by the time I am____years old:

_____

Client notes: _____

_____

"The best way to predict your future is to create it." — Abraham Lincoln

3

**Figure 23.4** (cont.)

**Key Point:** The SE-AN BA can be completed at all levels of care and in individual or group therapy settings.

# Why Use the SE-AN BA?

Persons with severe-and-enduring AN have long practiced ED behaviors, restrictive patterns, and well-ingrained tendencies developed over many years of the illness. This document was developed to match the need for rules, structure, detail, clear options (versus open-ended questions), and collaboration. ED clinicians should not function as "the Support" for the SE-AN client. It sets clinicians up to be what they are not. Clinicians facilitate the process to identify Supports with the client. This may take a few sessions. It forces and breaks down the avoidance walls that the client has built and creates new and renewed connections. If a client's AN symptoms are acute and treatment is in a higher level of care, then the treatment team serves as Supports. When the client transitions to a lower level of care, Supports outside of the therapy session need to be identified and incorporated into designated sessions to complete the BA together.

The client's need for assistance is greater than any one clinician can offer. Acknowledging that Supports are necessary for AN treatment is a core principle of TBT-S. Supports want to know what to do, when and how to do it to help their loved one and not burn out themselves. The SE-AN client holds the reins in identifying who, what, when, and where assistance is needed, through the structure of the BA. The clinician can supplement the BA in ongoing therapy by offering TBT-S experiential activities that help the client and Supports experiment with solutions that clarify the what, when, and how of recovery.

> **Key Point:** The SE-AN BA is structured to maximize AN temperament traits and allow the client to be the lead in identifying goals/objectives with their Supports.

# How to Use the SE-AN BA

There are multiple options for implementing the SE-AN BA. Outpatient clinicians could identify sessions for the BA development. Another option is for the clinician to assign the worksheets and/or the Trait Profile Checklist as homework. The clinician could schedule multi-hour sessions to complete the documents together, virtually or face-to-face, with 1- or 2-hour sessions to complete the SE-AN BA. The clinician facilitates the complete process, identifying the sessions for BA completion and when to include Supports. Whatever the treatment variables, the order of implementation is the same:

1. Give the Trait Profile Checklist to the adult client and Support(s).
2. Adult client and Support(s) complete Worksheet 1 for the BA.
3. Adult client and Support(s) complete Worksheet 2 of the BA, with the dietitian included in Goal 2, developing and committing to a meal plan.
4. Adult client and Support(s) and clinician complete the SE-AN Behavioral Agreement Summary with the clinician.

> **Summary Key Points**
>
> - The Behavioral Agreement for clients with severe-and-enduring AN and its preparatory worksheets provide a structured strategic plan of action for adult clients to develop and implement collaboratively with their Support(s).
> - It incorporates client and Support traits to determine what is realistic and unrealistic for long-term change.

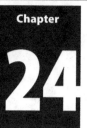

# Tailoring TBT-S Treatment Modules into All Levels of Care

TBT-S is offered in module format. Clinicians can use one module or dozens of modules to integrate with and augment ongoing eating disorder (ED) therapy, or to create a stand-alone program that adult clients and Supports enter into and then use when reentering ongoing care. A TBT-S program could be one-day through a one-week program or a one-hour session to multiple hours per week throughout treatment. TBT-S is the neurobiologically based "seasoning" for ongoing ED therapy.

## Examples of TBT-S Module Combinations

### Five-Day Young Adult (YA) TBT-S Schedule

YA TBT-S was developed in a modular format so that activities and modules can be selected and applied as needed by clinicians to augment other types of treatment. The activities in this book can be applied over a varying time course in sequence or singularly.

YA TBT-S was developed and tested in a 5-day format, where YA and parents receive all TBT-S modules in a multi-family group format. In this model, YAs and parents attend treatment for roughly seven hours per day (Monday–Friday) over the course of one week. This format holds a variety of benefits, including allowance for massed practice; *in vivo*, clinician-assisted skills coaching during therapeutic meals and snacks; and peer-to-peer consultation and assistance facilitated by the group members. Table 24.1 summarizes the YA TBT-S schedule over the 5-day format. It is important to note that the experiential activities may vary based on the particular group, in line with the TBT-S modular format.

### Six-Session TBT-S Series

Table 24.2 describes YA TBT-S modules delivered in a six-session weekly series. This series was conducted in a multi-family group format with clients and Supports receiving traditional ED treatment.

○  This series can be inserted into ongoing eating disorder treatment
○  Group settings

### Five-Day Severe-and-Enduring Anorexia Nervosa (SE-AN) TBT-S Schedule

There are many ways to apply a multi-day TBT-S modular schedule to augment ongoing eating disorder programs and treatments. For example, an eating disorder residential or partial hospital treatment program could hold one week every month or each quarter to insert a week of TBT-S, inviting Supports to join the program during that time period.

**Table 24.1** 5-day YA TBT-S program schedule

| | | | UCSD Young Adult Temperament Based Therapy with Support (YA TBT-S) | | |
|---|---|---|---|---|---|
| | Monday | Tuesday | Wednesday | Thursday | Friday |
| 8:00–9:00 | | BREAKFAST | BREAKFAST/Dietary Feedback Vitals | BREAKFAST | BREAKFAST Vitals |
| 9:00–9:45 | Orientation Multi-Family Therapy: Mixed Family Introductions/Goals | Neurobiology Psychoeducation: Traits, Interoception, and Anxiety | Neurobiology Psychoeducation: Reward & Inhibition | Neurobiology Activity: Yes/No Game | Multi-Family Therapy: Mixed Family Groups |
| 9:45–10:00 | Dietary Orientation. | | | | |
| 10:00–10:30 | SNACK | SNACK | SNACK | SNACK | SNACK |
| 10:30–11:00 | Skill: Training: Young Adult/Parent Group | Neurobiology Activity: Nondominant Hand Activity | Experiential Activity: Communicating and Listening | Multi-Family Therapy: Ask the Expert | Neurobiology Activity: Wire-Re-wire |
| 11:00–11:34 | | Experiential Activity: Family Wise Mind | | | |
| 11:30–2:30 | | | | | Dietary Q & A |
| 12:30–1:30 | Lunch | Lunch | Lunch | Lunch | Lunch |
| 1:30–2:30 | Intensive Skills Training (YA only) | Neurobiology Activity: Anxiety/ Brain Sculpt | Skill Training: Young Adult/Parent Group | Behavioral Agreement | Group Closing Feedback & Evaluations |
| 2:30–3:00 | Family Dietary Meeting/ Psychiatry Evaluations | | | | |
| 3:00–3:30 | SNACK | SNACK | SNACK | SNACK | SNACK |
| 3:30–4:00 | | | Nutrition Education Group | | |

**Table 24.2** Six-session YA TBT-S series

## 6-session TBT-S series inserted into eating disorder treatment as usual (TAU) group setting

| Session | Topic | Client–parent group activity | Client group activity | Parent activity |
|---|---|---|---|---|
| 1 | Anorexia is a brain illness | • MFT introductions<br>• Nondominant hand activity | Identifying traits | Introduction to dialectical model of support |
| 2 | Anxiety/interoception | • Anxiety brain sculpt<br>• MFT Debrief | None | None |
| 3 | Targeting anxiety & interoception: skills and strategies | • Practice: distract redirection<br>• Mixed client–support feedback group focused on how to manage anxiety<br>• Anxiety wave<br>• Summary of skills (based on group discussion):<br>• Distraction/reroute<br>• Structure/predictability<br>• Effective prompting support | • Create a pre-, mid-, and post-meal distract routine<br>• My recovery rules | • Creating structure and predictability as a Support via rules/guidelines<br>• Effective responses and prompting |
| 4 | Altered reward sensitivity | • Yes/no game | Establishing recovery guidelines and motivators | • Utilizing rules and contingencies |
| 5 | Behavioral agreement | • Behavioral agreement | | |
| 6 | Wire-re-wire activity | • Behavioral agreement (continued) | | |

TBT-S modules are like building blocks, with a neurobiological substance, that can be selected, inserted, and combined in a manner that complement ongoing ED therapies. A 1-week, 40-hour TBT-S program for SE-AN clients and their Supports was offered in a freestanding format during the open trials. Clients were referred back to their appropriate levels of care after the TBT-S treatment. Table 24.3 describes the modules used for the 5-day,

**Table 24.3** 5-day SE-AN TBT-S program schedule

| | Monday | Tuesday | Wednesday | Thursday | Friday |
|---|---|---|---|---|---|
| 8:00 | Medical Check-in | Medical Check-in | Medical Check-in | Medical Check-in | Medical Check-in |
| 9:00 | **Dietary Coached Breakfast**, Pre-meal: Deep breath 4 × 4 Post-meal 10 minutes "Walking tall" tool | **Dietary Coached Breakfast**, Pre-meal: Deep breath 4 × 4 Post-meal 10 minutes "Walking tall" tool | **Dietary Coached Breakfast**, Pre-meal: Deep breath 4 × 4 Post-meal 10 minutes "Walking tall" tool | **Dietary Coached Breakfast**, Pre-meal: Deep breath 4 × 4 Post-meal 10 minutes "Walking tall" tool | **Dietary Coached Breakfast**, Pre-meal: Deep breath 4 × 4 Post-meal 10 minutes "Walking tall" tool |
| 10:00 | Lessons Learned among Clients and Supports: **TBT-S Experiential Activity**: Interactive ED Information Question/Answer Game, and Listening to ED "Noise" | Lessons Learned among Clients and Supports: **TBT-S Tool**: Self-Critique Tool practice from previous night meal | Lessons Learned among Clients and Supports: **TBT-S Experiential Activity**: Expert advice from the client | Lessons Learned among Clients and Supports: Neurobiology **Psychoeducation**: Medical Q and A with medical professional | Lessons Learned among Clients and Supports: **Experiential Activity**: Drawing upon one another as experts: "What will you do?" activity. |
| 11:00 | **Neurobiology Psychoeducation on Trait:** Interoception **Experiential Activity**: Telephone | **Neurobiology Psychoeducation on Trait**: Anxiety **Experiential Activity**: Anxiety Wave, Stop, Reboot, Reroute | **Neurobiology Psychoeducation on:** Reward & Punishment **Experiential Activity**: Landmine | **Neurobiology Psychoeducation on:** Decision-making **Experiential Activity**: Wire/Re-wire | **Neurobiology Psychoeducation on:** Overview Review **Experiential Activity**: Brain Wave |
| 12:00 | **Dietary Coached Lunch**, Pre-meal: Deep breath 4 × 4 Post-meal 10 minutes "walking tall" tool | **Dietary Coached Lunch**, Pre-meal: Deep breath 4 × 4 Post-meal 10 minutes "walking tall" tool | **Dietary Coached Lunch**, Pre-meal: Deep breath 4 × 4 Post-meal 10 minutes "walking tall" tool | **Dietary Coached Lunch**, Pre-meal: Deep breath 4 × 4 Post-meal 10 minutes "walking tall" tool | **Dietary Coached Lunch**, Pre-meal: Deep breath 4 × 4 Post-meal 10 minutes "walking tall" tool |
| 1:00 | **Behavioral Agreement:** Worksheet 1 & Trait Profile Checklist | **Behavioral Agreement:** Worksheet 2 & first two pages | **Behavioral Agreement:** Worksheet 3 & last two pages | **Behavioral Agreement**: SE-AN BA Handout | **Behavioral Agreement**: SE-AN BA Handout to sign and copy to treatment team |
| 2:00 | **TBT-S Toolbox**: Ask for 3 Options, Active Listening Offer Compliment | **TBT-S Toolbox**: Wise-Mind Offer Support | **TBT-S Toolbox**: "Ground Myself" **Experiential Activity**: Red Rover or WW-D | **TBT-S Toolbox**: Accepting My Traits: What I can do/what I cannot do | **TBT-S Toolbox**: **Experiential Activity**: Charades |
| 3:00 | **Snack** | **Snack** | **Snack** | **Snack** | **Snack** |
| 3:00 | **Experiential Activity**: Nondominant Hand Day Summary: What helped? What didn't help? Take home message | Day Summary: What helped? What didn't help? Take home message | Day Summary: What helped? What didn't help? Take home message | Day Summary: What helped? What didn't help? Take home message | Day Summary: **Experiential Activity**: Social Gauntlet What helped? What didn't help? Take home message |

40-hour, 1-week open trial SE-AN studies.[9, 79] Treatment teams may choose to insert modules described in Chapters 9–12 or change the daily schedule to fit ongoing program needs. Two examples are outlined in Tables 24.4 and 24.5. Details of the skills are described in Chapters 16–19, and experiential activities are described in step-by-step detail in Appendices 1–27.

Treating to client traits is the complementing aspect of TBT-S with other treatment approaches. Behaviors, cognition, and emotional experiences trace back to the client's temperament. Client temperament traits are the underlying triggers that influence these outward expressions. Helping clients identify and understand their traits allows them to manage their symptoms and improve their health. SE-AN clients also realize that if they do not have specific traits or abilities needed to carry out identified goals, they need to practice asking Supports for assistance.

> **Key Point: TBT-S modules can be selected and arranged to supplement outpatient sessions or create multi-day neurobiologically based interactive programs that can be inserted into ongoing ED residential, partial hospital, or freestanding treatment programs.**

Table 24.4 is an example schedule of inserting TBT-S modules into intensive outpatient programs.

**Table 24.4** Examples of TBT-S modules added to intensive outpatient eating disorder program

| | | |
|---|---|---|
| ED IOP program offering cognitive and behavioral intervention with issue raised on why ED symptoms develop | TBT-S Neurobiological Psychoeducation on Traits, Anxiety and Interoception | TBT-S Module on Trait Profile Checklist |
| ED IOP Program offering treatment as usual, with issue raised on how to reduce ED symptoms | TBT-S Toolbox | Continue with treatment as usual |

Note: These are conceptual examples that have not been studied formally to determine module impact in variations of ED treatment.

Table 24.5 are examples of inserting TBT-S modules into outpatient weekly treatment as usual.

> **Summary Key Point**
>
> - **TBT-S modules can be delivered in whatever format clinicians choose to design, ranging from one-hour one time during treatment to a five-day, one-week format, with modules inserted into ongoing outpatient eating disorder treatment sessions.**

**Table 24.5** Examples of TBT-S modules added to outpatient eating disorder treatment as usual

### Individual therapy setting

| | | | |
|---|---|---|---|
| ED Assessment Treatment rules, identify and include Supports in selected sessions | **SE-AN Behavioral Agreement Worksheets 1 and 2** assigned as homework for client and Support(s) | TAU with client and homework assigned to take the **Trait Profile Checklist** | **SE-AN Behavioral Agreement handout** used to develop treatment goals and strategies, with clinician as coach for client and Support in virtual session | Complete the SE-AN and continue TAU |

### Group outpatient therapy setting

| | | | |
|---|---|---|---|
| SE-AN clients receiving TAU, issue raised on what to do in unexpected situations without triggering ED symptoms | **Experiential problem-solving activity:** Landmine is played with all SE-AN clients, option to include Supports | TAU | TAU with issue raised regarding anxiety | **TBT-S Neurobiological psychoeducation** on anxiety module, followed by **TBT-S experiential activities:** stop–reboot, reroute, and anxiety wave |

*Note:* These are conceptual examples that have not been studied formally to determine module impact in variations of ED treatment.

# Chapter 25

# How to Apply TBT-S in Diverse Settings

TBT-S can be applied to diverse treatment settings for both young adults (YA) and adults with severe-and-enduring anorexia nervosa (SE-AN) to augment ongoing eating disorder (ED) treatment. Core TBT-S principles (see Chapter 2) and its methods of application could be integrated into ongoing treatments across levels of care. As stated, open trials have been studied in a face-to-face format showing significant impact for both YA and SE-AN.[9, 79] The YA TBT-S 5-day program is also being explored in a virtual treatment format as well. The effects of TBT-S components separated and integrated into outpatient ED treatment settings is yet to be determined. This manual serves as a primary resource for those studies.

## The 5-Day TBT-S Program: YA TBT-S and SE-AN TBT-S

TBT-S continues to be actively studied in a 5-day, 1-week format conducted in person and virtually. It consists of introducing and applying all TBT-S core principles and interventions that are practiced hour after hour within one week. It is an immersion into the biological nature of the illness. TBT-S recalibrates and shifts the paradigm of treatment to supplement other ED programs and ongoing therapies that focus on cognitive, behavioral, and interpersonal (nurture) perspectives of the illness.

## The TBT-S 5-day Program Composition

- Consists of a group of up to seven adult clients, each with a minimum of one Support, two clinicians, a dietitian, and a medical professional.
- Includes two meals and two snacks daily, with food recommended by the dietitian and prepared by the adult clients and their Support (see Chapter 20).
- Provides neurobiological and temperament psychoeducation on AN (see Chapter 10).
- Integrates temperament into all interventions and treatment goals. See Trait Profile Checklist in Appendix 2 and Chapters 10–13.
- Offers experiential activities that metaphorically explain neurobiological AN dynamics (see Chapter 19).
- Offers experiential problem-solving activities that trigger each client's unique trait profile to play out solutions for their ED symptoms (see Chapter 19).
- Provides skills/tools to practice reshaping ED symptoms into productive actions that strengthen client health and lifestyle (see Chapters 16–18).
- Has two versions of treatment activities. A young adults (YA) version, for clients ranging in age from 18 to 27 and the SE-AN version, for clients ranging in age from 18 to age 60 and older who have had the illness for five years or more. (see Chapters 14 and 15).

- Has two versions of the TBT-S Behavioral Agreement, one for YAs and one for SE-ANs (see Chapters 22 and 23).

  There is an hour-by-hour, daily schedule for the YA and SE-AN versions in Chapter 24.

> **Key Point:** TBT-S has been studied in a 40-hour, 1-week group format that consists of novel interventions that integrate temperament and Supports in structured interactive treatment approaches for YA and SE-AN.

## Integrating TBT-S into Outpatient Levels of Care

TBT-S core principles (see Chapter 2) and treatment components could be selectively offered to augment other ED therapies in multiple levels of care:

- Outpatient (OP) weekly individual and groups settings.
- Intensive outpatient programs (IOP).
- Partial hospital programs (PHP).
- Residential level of care.

The temperament bases of AN and involvement of Supports could be "seasoned" into each session or offered in segments augmenting ongoing ED therapies. Providing TBT-S balances ED treatments with the biological bases of why AN develops and why ED symptoms are maintained. It also provides temperament bases of what to do and how to do it. How to initiate TBT- S into multiple levels of care is described in Chapter 24.

TBT-S acknowledges and utilizes the fact that temperaments initiate solutions as well as trigger problems. If outpatient clinicians are implementing TBT-S into their treatment settings, TBT-S advocates that clinicians utilize treatment interventions that draw upon the client's temperament, not the clinician's temperament. (See Trait Profile Checklist in Appendix 2.) What the clinician says, how it is said, and how interventions are applied should be grounded in the client's AN temperament to maximize empathy, understanding, and motivation. This impacts both short- and long-term change.

TBT-S advocates that clinicians include Supports in identified segments of treatment. Supports often initiate the request for TBT-S treatment for YA clients with AN, while clients with SE-AN tend to need coaching to identify and include Supports. Why Supports are needed and how to explain this is described in Chapter 7.

> **Key Point:** TBT-S neurobiological information and temperament approach could be "seasoned" into segments at multiple levels of ED treatment.

## How Often Do Supports Attend Outpatient Treatment Sessions?

Clinicians schedule Supports to attend specified appointments or segments of treatment. Supports could attend virtually or face-to-face; with different Supports living at different locations, each may have a different role in assisting the adult client. Actively bringing Supports into designated treatment sessions ensures consistency inside and outside of treatment. Clinicians work with Supports and adult clients to address the following:

- Meal and snack planning from food recommendations by the dietitian.
- Neurobiological and temperament psychoeducation on AN.
- Identification of the adult client temperament (see Trait Profile Checklist, Appendix 2).
- Experiential activities that metaphorically explain neurobiological AN dynamics.
- Experiential problem-solving activities that trigger the client's unique trait profile to develop solutions for their ED symptoms.
- Skills/tools that both clients and Supports can practice to reshape ED symptoms into productive actions that strengthen the client's health and lifestyle.

The number of sessions devoted to each area depends upon the clinician, client, and Supports. Scheduling possibilities seem endless based on clinician creativity, amount of structure provided, and client and Support needs. For example, an adult client with SE-AN identifies three Supports who could provide assistance in different ways. The clinician identifies and explains the neurobiological bases of AN to the client and Supports together. The clinician may decide that two sessions are needed to share temperament based research findings and answer questions. There could be a one-on-one session with the client to process the experience.

In another segment of a virtual session, the clinician could schedule the client and all three Supports to complete the SE-AN Behavioral Agreement (BA) together. The client and Supports could complete portions of the BA outside of treatment, and other portions completed during the treatment session to ensure that all parties are clear on their roles based on the client's expressed instructions outlined in the BA.

The clinician and/or dietitian may choose to practice specified skills/tools (based upon the client's temperament) with the client and Support designating sessions when all persons can be together face-to-face or virtually. Clinicians who are starting TBT-S could identify what components of TBT-S they need with a YA or SE-AN client in the upcoming six months. The clinician needs to identify the number of sessions to hold for TBT-S neurobiological information, the BA, and skills/tools and schedule them into sessions during the designated time periods. For example, the clinician may identify three skills/tools relevant to the client's temperament and portions of neurobiological information relevant to the SE-AN client. The order of which intervention to offer first or last can vary. There is no one right way. The more the clinician experiments with different clients, one series of TBT-S interventions may appear better for one client and a different series for another client.

For example, a client may need to begin practicing specific TBT-S skills/tools immediately; so a session is scheduled with the client and identified Supports to train and practice a tool. Both Supports and the client are assigned to practice a tool outside of therapy. The clinician may decide to schedule the BA in the following three sessions with the client and all Supports. The SE-AN BA Worksheets 1 and 2 could be handed out for the client and Support to fill out in preparation before the designated session. The BA serves as a detailed road map of who does what and when. The "how" is scheduled with the client and Supports by offering specific skill/tool trainings. Segments of neurobiological information could be sprinkled into sessions. It is ideal to have all Supports and the client present when sharing the underpinnings of the illness, but this is not always practical in outpatient settings. The decision lies with the clinician. Note that it is important that clinicians not expect themselves to be expert neuropsychologists. See the *script* that follows.

The new TBT-S clinician may be nervous about offering TBT-S interventions and information. That is normal. We recommend that clinicians own their feelings and move forward, just as moving forward toward eating one's meal plan is expected of the client.

**Script**

*I would like to schedule your identified Supports to be a part of the next three virtual sessions.*

*I will email you and each Support a copy of the Worksheets and Behavioral Agreement. I would like you to fill out Worksheet 1 and the Trait Profile Checklist before our session together next week.*

*I need your help. Please fill in your answers on both forms. There are no "right" answers. The best answers are one that match your traits and work best for you. I will ask your Supports to fill out the questions identified for them in Worksheet 1 and be prepared to share their responses during next week's session.*

*I am a bit nervous to do this because it is my first time and yet, if I can't wade through my hesitations, I can't expect you to wade through your hesitations to reduce your ED symptoms. The forms will indicate what we need to clarify and discuss together. There may be other issues that arise, that your Supports may bring up, but I am going to hold us to the worksheets while we are identifying core treatment issues. The worksheets tend to answer most of the Supports' questions.*

The BA and skill/tool descriptions could be entered into the client's electronic or paper file. The information on the signed BA can serve as the primary treatment plan or as clinical notes that augment the electronic treatment plan. Whether offered in a group or individual session, the TBT-S forms are structured, detailed, and highly individualized. The structure can help the clinician who is new to a TBT-S approach, simultaneously helping the client who is learning to acknowledge the need for structure due to their temperament.

> **Key Point:** The clinician schedules members of the ED treatment team, such as dietitians and medical professions, and Supports to participate with the adult client in various combinations of ways to address key aspects of treatment planning and skill/tool development. This ensures consistency inside and outside of treatment.

## How to Flexibly Use TBT-S Modules

TBT-S can be integrated into ongoing ED treatments from outpatient to PHP and potentially residential ED programs. It can also be offered as a short-term treatment multiday program to establish a foundation for ongoing treatment. This could include a 5-day series or offered in segments over several months. TBT-S could be offered in outpatient group settings with the clinician inviting Supports to attend designated sessions.

As stated in earlier chapters, TBT-S has been studied in open trials that measured the effect of the treatment on both YA and SE-AN groups consisting of clients and their Supports in five consecutive day-long treatment programs. The YA and SE-AN TBT-S Programs were implemented differently. Both drew upon TBT-S core principles, neurobiological themes, and temperament. They selected skills/tools relevant to the group members in each program. The arrangement and the inclusion of some information and exclusion of other neurobiological information were experimented with to clarify if any one theme impacted change. It did not. Significant psychological and behavioral changes occurred in clients and Support persons in both YA and SE-AN programs. Improvement was maintained for both YA and SE-AN programs at three to six months follow-up to treatment.

While the effect of introducing portions of TBT-S by integrating it into ongoing ED therapies is not yet known, it appears that combinations of TBT-S interventions can be implemented to enhance and/or fill the temperament gap in ongoing therapies. For example, clinicians who know little about neurobiological research may choose to begin with the TBT-S handout titled "Ten Biological Facts about Anorexia Nervosa" (Appendix 1) to address underpinnings of the illness, instead of trying to summarize temperament bases on their own. The TBT-S approach varies. It is not a single step-by-step approach.

### Summary Key Point

Clinicians and programs could flexibly augment TBT-S core principles and components into ongoing ED treatment in varying ways.

# How to Interface TBT-S Treatment with Ongoing Providers and Eating Disorder Programs

**Chapter 26**

## How to Interface TBT-S Modules into Ongoing ED Therapy

If a client is referred to a young adult (YA) TBT-S or a severe-and-enduring anorexia nervosa (SE-AN) TBT-S virtual or face-to-face program, the interfacing process is similar to any other treatment referral between levels of care. Possible referral combinations could include the following:

- Outpatient clinicians IOP, PHP, or inpatient eating disorder (ED) programs referring clients to a YA or SE-AN TBT-S Program.
- TBT-S Program referring client up to inpatient, to a PHP, IOP, or outpatient clinician.
- Outpatient levels of care that have integrated TBT-S into ongoing treatment referring to a PHP program that has integrated TBT-S into its program and vice versa.

When clients receive treatment in a TBT-S Program, we have found client's primary posttreatment requests are to continue a temperament based approach in their ongoing recommended level of care. This has been exceedingly difficult to offer in the past. As ED staff become increasingly trained in a TBT-S approach, transferring from a TBT-S Program to different levels of care with TBT-S integrated into ongoing treatment, becomes more realistic.

Each ED treatment program determines its own protocols based upon their facility requirements. When referring clients into a YA or SE-AN TBT-S Program, it is common to request current client physicals, past treatment, hospital stays, suicidal history, and a complete psychological and psychiatric history. We found offering weekly scheduled question-and-answer phone meetings before 5-day TBT-S programs allayed many concerns. Potential clients and referring clinicians/dietitians could obtain information about the treatment program. The callers are invited to ask questions about a variety of concerns, including treatment approach, structure, and who is included when. It is a proactive opportunity for clients and Supports to discuss concerns and hear what other callers ask or share before entering the treatment program. This was relevant, whether for a YA or an SE-AN TBT-S Program. Question and answer (Q and A) phone meetings allow clients and Supports to be anonymous while exploring treatment options.

Clients and/or Supports may initiate treatment. YAs are always the primary participants in the admissions process; however, for many YAs, parents participate in the phone meetings and can serve as a motivating force for their loved ones to enter the program. For those with SE-AN, we found that it was the clients who were more likely to participate by listening to other persons' questions and answers. Upon hearing that they were leaders in the treatment process, many SE-AN clients followed the Q and A phone meetings with a request for admission into an upcoming TBT-S Program. A TBT-S staff person was trained in how to ask questions necessary to help an SE-AN client identify at least one Support person to join the client virtually or face-to-face for all five days of the program. Additional Supports could attend at various times during the program.

A phone meeting with the SE-AN client and the identified Support(s) is helpful prior to the program start date because the closer the entry date, the higher the clients' fear to enter the program as avoidance tendencies increase. It is at that point, the week prior to the TBT-S Program, that Supports are encouraged to step in and step up to encourage the client to begin the brief treatment, even for only one day. Now that treatment can be virtual, the fear remains high, but the ability to enter treatment from the client's home reduces avoidance tendencies.

Many higher levels of care programs require pretesting for DSM-5 diagnoses, ED assessments, such as the Eating Disorder Examination Questionnaire (EDE-Q)[188] to be administered by phone, online, or face-to-face. PHP levels of care usually require a clinical and medical assessment within 24 hours of the first day of the program. Pretesting of traits, ED symptoms, depression, and anxiety are also commonly assessed prior to the entry point of the program.

Upon completing the TBT-S Programs (its open trials had 99 percent retention rates) post-testing is administered with follow-up testing at three months, six months, and one year to both YA and SE-AN clients and their primary Support. Other ED facilities and treatment programs that administer TBT-S internationally decide upon their battery of pre-post testing and program admission criteria based on their protocols.

> Key Point: Entry and exit into and out of TBT-S Programs are similar to other treatment transfers from one level of care to another. Scheduled phone sessions open to clients, Supports, and clinicians to address questions are recommended for multiday TBT-S programs to dispel anxiety or confusion, with additional recommended phone sessions scheduled for questions and answers with clients.

# TBT-S Promotes Seamless Transitions of Care

It is important to ensure a seamless transition of care for all clients who transfer from one level of care or program to another. Working to use the same treatment language, skills/tools, Behavioral Agreements, and understanding of the illness promotes longer-term progress in reducing relapse potential. Waiting weeks, instead of days, to enter into the next level of care treatment promotes the resurfacing of ED symptomatic habits. This is especially true when treating AN due to the neurobiological circuit alterations and traits that defend ED symptom expressions. Newly identified client trait-related rules and rituals as well as detailed planning can prevent relapse. If clients receive treatment in a TBT-S Program, they step into ongoing clinically appropriate levels of care after the multi-day program. The TBT-S Program could be in the same system as the ongoing care, making the transition easier after the TBT-S Program.

> Key Point: The more detailed the planning and passing of the baton, from a TBT-S Program to ongoing ED treatment settings, the more seamless the care, thus-reducing vulnerabilities for relapse.

# What Materials Are Sent to Ongoing Providers?

The YA and SE-AN Behavioral Agreements are a central TBT-S tool that schedules, organizes, and identifies the who, what, when, and where of client goals with the current and upcoming treatment team. These documents allows everyone on the TBT-S and future treatment teams to be fully informed. This includes the clinician, client, Supports, dietitian, and medical professionals at both the TBT-S and ongoing treatment team settings. It may be unrealistic for ongoing programs and outpatient clinicians to use the BA as the sole treatment plan, due to program electronic medical records (EMRs), which have treatment plans integrated in the software, or due to clinician preference to use their own treatment plan. The TBT-S BA, however, is a critical document that can be entered into the client's EMR or clinical notes and utilized during weekly sessions to carry out the detailed plans that the clients and Supports created together to ensure continuity in actions. The BA serves to make continuity of care seamless.

Medication and post-testing of anxiety, depression, and ED symptoms are examples of information that is needed when transferring clients to different settings for ongoing treatment. Authorization consenting to the release of clinical information is required and signed by adult clients. The Trait Profile Checklist and skills/tools that each client has identified as important in helping them manage their ED symptoms are also helpful to send to an ongoing ED level of care treatment. The client TBT-S Toolbox is a form that clients may want transferred and ongoing clinicians to continue to practice identified tools seen as helpful by the client.

---

**Summary Key Point**

The Behavioral Agreements, and Toolbox are examples of TBT-S documents sent to ongoing treatment settings to ensure continuity of care and adult clients' goals of who does what, when, and how for the following weeks and months of treatment.

# Chapter 27

# Summary of Temperament Based Therapy with Support

Treat to the traits

to manage symptoms

with Supports

for clients of all ages

# Appendix 1  Ten Biological Facts about Anorexia Nervosa Handout

Laura Hill

1. **Anorexia nervosa is dangerous and deadly.**

   - Anorexia nervosa is a serious, life-threatening condition that has one of the highest death rates of all mental illnesses.[1-3]
   - The mortality rate of anorexia nervosa is about 12 times higher than the annual death rate for all causes of death among females ages 15–24 in the general population.[156] The mortality rate for AN in British Columbia was 10.5 percent assessed over a 20-year period.[1]
   - One study found that midlife adults with AN had the highest rates of poor outcome or death.[157]
   - Prediction of poor outcomes or death is worsened if there is a history of alcohol and/or drug misuse and endocrine concerns.[157]
   - Estimates suggest that persons with AN are more than five times more likely than age-matched controls to die of any cause, with one in five of the deaths resulting from suicide.[158]

2. **Anorexia nervosa is heritable.**

   - Once described primarily as a disease with psychological underpinnings, AN is now known to be a biologically based, heritable illness.[6, 160, 161]
   - Heritability estimates for anorexia nervosa, bulimia nervosa, and binge eating disorder range from 40 percent to 65 percent.[33]
   - Recent genome-wide associated studies (GWAS) findings report that female relatives of individuals with AN are 11 times more likely to develop AN than relatives of individuals who do not have AN.[6]
   - There may be heightened self-reported symptoms of AN among college students marginalized by gender and/or sexual orientation.[162]

3. **Anorexia nervosa is not a choice. It is a biological and brain-based illness.**

   - We do not get to choose our genes. We inherit them and must work with what we have throughout life. Is there one anorexia nervosa gene that causes the illness? No.
   - Eight chromosome loci have been identified thus far that appear to be associated with anorexia nervosa.[91, 140]
   - AN is polygenetic. Findings indicate that AN-associated genes impact brain, gut, and metabolic factors,[6, 141, 142] and temperament traits that are linked to the development and maintenance of anorexia nervosa.[78, 110, 143-146]

- AN-associated genes code brain circuits and body functions that respond differently in persons with AN compared with persons without the illness. Anorexia nervosa is not a consequence of choice.
- Genes begin trait formation during the second trimester of fetal development influencing brain structure and function.[6, 140]
- Environmental factors can magnify the temperamental change process.[35]

4. **Anorexia nervosa involves altered brain circuits that contribute to difficulty sensing reward and interpreting body signals to inform decisions.**

- AN is an illness that diminishes one's ability to trust everyday decisions due to genetically influenced reduced sensitivity to primary internal cues that instinctively guide us.[35, 100]
- Altered brain circuit responses impact daily thoughts, feelings, and actions for those with AN.
- Those with AN have altered brain circuits that impact interoception,[45, 149–151] which is one's ability to *sense* (not think about) internal sensations such as hunger, fullness, taste, or pain, disrupting their ability to accurately predict how the body will respond to external stimuli.
- Diminished interoception interferes with *knowing* or trusting hunger or fullness signals and may alter pain thresholds. Altered interoceptive signaling coupled with possible avoidant and inhibited AN traits may underlie the seemingly natural tendency to not eat.
- Persons *with* AN tend to experience reduced pleasure from eating.[107] This may be related to altered dopamine function, which is associated with experiencing pleasure. Paradoxically, dopamine release in persons with AN has been associated with anxiety which may contribute to food avoidance. [46, 52, 153]
- "Blinded" interoception may increase anxiety and the ability to intuitively know when and how much to eat.[154, 155]
- Altered interoceptive and reward signaling may interfere with one's ability to trust when to eat, when to stop eating, and how much to eat.
- Together these alterations contribute to an altered motivation to eat. Thus, there is a biological basis for many of the symptoms experienced by individuals with AN.

5. **Anorexia nervosa shares genes and neurodevelopment processes with other psychiatric illnesses, such as obsessive-compulsive disorder (OCD) and anxiety disorders.**

- Genome-wide associated studies are finding that genetic influences cross diagnostic boundaries.[140, 160] Results show that AN is significantly correlated with other psychiatric diagnoses such as obsessive-compulsive disorder (OCD), major depression, and anxiety.[91]
- The genetic correlation between AN and OCD is stronger than with other psychiatric illnesses indicating common traits in both disorders.[140]

6. **Temperamental traits increase one's vulnerability to and contribute to the maintenance of anorexia nervosa.**

   - Temperamental traits that increase vulnerability and maintenance of AN are passed down to offspring.[21, 30, 48, 116, 145, 151, 159, 164–167]
   - Common temperament traits that increase AN vulnerability include difficulty trusting decisions, altered sensitivity to reward, difficulty clarifying pros/cons (reward valuation), interoceptive awareness deficits, anxiety, behaviorally inhibited, harm avoidant, perfectionistic, high achievement orientation, detail oriented, obsessive (symmetry, exactness) thoughts, compulsive actions, and sensitivity to criticism and punishment.
   - *Note the difference between symptoms and traits*:
     - Symptoms are indicators or reactions to illnesses and have the potential to be reduced and eliminated.
     - Traits are genetically programmed innate features that can be altered via *intentionally* shifting expressions but cannot be eliminated.

7. **The environment supersedes genetic influences on trait expressions during childhood, while genes supersede environmental influences after puberty. Preventive efforts have greater potential impact during childhood based on biological influences.**

   - Genetic influences are modest during childhood but increase during early adolescence through mid-adulthood.[68]
   - Genes modulate hormonal changes during puberty. It appears that lower levels of estrogen impact certain genes to change, increasing traits to shift and intensifying AN symptoms, resulting in destructive thoughts and behaviors.[7, 148]
   - The same personality traits that are strengths in character in childhood are simultaneously vulnerable to triggering the illness.[6, 32, 35, 140]
   - Genetic influences "tip the scale" toward AN during and after puberty for those who have a temperament profile that increases this vulnerability.[168] This biological tendency is magnified by pressures to diet and other environmental stressors. Increased genetic influences during puberty also appear to be true for binge eating.[169]
   - This impacts timing for ED prevention. Clinicians who work with children and adolescents can assess for AN traits and advise parents to establish structures that reroute trait expressions from becoming problematic and help shape trait expression to remain productive.

8. **Genes trigger an increased risk for lower percentage of body fat, fat-free mass, and body mass index and increased physical activity among males and females with anorexia nervosa.**

   - GWAS findings report that AN and OCD positively correlate with measured physical activity.[170]
   - Genetic influences have an impact on lower percentages of body fat, lower fat-free mass, and lower body mass index (BMI) in both men and women.[170] Findings indicate women have a greater genetic influence toward percentage of

body fat and increased physical activity than men. Nevertheless, both sexes have significant propensities toward these biological trait expressions in contrast with those who do not have AN.[170]

- Individuals with AN have behavioral traits associated with higher educational attainment, possibly driven by high achievement and perfectionistic traits.[91] It has been assumed in the past that BMI is a consequence of AN and higher physical activity is a choice utilized to reduce anxiety and weight. GWAS findings indicate the opposite is true.[170]

- Biological traits become entwined with temperamental traits such as perfectionism, competitiveness, and low interoception. This is demonstrated when, for example, persons who have a genetic tendency to have a lower fat mass and be more physically active becomes entwined with competitive and perfectionistic tendencies that drive persons to excessive exercise and feelings that a set amount of exercise is never good enough.

9. **Faulty interoception (internal physical sensations) in persons with anorexia nervosa may contribute to body dissatisfaction.**

- Anorexia nervosa fundamentally involves disturbances in the experience of physical sensations in one's body. This is called *interoception*. Interoception includes internal physical experiences such as hunger and fullness, taste, pain, touch, heartbeat, breathing, and gastrointestinal sensations. Altered interoception has been posited to contribute to body image disturbances.

- Body distortion appears to be regulated by genetically coded traits, not solely by the illness.[171] It occurs before, during, and after the illness.[172]

- Self-awareness can be clouded by heightened anxiety, but lowered anxiety does not necessarily restore neural function to signal a positive body perception for those with AN.[21]

- Many other AN symptoms relate to altered interoceptive experiences, including increased gastric/intestinal discomfort/distress, a reduced ability to sense hunger or fullness or feel pain until the sensations are extreme.

10. **Persons with anorexia nervosa tend to process information in detail and see errors over successes.**

- Many persons with AN tend to experience a high need for certainty, have high error detection, prefer repetition and routine, and experience a mismatch between what they expect and experience (i.e., prediction error).[105, 106, 118–120] Treatment structure helps manage these responses by offering consistency and mutually agreed limits.

- Persons with AN tend to focus on details rather than see the big picture (i.e., they have low central coherence). This can be a productive ability, strengthening when, for example, editing papers, working in IT, or managing a schedule.[145]

# Appendix 2  TBT-S Trait Profile  Checklist

Laura Hill

## Trait Profile Checklist

**1st: Check the traits that characterize me.**
**2nd: Circle how I have expressed those traits <u>on average</u> over the past few months, on the continuum:**

*"I have <u>tendency</u> to ..."*

*<u>How I am currently expressing this trait</u>*
More productive          More destructive

| Trait | 5 | 4 | 3 | 2 | 1 |
|---|---|---|---|---|---|
| ☐ Be perfectionistic | 5 | 4 | 3 | 2 | 1 |
| ☐ Be determined | 5 | 4 | 3 | 2 | 1 |
| ☐ Be anxious, worry | 5 | 4 | 3 | 2 | 1 |
| ☐ Be cautious | 5 | 4 | 3 | 2 | 1 |
| ☐ Have low self-esteem, see what's wrong in me | 5 | 4 | 3 | 2 | 1 |
| ☐ Want similarity and routine | 5 | 4 | 3 | 2 | 1 |
| ☐ Be Introverted, energized when alone/few people | 5 | 4 | 3 | 2 | 1 |
| ☐ Be high-achieving | 5 | 4 | 3 | 2 | 1 |
| ☐ Think the same thoughts repeatedly (obsessive) | 5 | 4 | 3 | 2 | 1 |
| ☐ Do the same things repeatedly (compulsive) | 5 | 4 | 3 | 2 | 1 |
| ☐ Be extroverted, energized being with others | 5 | 4 | 3 | 2 | 1 |
| ☐ Be optimistic, tend to see the best in things | 5 | 4 | 3 | 2 | 1 |
| ☐ Be pessimistic, tend to see negative in things | 5 | 4 | 3 | 2 | 1 |
| ☐ Avoid what seems harmful or uncomfortable | 5 | 4 | 3 | 2 | 1 |
| ☐ Prefer novelty, new or different | 5 | 4 | 3 | 2 | 1 |
| ☐ Be agreeable, or cooperative, or kind | 5 | 4 | 3 | 2 | 1 |
| ☐ Be aggressive, antagonistic, or hostile | 5 | 4 | 3 | 2 | 1 |
| ☐ Be physically active | 5 | 4 | 3 | 2 | 1 |
| ☐ Be conscientiousness, dutiful, or deliberate | 5 | 4 | 3 | 2 | 1 |
| ☐ Be stubborn | 5 | 4 | 3 | 2 | 1 |
| ☐ Be shy, timid | 5 | 4 | 3 | 2 | 1 |
| ☐ Be attentive, focused | 5 | 4 | 3 | 2 | 1 |
| ☐ Pursue pleasure or rewards | 5 | 4 | 3 | 2 | 1 |
| ☐ Be adaptable or flexible | 5 | 4 | 3 | 2 | 1 |
| ☐ Be reactive | 5 | 4 | 3 | 2 | 1 |
| ☐ Be assertive, speak out for self | 5 | 4 | 3 | 2 | 1 |

1

| "I have <u>tendency</u> to ..." | How I am currently expressing this trait | | | | |
|---|---|---|---|---|---|
| | More productive | | | More destructive | |
| ☐ Be curious | 5 | 4 | 3 | 2 | 1 |
| ☐ Be imaginative, creative, esthetic | 5 | 4 | 3 | 2 | 1 |
| ☐ Be altruistic or concerned for others' well-being | 5 | 4 | 3 | 2 | 1 |
| ☐ Be dutiful, following rules or principles | 5 | 4 | 3 | 2 | 1 |
| ☐ Be disciplined | 5 | 4 | 3 | 2 | 1 |
| ☐ Be impulsive, act on urges in the moment | 5 | 4 | 3 | 2 | 1 |
| ☐ Be detailed | 5 | 4 | 3 | 2 | 1 |
| ☐ Be committed | 5 | 4 | 3 | 2 | 1 |
| ☐ Be independent or self-directed | 5 | 4 | 3 | 2 | 1 |
| ☐ Be uncertain or not trust my decisions | 5 | 4 | 3 | 2 | 1 |
| ☐ Be persistent | 5 | 4 | 3 | 2 | 1 |
| ☐ Be competitive | 5 | 4 | 3 | 2 | 1 |
| ☐ See errors over successes | 5 | 4 | 3 | 2 | 1 |
| ☐ Be hesitant, concerned about consequences | 5 | 4 | 3 | 2 | 1 |
| ☐ Be sensitive (emotionally, smells, sounds, etc.) | 5 | 4 | 3 | 2 | 1 |
| ☐ Be diligent or thorough | 5 | 4 | 3 | 2 | 1 |
| ☐ Be inhibited, hold back, or procrastinate | 5 | 4 | 3 | 2 | 1 |
| ☐ Have thoughts get stuck on something | 5 | 4 | 3 | 2 | 1 |
| ☐ Be empathic (aware of the needs of others) | 5 | 4 | 3 | 2 | 1 |
| ☐ Be social, interactive | 5 | 4 | 3 | 2 | 1 |
| ☐ Be uncertain | 5 | 4 | 3 | 2 | 1 |
| ☐ Be reliable or dependable | 5 | 4 | 3 | 2 | 1 |
| ☐ Plan ahead or prefer structure or organization | 5 | 4 | 3 | 2 | 1 |
| ☐ Be addicted to_____ | 5 | 4 | 3 | 2 | 1 |
| ☐ Be hard-working | 5 | 4 | 3 | 2 | 1 |

I tend to sleep less than 6 hrs. a night: ☐ Yes ☐ No

I tend to have difficulty falling asleep: ☐ Yes ☐ No

2

[1] Traits listed are from Temperament Personality Models by, e.g., Costa et al.; Cloninger; Zuckerman et al.; McCrae and Costa; Quantitative and Molecular Genetic Studies of Temperament by J. Saudino & Wang; and eating disorder research, e.g., Levallius et al.; Kaye et al.; Frank et al; Wierenga et al. See References in the text, *Temperament Based Therapy with Supports for Anorexia Nervosa: A Novel Treatment,* for full citations.

To what degree do I *sense* (not think about, but internally sense) the following?

### Degree of Average Sensation

| | Highly Sensitive | | | | No sensation |
|---|---|---|---|---|---|
| Hunger | 5 | 4 | 3 | 2 | 1 |
| Pain | 5 | 4 | 3 | 2 | 1 |
| Physical touch | 5 | 4 | 3 | 2 | 1 |
| Taste | 5 | 4 | 3 | 2 | 1 |
| Fullness | 5 | 4 | 3 | 2 | 1 |
| Need to urinate | 5 | 4 | 3 | 2 | 1 |
| Pleasure | 5 | 4 | 3 | 2 | 1 |

☐ Other trait tendencies: _____

### Scoring:

1. Count the number of traits I identified _____
2. Count how many traits I have been expressing productively (4 or 5) _____
3. Count how many traits I have been expressing destructively (1 or 2) _____

### Scoring interpretation:

a) If the productive number is higher, I can use the momentum of these traits to reduce my eating disorder symptoms.

b) If the destructive trait number is higher, I can use tools to assist my productive traits to *shift* my destructive traits toward productive expressions. Practice will hold the productive expressions in place.

c) If the numbers are equal, I can use tools and my productive traits to eliminate my symptoms.

**Four** productive traits I have (scored as 4 or 5) that I can use to help manage my symptoms are:

_____

_____

_____

_____

**Three** destructive traits I have (scored as 1 or 2) and want to shift to be less destructive and more productive are:

_____

_____

_____

# Appendix 3 Young Adults: Emerging Adulthood Handout

## Stephanie Knatz Peck

Young adulthood (YA) is a unique developmental stage with distinctive developmental milestones. Assisting healthy growth through this stage requires a fluid style of parenting and awareness of specific developmental challenges that YAs experience.

Our goal is to assist in recovery in a way that converges with this developmental stage.

## Developmental Life Stage: The In-Between Ages of 17–27 Years
### Developmental Challenges
- YAs feel in-between. They are pulling away from adolescent struggles and want to be responsible for themselves while they often remain closely tied to their parents and/or family.
- YAs are exploring their personal identity.
- YAs are transitioning/launching into autonomy.

### Key Features
- **Age of Identity and Exploration.** Young adults enter into a changing process of deciding who they are and what they want out of life.
- **Age of Instability.** This developmental time is marked by changes in residence, friends, and work or school demands.
- **Age of Self-Focus.** Freed of parent- and society-directed routines of school, young adults begin to autonomously decide what they want to do, where they want to go, and whom they want to be with.
- **Age of Feeling In-Between.** Some emerging young adults assume increasing responsibilities without yet feeling or experiencing themselves as a responsible adult.
- **Time for New Possibilities.** For those with novelty-seeking, impulsive, and curious traits, this can be a time filled with new adventures either for the good or at the expense of their well-being. If the YA has an optimistic trait, it is a time of hope for new self-fulfilling, life opportunities.

# Appendix 4 Parenting Young Adults with Anorexia Nervosa: Providing Parental Assistance in Developmentally Appropriate Ways Handout

Stephanie Knatz Peck

### Match Level of Challenge with Parental Ability

What level of ability does your loved one have to participate in recovery? Your efforts and involvement will be matched accordingly. For example, if your loved one is consistently demonstrating an ability to plate and complete meals without help, then encourage more independence and self-reliance. Alternatively, if your loved one is consistently unable to plate appropriately, then step in and provide more assistance. Despite their age and their legal status as an adult, you still maintain your role as a parent.

Parents can provide assistance by

- **Balancing Structure and Flexibility**
  - Establish a mutually agreed platform of expectations necessary to restore health.

- **Creating a Safety Net**
  - You still hold responsibility for ensuring your young adult's health.
  - Discuss and agree in advance on a plan of assistance if progress isn't being made. This is completed in the YA Behavioral Agreement (Chapter 22).

- **Monitoring**
  - Parental involvement is needed.
  - TBT-S includes parents/Supports as part of the treatment team. Your input and interventions outside of treatment are critical to move forward.
  - Know treatment recommendations and find a way to discuss progress regularly so you can provide assistance.

- **Fostering interdependence versus independence or dependence**
  - Have a collaborative relationship and make commitments to each other. Your young adult will have expectations of you through this process also. Making commitments solidifies the growth process for all involved.
  - YAs have needs for assistance that will continue throughout life. The types of assistance morph and change based upon illness acuity, stages of life development, or wellness.

- **Being a mentor not a manager**
  - Your young adult may have valuable insights and can think through their own problems.

- If/when your young adult has a problem, listen attentively for cues if the YA is seeking advice or unsure of what to do. Offer advice if asked but allow your young adult to engage in problem solving on their own.
- When YAs are debating or hesitating and seem uncertain about what to do or are unable to trust their decisions, offer multiple-choice possibilities for decisions. This approach assists them in exploring their own solutions with their trait abilities.
- If the YA does not have problems trusting their decisions, then ask open-ended questions intended to help guide them to identify their own solutions.

- **Being a collaborator not a commander**
  - Be a member of the recovery team. Parents can provide emotional assistance and guidance in addition to holding young adults accountable. The YA Behavioral Agreement provides the framework for both the parents and YA to identify what assistance is needed, how, and when it is offered.

## Homework

1. Practice asking your loved one reflective questions directing them to find their own solutions. *If* they are unable to do this, present multiple-choice questions to provide scaffolding for them to identify productive solutions to problems.
2. Ask your loved one what assistance they need to follow their prescribed energy plan.

# Appendix 5 Dialectical Model of Parental Support

Stephanie Knatz Peck

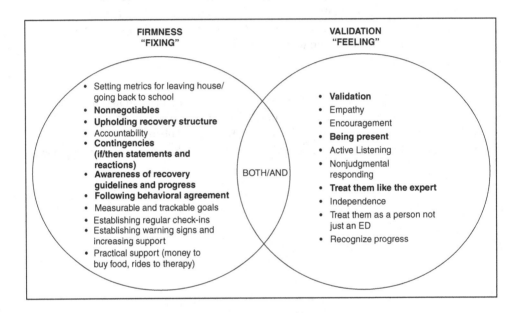

**FIRMNESS "FIXING"**

- Setting metrics for leaving house/ going back to school
- **Nonnegotiables**
- **Upholding recovery structure**
- Accountability
- **Contingencies (if/then statements and reactions)**
- **Awareness of recovery guidelines and progress**
- **Following behavioral agreement**
- Measurable and trackable goals
- Establishing regular check-ins
- Establishing warning signs and increasing support
- Practical support (money to buy food, rides to therapy)

**BOTH/AND**

**VALIDATION "FEELING"**

- **Validation**
- Empathy
- Encouragement
- **Being present**
- Active Listening
- Nonjudgmental responding
- **Treat them like the expert**
- Independence
- Treat them as a person not just an ED
- Recognize progress

# Appendix 6 Young Adult Client Rules and Framework for Meals and Snacks Handout

Stephanie Knatz Peck

---

**Young Adult Behavioral Agreement Template: Meals and Snacks, by Stephanie Knatz Peck**

☐ Eat 3 meals and____snacks every day following the schedule below:
  ☐ Breakfast at____AM
  ☐ AM Snack at____AM
  ☐ Lunch at____PM
  ☐ PM Snack at____PM
  ☐ Dinner at____PM
  ☐ Evening Snack at____PM
☐ Complete 100% of meals and snacks
☐ SUPPLEMENTING: Supplement drinks (or bars) will be used if meal/snack is not completed.
  ☐ If more than 50% but less than 100%, 1 supplement will be consumed.
  ☐ If less than 50%, 2 supplements will be consumed.

☐ Meals follow the USDA plate model. Examples that could be default meals:

| BREAKFAST EXAMPLES | | |
|---|---|---|
| | | |

| LUNCH EXAMPLES | | |
|---|---|---|
| | | |

| DINNER EXAMPLES | | |
|---|---|---|
| | | |

1

☐ Snacks will be based on approved snack list. Default snacks include:

_____      _____

_____      _____

_____      _____

☐ Meals will be eaten in____minutes and snacks will be eaten in____minutes.

☐ I will remain in the presence of a Support for 60 minutes following meals and snacks to avoid purging.

☐ Bathroom visits will be supervised by a Support.

☐ Support persons,_____and_____,will remain informed of meal plan and any changes.

☐ Supports will attend the following regular appointments:_____

_____

☐ Supports will be present for the following meals and snacks regularly:

   ☐ Breakfast at____AM

   ☐ AM Snack at____AM

   ☐ Lunch at____PM

   ☐ PM Snack at____PM

   ☐ Dinner at____PM

   ☐ Evening Snack at____PM

☐ When Supports are not present, I commit to:

   ☐ Having meals with others who can assist me (Name:_____)

   ☐ Reporting back to Supports by: (describe how you will keep them updated).

   ☐ Video chatting during meals and snacks (list which ones).

   ☐ _____

   ☐ _____

☐ When Supports are present, I will:

   ☐ "Check off" that my meals/snacks meet dietary requirements.

   ☐ Assist with distractions.

   ☐ Provide the following feedback if I am having difficulty initiating/completing my meal:

   Discuss and write strategies you would like your Support to use:

_____

_____

_____

   ☐ Provide the following feedback if I am engaging in any ED behaviors during meals/snacks:

_____

_____

_____

2

# Appendix 7 List of Distraction Activities Handout

Choose distraction activities that can be used before, during, and after meals
- Listening to music with headphones
- Playing a table game, card game, or board game
- Using table topics cards for interesting conversations
- Watching Youtube, favorite Netflix series, favorite show or movie
- Crossword puzzle
- Picture find
- Word search game
- Making a list
- Listening to a conversation
- Engaging in conversation with others at the table on an interesting topic
- Sewing
- Knitting
- Adult coloring/mandala coloring
- Playing an instrument
- 5 minute walk
- Doodling/drawing books
- Iphone games
- Video games
- Math worksheets (long division and multiplication)
- Sudoku
- Brain teaser books/games
- Reading comics
- Origami
- Clean room
- Finish a task
- Surf the internet
- Write emails
- Call a friend
- Build/legos

# Appendix 8 Young Adult Client "RAD" Skills Handout

Stephanie Knatz Peck

## Anorexia Nervosa Involves Faulty Internal Physical Sensations

- Anorexia nervosa fundamentally involves disturbances in the experience of physical sensations in their body. This is called *interoception*.
- Interoception includes internal physical experiences such as hunger and fullness, taste, pain, touch, heartbeat, breathing, and gastrointestinal sensations.
- Many AN symptoms related to altered interoceptive experiences include increased gastric/intestinal discomfort/distress, a reduced ability to sense if hunger or fullness or inability to feel pain until the sensations are extreme.
- Faulty interoception is like a faulty gas gauge in a car.
- When a "gauge of hunger or fullness" is faulty, external requirements are needed to compensate, such as adjusting the prescribed "fuel" plan.
- Clients can work with the dietitian to shift fuels to a "higher octane" that offers more energy and less volume if they experience pain when eating high-volume foods.
- During recovery, it is more effective to use external guidelines (such as a meal plan) to meet your body's needs since the internal gauge is not working properly.

## Skill 1: Turning UP the Volume on External Signals

External guidelines compensate for internal faulty gauges. Your energy needs, determined by your treatment team and family, provide a road map to strengthen your body and mind. Using a structure helps reduce eating disorder fears. Your energy plan is a treatment prescription, just as a physician would give you a prescription for medications, if you had dangerously high blood pressure. (We wouldn't expect someone with high blood pressure to rely on being able to FEEL when they needed to take their medications.)

Allowing external guidelines to manage your energy intake will help by

1. Ensuring you are meeting your body's energy needs.
2. Reducing your uncertainty since your body is not currently able to accurately gauge how hungry or full or in pain you are.
3. Providing enough fuel to "not run out of fuel," and giving you enough energy to carefully restore your strength. This comes from your individual meal plan prescribed by the dietitian.

### External Guidelines

1. **Know your meal plan**. Commit to following it. Make sure your Supports know your meal plan so that they can assist you.

2. **Commit to set times for meals/snacks.** Since your body may not be sending you accurate alarm signals for when to start and stop eating, use external alarms.

3. **Set reminders on your phone** for meal and snack times and keep the same schedule every day. **Block out times for meals and snacks** in your planner or calendar.

4. **Pre-plan meals and snacks instead** of relying on deciding in the moment. Commit to sticking to the designated plan.

5. **Plan for new foods that are difficult to eat but you want to eat** (challenge foods). Make a list of foods you used to eat (pre-ED) and are currently avoiding. Work them into your meal plan. Ask your Supports how your ED has changed and identify which foods you want to incorporate back into your meal plan.

6. **Plan how to eat your meals in different social situations.**

## RAD Skill

RAD is a dialectical behavioral therapy skill to assist the client in becoming aware and nonjudgmentally acknowledge what they experience or don't experience.

### Recognize

- Recognize a sensation you experience in this moment.
  - ○ Recognize if you are *not* experiencing a sensation that should be occurring in this moment (for example, hunger if you have not eaten for three or more hours; pain if you are running).
  - ○ Name the sensation in a descriptive, nonjudgmental way, for example, "I am feeling full."

### Acknowledge

- **Acknowledge your actions** that may be at odds with your sensory experience.
  - ○ What is your meal plan?
  - ○ Why is it important for you to follow it?
  - ○ What would be the most effective action to take right now?
  - ○ Acknowledge and allow the feeling or sensation to be valid. Allowing doesn't mean you have to *like* the situation. It means you are no longer resisting what is happening.
  - ○ Acknowledging the experience lets you choose a conscious response to it, rather than getting "caught up " in the sensation.

### Deidentify

- Distract your attention to the realization that YOU are not your sensory experiences. YOU have the power to decide how to react to your sensory experiences, versus allowing the high intensity or lack of sensory experiences controlling you.
- No matter how intense, uncomfortable, or minimal your sensation experiences are, there are parts of you that are still, silent, and untouched.
- Think of the sensation as a "false alarm" that you choose not to act on because you have identified it is a faulty alarm.
- What strategies would you use to avoid acting on the following urges?
  - ○ Urge to scratch a rash that you can't per MD's orders.

- ○ Urge to move/leave when you are asked to stay still in an MRI/X-ray machine or a small elevator.
- ○ Urge to move when you are sitting in an uncomfortable position.
- ○ Urge to leave when you are
  sitting in a building when a false alarm goes off and you need to ignore it.
  - • Distract
  - • Nonjudgment
  - • Deep breathing
  - • Refocus on external goals

## When Internal Signals Contradict External Messages: BE RAD!

In recovery, there are times that your internal signals (your body's signals of fullness or hunger, or even emotions) are at odds with your needs for recovery (and what your treatment team recommends). This can be EXTREMELY uncomfortable. These uncomfortable signals are designed to get your attention. From a young age, you have learned to listen to and rely on your body's signals to guide your actions. Learning how to recognize that your signals may be faulty and not letting them guide your actions requires advanced practice.

Practice Being **RAD!**

# Appendix 9  TBT-S Toolbox

## Toolbox Instructions

This appendix includes a toolbox for SE-AN clients and Supports. The border or "container" of the toolbox represents each client's traits. Before tools are identified, client traits need to be identified so that traits and tools can work hand-in-hand.

1. Administer the Trait Profile Checklist handout, in Appendix 2. Instructions are included on the form.

    a. After clients score their checklist, they are asked to identify four current productive and three destructive traits.

    b. Identifying their productive and destructive traits allows them to acknowledge their innate strengths and weaknesses.

    c. Hand out the TBT-S Toolbox worksheet.

    d. Ask the client(s) to choose four productive traits and write them in the borders of the toolbox. Just as a toolbox contains or holds tools, client traits are the "container" of who they are and how they could use the tools.

2. Review each of the tools in the toolbox with the client(s).

    a. Have each client fill in the blanks and actively "try on" each tool.

    b. A tool may look interesting or seem relevant, but test this possibility by having the client try on the tool to determine if it is a "good fit."

3. Optional: Have clients practice the tools with other clients by playing the TBT-S experiential activity, "Charades" (see Appendix 21).

4. After all tools have been "tried on," have clients circle the tools that reflect or fit with their own traits. This increases the potential they would use the tools.

5. Have each client choose three tools.

    a. These tools should be actions that are congruent with their traits, not incompatible with their temperament.

    b. Tools that work *with* their traits are easier to adopt.

6. Point out that it may take two or three tools to manage one ED symptom.

    a. One tool alone may not interrupt or be able to redirect an ED behavior.

    b. Some tools may work better as a set when interrupting an ED symptom.

7. Ask Supports to identify tools for themselves.

    a. Have Supports share which tools they have chosen to assist in helping their loved one.

    b. Have Supports affirm with the client if they would find those tools helpful or unhelpful.

    c. Supports may use the same tools that the client identifies.

## TBT-S Toolbox

## TBT-S Toolbox

**List 4 traits that I express productively** (from Trait Profile Checklist)

My Trait:

My Trait:

My Trait:

My Trait:

Say, **"Give me two/three options"** when others ask me open questions, e.g., "What do you want to do?"

**Delay** ED behaviors by doing: _____.

**Give a compliment** to another person via text: ID one _____.

**Walk ____ minutes.**

**Actively listen and participate in a conversation**

**Do one hour of a project that takes my concentration**_____.

**Deep breathe** – inhale 4 seconds, exhale 4 seconds.

**Distract** by: Fill in two actions:_____   _____

**Ground myself** to this moment. ID: 2 things I see; 2 things I hear; 2 things I can touch; 2 things I smell.

**Walk Tall** (Stretch up as much as possible as walk).

**Hold myself accountable** by telling (ID the person) ____ if I act on a destructive behavior.

**Stop, reboot, reroute:** If waking toward destructive action, "Stop," turn 180° Walk in new route.

**WW ____ D?** Ask self, "What would ____ Do? ID person I admire _____, Then do it.

**WWID4 ____?** "What would I do for_____?) ID the person_____, Then do it.

**Ask for help** ID 2 people _____.

**Use my wise mind** using the dialectic "I think/or feel_____ AND I think/feel:_____."

**Earphones with music** of my playlists

**Food is my medicine:** I will eat my planned breakfast, lunch, dinner, snacks.

**Take my prescribed medication:** food, pills/supplements

**Restorative Yoga** with ID person _____ when, ID days _____.

**Self-Critique** an action/interaction/event: In this order: What would I do the same? What would I do differently? How would I do it differently?

**Use a premeal routine.**_____.

**Help another person by doing** _____.

**Accept myself for who I am** and use my traits in the current situation.

Instead of **walking toward a** destructive action, I will **walk to** _____.

Instead of **counting** _____ to restrict, I **will count** _____.

Instead of holding back on (food or interactions), I will hold back on _____ to focus on _____.

**Choose three tools/skills that work WITH my traits.**

# Appendix 10  YES/NO Game: TBT-S Neurobiological Experiential Activity

Stephanie Knatz Peck and Hannah Patrick

## Neurobiological and Trait Targets
- Alterations in reward processing
- Excessive inhibitory control
- Harm avoidance
- Punishment sensitivity
- Uncertainty intolerance

## Objective
The YES/NO activity specifically highlights our brain's innate reward circuit and its opposing system, the inhibitory control system. The purpose of this exercise is to highlight how alterations in reward processing in AN may affect decision-making around food and other domains. To do this, this game is an activity and a live demonstration that represents how these alterations affect decision-making.

## Who Is Involved?
- This exercise was designed as a group exercise.
- A minimum of six people are needed, including clients and Supports.
- This exercise can be implemented with a group of clients or a group of Supports.

## Materials and Time Needed
- A room large enough to walk around in.
- 45–60 minutes.

## What Does the Research Say?
- What is reward processing? The *reward processing system* is the brain circuit responsible for how the brain responds to rewarding stimuli. This includes how the brain learns from receiving reward, including anticipating future rewards, and how reward motivates action and goal-directed behavior.
- The opposing system is the *inhibitory control system*, which allows a person to inhibit their impulses or natural response to something.
- These two systems are the brain's green light (to motivate to engage in an action) and red light (to stop or avoid engaging in an action).
- How do reward and inhibition relate to AN?

People with AN may be more sensitive to punishment or avoiding punishment or consequences than they are to reward. This means that their brains may be more responsive to a punishment signal than they are to a reward signal. For example, the anticipated consequence of gaining weight or feeling fat after a meal may feel stronger or more important than the rewarding taste of food, and therefore people with AN choose not to eat. This can be true for more than just food. Thus, in AN, there is a risk-reward imbalance where potential risks outweigh potential rewards. It is the difference between the brain signaling, *"Yes that look's fun, do it!"* (Reward system) versus *"That may be dangerous, What if XXX happens?! If I do that, I will (insert negative consequence)."*

This brain "bias" means that people with AN are often *harm avoidant,* or *punishment sensitive* by nature/temperament.

- According to personality assessments, people with AN tend to be harm avoidant and punishment sensitive.
- Studies suggest that compared with healthy controls, AN (even recovered) do not show a reward response to hunger (tested with both food and monetary rewards).
- In a gambling task meant to assess reward processing, ill adolescents with AN show exaggerated responses to loss compared with wins – their brain is more sensitive to punishment than to reward.
- People recovered from AN show failure to differentiate between wins and losses (in a gambling task) – so there is a failure to appropriately scale or identify the emotional significance of a stimuli.

### Key Points

- **Reward centers in our brain guide our actions by signaling reward and potential harm.**
- **People with anorexia nervosa may be more motivated to avoid negative consequences than to obtain rewarding outcomes.**
- **Persons with AN may have trouble differentiating between pro (rewarding) and con (harmful) signals.**
- **This brain bias leads to harm avoidance and/or difficulty trusting decisions.**

## Clinician Checklist

⇒ Completed all three versions of the game.
⇒ Reviewed what each game condition represented with group (after the game).
⇒ Provided psychoeducation on temperament/neurobiology.
⇒ Orchestrated group discussion using Activity Discussion Points.
⇒ Assigned Homework.

## Experiential Activity Instructions

### Rules

1. This game is an adaptation of the classic "Hot/Cold" game, where participants are guided by "hotter and colder" responses to find an object in the room.
2. In this game, the "hot" message is Yes, which represents the reward system response of affirmation. The "cold" is a No response representing the brain's inhibition system.
3. There are three iterations of this game to play:
   ○ "A "balanced brain" receiving well-adjusted YES and NO responses.
   ○ An "AN brain" receiving only NO (stop signals) from the inhibitory control system.

- An "AN brain" receiving unclear signals (maybe's and other ambiguous signals instead of clear Yes's and No's).

- The clinician chooses three *clients* from the group and asks them to leave the group room (one client for each version).
- The clinician informs them that they will play a game and that their team (the group at large) will help them to "complete a task."
- Group preparation: the group at large is instructed to identify an object or a simple action to do in the room. (Ex: serving a cup of coffee, organizing markers, writing something on the board.)
- ONLY verbal Yes's and No's can be said by the group members as prompts to assist the participant with completing a task.
- The Yes's and No's represent the reward and inhibition circuits, respectively.
- The group guides the client by using verbal:

  - *YES prompts*: "YES's" are used as a proxy for the reward system because Yes's often elicit a sense of being praised and feeling encouraged to continue to pursue an action.
  - *NO prompts*: No's represent the inhibition system, as they typically elicit a strong sense of stopping an action and feeling of doing something wrong.

- Upon completion, each of the three chosen clients joins the larger group and is asked to share their experience, to be shared with the group at a later time.

## Condition 1: The Balanced Brain

1. In this version of the game, the volunteer receives an equal amount of both Yes and No prompts guiding them to complete the task.
2. This is designed to represent a brain that is receiving appropriate signaling from both the reward (Go!) and inhibition (Stop!) systems.
3. Three volunteers (one for each condition) are chosen and asked to leave the room.
4. The task to complete is chosen by the group.
5. Group members are instructed to ONLY use Yes's and No's, or the game will start over.
6. No other words can be used. If a group member violates this rule, the volunteer must leave the room again and start the game over.
7. Volume and enthusiasm are allowed to vary to guide the volunteer.
8. Group members are instructed to cheer and clap loudly and provide congratulations when the task is completed.
9. The first volunteer is invited back into the room. They are told: *You have a task to complete in the room and your team* (the group) *will help you complete the task.*
10. Once the task is completed, the volunteer joins the rest of the group for the remainder of the game. They are asked to remember their experience to share later.

### Notes for the Clinician

- The swift completion (which is in contrast to the next two conditions) highlights the utility of both the reward and inhibition systems and how, when used in tandem, a person can efficiently make and trust decisions and take action.

- Once the volunteer has completed the task, the group cheers, making it clear that the task was successfully completed. Reward experienced!
- This condition mimics decision-making abilities controlled by these two systems. When a person receives clear signals from the reward system, it guides them to a valued action, and inhibitory signals to divert unproductive or destructive actions.
- When the action is completed, the group cheering represents the endogenous dopamine response that affirms an action, the brain's metaphorical pat on the back.
- It becomes clear why both prompts are necessary to navigate decision-making.

## Condition 2: Excessive Inhibition (No's Only)

1. In this version of the game, the volunteer receives only No prompts guiding them to complete the task.
2. This represents a brain that has no reward responses and excessive inhibition.
3. The same task is to be completed by the second volunteer (who has been waiting outside the room).
4. Volunteer two is invited back into the room. They are told, *You have a task to complete in the room and your team* (the group) *will help you complete the task.*
5. Group members are instructed to use ONLY No's or the game will start over. No other words can be used. If a group member violates this rule, the volunteer must leave the room and the game starts over. Volume and enthusiasm are allowed to vary to guide the volunteer.
6. When the task is completed, the participants do not cheer or clap or make any signal that the task is completed.
7. Once the task is completed, the volunteer joins the rest of the group for the remainder of the game. They are asked to remember their experience to share later.

## Condition 3: Ambiguous Signals

1. In this version of the game, the participant receives only ambiguous signals, instead of clear Yes's and No's.
2. This is designed to represent a brain that cannot differentiate between reward and inhibition signals, which occurs for many with AN.
3. The same task is to be completed by the third volunteer (who has been waiting outside the room).
4. Volunteer three is invited back into the room. They are told, *You have a task to complete in the room and your team* (the group) *will help you complete the task.*
5. Group members are instructed to use ONLY unclear and ambiguous responses. Examples include: *Maybe, I'm not so sure; Are you sure; That could be right.* Allow the participants to be creative to generate any ambiguous responses, except they must be accurate in still leading the participant to solve the game. No other words can be used. If a group member violates this rule, the volunteer must leave the room again and start the game over. Volume and enthusiasm are allowed to vary to guide the volunteer.
6. One person in the group is nominated to give clear Yes's and No's periodically when the participant is really stuck and unable to figure out the task.
7. The clinician gives a time limit of 5–10 minutes. It is important to note that this task may not be completed, which will emphasize the meaning of this game.

8. When/If the task is completed, the participants do not cheer or clap or make any signal that the task is completed.
9. Once the task is completed, the volunteer joins the rest of the group for discussion. They are asked to remember their experience so that they can share it later.

## Discussion Points

- After the exercise, clinicians should facilitate a group discussion to explain how the exercise represents alterations in reward and inhibition processing and to elicit feedback from the group about their experiences.
- Yes and No Condition

  o *The Yes and No condition represents a "balanced" brain demonstrating the volunteer getting both "Stop" signals, from the inhibitory control system, and "Go" signals from the reward system.*
  o *Both of these systems are necessary guide actions. Notice how the task was completed quickly and the volunteer was guided with clarity.*
  o *This is how the brains of those without anorexia nervosa respond.*

- No Only Condition

  o *The No condition represents a brain that responds with excessive inhibition. It is more responsive to "NO" signals.*
  o *Studies suggest that those with anorexia nervosa may have excessive inhibitory control.*
  o *Notice how the task was harder to complete. The participant was more "frozen" and unable to move.*

- Ambiguous Condition

  o *The ambiguous condition represents a brain that cannot differentiate between reward and punishment signals.*
  o *A study conducted with people recovered from anorexia nervosa suggests that they could not differentiate between these reward and inhibition signals.*
  o *This impacts one's ability in knowing the significance of something, taking an appropriate action, or trusting decisions.*
  o *Pros and cons were indecipherable.*
  o *Notice how the person in this version was unable to figure out how to complete the task.*

- Post-Activity Questions:
- To the three volunteers:

  o *What was helpful?*
  o *How did you feel during the exercise?*
  o *How did you feel once you completed the task?*
  o *How did this exercise relate to your experience with anorexia nervosa?*
  o *What does this mean for your recovery?*

Clients and Supports are also asked to share what is necessary for assistance and tools based on their experience. This discussion can be conducted in small interfamily groups.

## How to Treat to These Traits

### Targeting Harm Avoidance

Often those with high harm avoidance or excessive inhibition (a brain with only No's) benefit from clear and firm directions from clinicians and Supports.

### Targeting Reward Insensitivity

People who are not getting internal reward signals also benefit from clear directions and planning from clinicians and Supports. Those who are unable to sense reward signals are often more motivated to avoid negative consequences versus feeling good from a reward. If reward insensitivity is only related to eating, often setting up external privileges and motivators for food completion can assist in motivating eating.

### Targeting Decision-Making

Clear and specific directions that are consistent and predictable are needed. This includes offering "pros and cons" instead of the client, since the client is unsure what is a pro/con based on reward and inhibition responses. The client could reason, or think through a response, but may not be able to "sense" whether or not it is rewarding. People who cannot differentiate between reward and punishment signals may not be able to assess the emotional valence of a stimuli and therefore feel unsure or unclear about decisions.

### Homework

- Clients practice asking "for a few options" to help think through decisions.
- Supports practice offering clear options, not open-ended questions, making it overwhelming for the client to know what to do.

## Clinician Notes

_____

_____

_____

_____

# Appendix 11  Nondominant Hand: TBT-S Neurobiological and Problem-Solving Experiential Activity

Laura Hill

## Neurobiological and Trait Targets
These traits could work *against* the client in this situation:
- Altered interoception
- Altered reward sensitivity
- Anxiety

These traits could work *for* the client in this situation:
- Determination
- High achieving (or achievement oriented)
- Attentive/focused
- Persistence

## Objectives
- Experience dominant destructive trait responses of ED thoughts and behaviors via a structured metaphorical activity.
- Experience how dominant destructive trait ED responses work against a person when overcoming ED symptoms.
- Identify what it takes to overcome dominant ED responses.
- Identify each client's traits that helped them shift destructive ED traits to dominant productive expressions.

## Who Is Involved?
- Clinician and ED client in one-on-one sessions virtually or face-to-face.
- Students in classroom.
- Clinician and ED clients and/or Supports in groups virtually or face-to-face.

## Materials and Time Needed
- Paper and pencil/pen (not iPad or computer).
- 15 minutes.

---

The Nondominant Hand was first published in the *Family Eating Disorder Manual*, by Hill, L. et al., 2012, The Center for Balanced Living, Columbus, Ohio. A variation of it was also published in *Brain-Based Approach to Eating Disorder Treatment*, by Hill, L., The Center for Balanced Living, Columbus, Ohio. 2017.

## What Does the Research Say?

- AN is associated with anxiety, decreased reward sensitivity, and altered interoception (i.e., experience of one's internal physical sensations, like hunger) that serve to decrease motivation to eat.
- It is a "dominant" brain response to enjoy food and eat with ease, for those who do not have eating disorders; it is "nondominant" to experience pleasure, motivation, and hunger/fullness for those with eating disorders.
- Altered brain circuits can be difficult to change, requiring that the brain re-wires new circuits from repeated healthy actions to create new productive trait expressions.

Key Point: Reducing ED symptoms is a nondominant brain response.

## Clinician Checklist

⇒ Have the four steps of the activity memorized, do not read them. Conduct playfully.

⇒ Draw upon client and/or Support answers; let them ID their own solutions.

⇒ Memorize and state the neurobiological and summary key points looking at the clients directly to enhance the points. Do not read them.

## Experiential Activity Instructions

### Rule

1. The goal of this activity is to experience body responses, thoughts, and feelings when an action is nondominant, by writing with the nondominant hand.

### Steps and Scripts

1. Clinician shares (does not read) the following instructions:
   1. *I would like you to try on an experience that has you acting against your dominant responses that your brain is wired to do.*
   2. *Please take out a piece of paper and pencil/pen.*
   3. *There are four steps to this activity.*
2. *Everything you write is to be with your nondominant hand.*
3. *First, write down, with your nondominant hand the following: "I am writing with my nondominant hand."*
   a. When completed: *"Now show your writing to the person next to you (or the clinician if one-on-one)."*
   b. Allow a couple minutes for each person to show what their writing looks like.
4. *Now fill in the blank, your answer to this question, while writing with your nondominant hand: "I feel _____ writing with my nondominant hand."*
   a. Wait while the client(s) and/or Supports write their "feeling words."
   b. No need to write the complete sentence.
5. *Now turn to a person beside you as your partner* (the partner would be the clinician in one-on-one settings). *One person is to be the person who writes, the other person will be the "talker."*
   a. When partners have identified their roles, present the following instructions:

b. *The person who is the talker is to speak to, interrupt, or disrupt in various ways the person who is writing. Pressure the person to write faster and get done sooner.*

c. *The person who is the writer is to write with their nondominant hand, the following statement, "I am still trying to write with my nondominant hand!"*

d. *You have 30 seconds to write this statement. Now begin.*

e. When completed, instruct everyone to answer the last question using their nondominant hand.

f. *The last question, still using your nondominant hand, is: "If I were to tell you that you had to write with your nondominant hand for the rest of your life, what would you do?"* (Note: not feel, or think, but do.)

g. Wait until everyone has completed their answers (about 1–2 minutes).

## How to Treat to These Traits

- Clinicians should use the client's own solutions to respond to their ED symptoms.
- What was it like to show your "nondominant" writing to another person (NOT what did you feel)?
  - This is similar to showing the results of your food logs to your clinician or dietitian.
- What did you "feel" when writing with your nondominant hand.
  - Share responses.
  - Empathically state out loud client and Support responses validating their voices; point out the feelings that are repeated, e.g., awkwardness.
  - Ask clients if the feelings described are similar to what they feel when they try to eat their healthy meal plan.
- When interrupted by your partner, what was it like to try to get the sentence written in a short amount of time?
  - Empathically state out loud client and Support responses validating their voices.
  - Ask clients if the responses are similar to what they experience when trying to eat their recommended meal when others are talking, interrupting, and pressuring them to hurry up.
- What did you write down that you would "DO" if told you had to use your nondominant hand for the rest of your life?
  - Empathically state out loud client and Support responses validating their voices.
  - Use the clients and/or Supports *own solutions*. Some responses may include the following:
    - ➤ I wouldn't write, I'd find another way. (This could be predictive of what the client is doing with food intake.)
    - ➤ I'd practice (the most frequent response). Practice is key.
- Clients want to eat and not feel upset, have fun and enjoy foods like others, exercise and not purge, but these are currently nondominant responses for them until they practice through or around them.
- Restricted eating, or binge eating, or purging or over-exercising are dominate, natural responses for those with ED.

- Every day requires ED clients to use *nondominant* actions to counter dominant brain responses. Not easy, not fun.
- *Solutions are found in YOUR solutions that you gave: e.g., to repeatedly practice.*
- The clients' own traits can serve to shift dominant ED symptoms to healthy eating and exercise that can become more dominant over time with practice.

Key Points
- **Altered ED brain circuits contribute to the cause of dominant ED symptoms.**
- **For someone with AN, it is nondominant to eat the needed amount of food.**
- **It takes intense focus, practice, determination, and assistance to get through the distress of not doing the neurobiologically dominant ED actions.**

## Homework
- Clients are to practice an action and their own productive traits identified earlier for one week and report back.

## Clinician Notes

_____
_____
_____
_____

# Appendix 12 Telephone: TBT-S Neurobiological Experiential Activity

Laura Hill

## Neurobiological and Trait Targets
- Brain circuits
- Neuron activity
- Altered interoception

## Objectives
- Experience how brain circuits respond in healthy brains.
- Experience how altered ED brain circuits respond.

## Who Is Involved?
- Clinician and clients with ED and/or Supports.
- This is a face-to-face group activity that needs a minimum of six people. Groups function well with up to ten people. Multiple circles of telephone can be set up simultaneously for large groups.
- Students in classroom.

## Materials and Time Needed
- No materials.
- 15–20 minutes.

## What Does the Research Say?
- Neurons are brain cells that transmit electrochemical messages throughout the brain and central nervous system.

  ○ The brain uses neurons instead of other types of body cells due to speed. The electrochemical signals in neurons are faster at communicating than cells in the body.
  See Figure A12.1.

  ○ A neuron consists of (a) a cell body, (b) dendrites, and (c) axons.*

---

A variation of this activity is in the electronic text by Hill, L. (2017). "*A Brain-Based Approach to Eating Disorders*" at www.BrainBasedEatingDisorders.org

---

* Cell bodies are the factory of activity where energy from food and minerals are transformed into electro-chemical messages relayed to other neurons. Dendrites are branches that bring messages into the cell body. Axons are short to exceedingly long cables that transmit messages out from the cell body to other neurons.

- Millions of brain circuits fire simultaneously communicating thoughts, feelings, actions, perceptions, and sensations to specified areas of the brain.
- When circuits become altered or skewed, they can distort thoughts, feelings, and actions.
- Interoception is one's ability to experience internal physical sensations, e.g., hunger, pain, fullness, touch. The insula is the hub for interoception. For those with ED, the insula often transmits altered signals causing aberrations in the ability to sense physical sensations accurately, such as hunger and fullness and pain signals.
- The insula communicates with cognitive control and reward circuits to evaluate and interpret physiological signals to guide decisions on what to do (e.g., drive to eat when hungry).
- Altered signals can miscommunicate messages and interfere with decisions on what to do. For example, reduced hunger signaling can lead to low motivation to eat; low fullness signaling can result in continuous eating, and low pain signaling can impact over exercising. See Figure A12.1

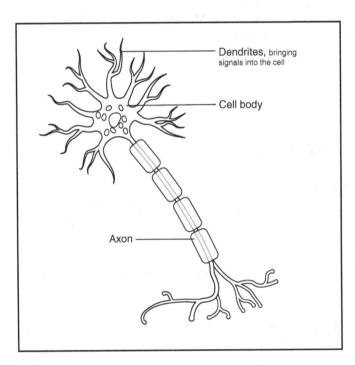

**Figure A12.1** Neuron

Key Point: Altered brain circuits pass their signals onto multiple brain areas that perpetuate inaccurate thoughts, feelings, and destructive ED symptoms.

## Clinician Checklist

⇒ Have the three steps of the Telephone brain activity memorized. Do not read them. Be playful.
⇒ Draw upon client and/or Support answers.
⇒ Memorize and state the key points directly to the group, do not read them.

## Experiential Activity Instructions

### Rules

1. Telephone is a child's game that has one person whisper a message to the next person, who whispers to the next until the message returns to the person who initiated it. The returning message is usually different from the original message. Messages get lost along the way.
2. This Telephone game is a metaphor for how altered ED brain signals miscommunicate along brain circuits causing incorrect conclusions.
3. Players can stand or sit in a circle.
4. Each person serves as a neuron passing messages to the next person in the game of telephone. See Figure A12.2.

   • The right arm is labeled dendrites, bringing brain signals to the cell body.
   • The head/chest is the cell body.
   • The left arm is the axon sending signals out to the next person or neuron.

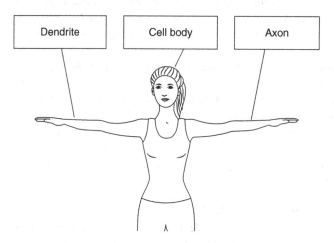

**Figure A12.2** Female with arms extended representing a neuron

## Steps and Scripts

1. *Who has played "Telephone"?*
2. Have a player describe the game rules.

3. *This is a variation of the child's game, a "brain game of Telephone." Instead of a verbal message passed to one another, you will send physical signals by squeezing your partner's hand. This is similar to brain neurons sending signals from one neuron to the next.*
4. *Each of you will be a neuron. Sending signals among you makes you a circuit.*
5. *I would like everyone to form a circle, with enough space between you to allow your arms to reach out and to hold the player's hand on each side of you.*
6. *I am going to have a player begin a brain signal that is to be passed onto the next player to the left, going clockwise. The signal goes around the circle, or circuit, and back to the "sender."*

## Round 1: Healthy Brain Circuits

1. Choose a person to start the message (#1).
2. Share with #1 (in front of the others): *I want you to squeeze the hand of the person to your left one time. One, medium squeeze. Because the brain uses signals, I will ask everyone to close their eyes, so you can "sense" the signal. Each of you is to pass on the squeeze as you experience it.*
3. *When the message gets back to #1, say, "Got it," and all can open their eyes.*
4. *Now everyone close your eyes . . . Go!*
5. After #1 says, "Got it," ask #1 the following question using three options: *Was the squeeze*

    a. *The same?*
    b. *Weaker?*
    c. *Or stronger compared to what you sent out?*

6. The facilitator interprets Round 1: If #1 says:

    a. **Weaker:** *This is similar to many circuits in the brain. It can begin with a clear signal but weakens as it passes from one neuron to the next, and eventually, the message may die out. This is what happens regularly for those who have eating disorders.*

    b. **Stronger:** *This is similar to some circuit signals in the brain. It can begin with an intense signal and gains momentum as it passes from one neuron to the next, with the message becoming stronger, dominating thoughts and actions. This is similar to those who have eating disorders.*

    c. **The Same:** *You are a healthy circuit! This circle represents a strong healthy brain circuit. A message begins with one neuron and travels to areas of the brain transmitting the signals accurately. This is like those who do not have eating disorders.*

## Round 2: AN Altered Brain Circuits

1. Identify the third person in the circle from #1 (#3). Call the person by name and in front of the others instruct the following: *"For round 2, when you receive the squeeze this time, no matter how you receive it, pass in on with one very weak squeeze."*
2. Identify the fifth person from #1 (#5). Call the person by name and in front of the others instruct the following: *"When and IF you receive the squeeze, then pass on several strong repeated squeezes."*
3. Turn to #1 and ask if they are ready to begin again with one medium squeeze.

4. *Everyone close your eyes. Go!*
5. Once it makes it around, the "sender" says, "Got it," or after a while if the signals do not get back to #1, ask everyone to open their eyes.
6. *What kind of squeeze, if any, did you receive this time?*
7. Integrate #1's answer with the following neurobiological interpretation:

   a. *For those with AN, there is an area in the lower (or ventral) part of the brain that appears to under-fire or not fire at all. That was #3's* (state player's name) response by giving a light squeeze.

   b. *There are also areas in the AN brain that won't stop firing intensely. That was what #5* (state player's name) *was doing upon receiving a signal by squeezing hard many times.*

   c. Use the brain picture and point as you share: "*The ventral/temporal area of the brain that includes the insula and nucleus accumbens areas that tends to under-fire for those with AN, while the dorsolateral prefrontal cortex, amygdala and orbitofrontal cortex tend to over-fire. For example, circuits affecting thoughts (running through the DLPFC) and feelings (from the amygdala) about body shape and weight become intensified, increasing their signals each time the circuit re-fires over and over.*

   d. *Just as with the squeezes, those identified areas of the brain appear to under-fire and over-fire repeatedly.*

8. *Was it possible to get the medium squeeze signal through the altered circuit accurately?*
9. *This is the same for those with anorexia nervosa. Due to brain circuits that under- and over-firing, the messages cannot get through accurately. This is a reason why some persons with AN are unable to sense if they are hungry or full (the weak message area) and are continuously think about their size and weight when the brain continues to over-fire in the dorsal prefrontal area.*
10. *If clients have avoidant and/or inhibited traits, additional brain signals may express thoughts and feelings to not eat, or hold back on food, or avoid many foods.*
11. *In this telephone game, each of you is a neuron and together make up a circuit. Your left arm is the axon that passed the message on. Your body is the cell body, and your right hand is a dendrite, receiving the incoming message.*
12. *There are about 100 billion neurons in the brain. Circuits switch neurons based on the messages sent. Millions of circuits fire simultaneously.*
13. *It's miraculous that as many signals function as well as they do. It is normal to have aberrations in circuits. Those with ED appear to have more significant alterations in circuit response compared with those without ED.*

## Discussion Points

- Figure A12.3 shows involved in eating areas.
- Experiencing AN and other ED-altered brain responses are part of the causes of ED symptoms.
- The Telephone game explores what clients with AN experience.

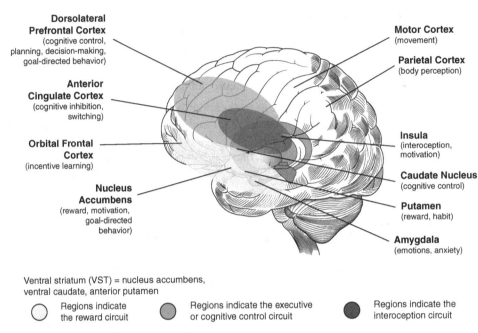

Ventral striatum (VST) = nucleus accumbens,
ventral caudate, anterior putamen

○ Regions indicate the reward circuit

◐ Regions indicate the executive or cognitive control circuit

● Regions indicate the interoception circuit

**Figure A12.3** Areas of the brain involved in eating

## How to Treat to These Traits

1. After experiencing Telephone, clients report relief and reduced guilt or shame for their ED symptoms, realizing through experience, the neurobiological bases.
2. Experiencing malfunction increases understanding in why ED symptoms occur, allowing clients and Supports to realize the biological influences of the illness, and that it is not the client's or family's fault.
3. You will be trying on another experiential activity that explores how to rewire new circuits to compensate for these faulty ones. (See Appendix 17.)

### Key Points

- There are altered brain circuits that under-fire and that over-fire in those with ED contributing to ED symptoms.
- There are neurobiological reasons why persons with ED think and feel as they do. It is not their choice.

## Homework

- None.

## Clinician Notes

_____
_____
_____
_____

# Appendix 13  Neuron Activity:  Why Food and Support Are Needed: TBT-S Neurobiological Experiential Activity

Laura Hill

## Neurobiological and Trait Target
- Brain circuit function

## Objectives
- Experience how brain circuits respond in healthy brains.
- Experience how and why brain circuits need food to function effectively.
- Experience how the brain uses cellular assistance to ensure effective neural function to indicate the normalcy of clients needing Support to ensure health.

## Who Is Involved?
- Clinician and clients and/or Supports.
- Students in classroom.
- This is a face-to-face group activity that needs a minimum of ten people.

## Materials and Time Needed
- Lots of paper wadded up in balls.
- 30 minutes.

## What Does the Research Say?
- Neurons are brain cells that transmit electro-chemical messages throughout the brain and central nervous system.

  ○ The brain uses neurons instead of other types of body cells due to speed. See Figures A13.1 and A13.2.
  ○ Electrochemical transmission is faster than blood circulation and other means of body cellular communication to accommodate fast responses to thoughts, feelings, and actions.[145]
  ○ A neuron consists of (a) a cell body, the factory of activity where energy from food and minerals is transformed into electrochemical messages relayed to other neurons; (b) *dendrites*, branches that *bring* messages into the cell body; and (c) *axons*, short to very long branches that *transmit messages out* to other neurons.
  ○ Circuits are neurons transmitting from one neuron to another, creating highways of neurochemical communication.
  ○ There are gaps between axons and dendrites, like intersections in a highway, called *synapses* where neurochemicals cross over to continue the neuron signal.

- Neurochemicals such as dopamine and serotonin, created from proteins and carbohydrates, are the chemical agents that travel across synapses.
- Circuits pass signals throughout the brain, simultaneously communicating thoughts, feelings, actions, perceptions, and sensations. It takes millions of circuits communicating at once. Depending on the topic/focus, messages are passed to specified areas of the brain.
- When the brain does not receive enough glucose from food intake, neurons are unable to fire adequately causing brain messages to be reduced and thoughts become more rigid or stuck.
- Playfully experiencing a metaphorical brain circuit in action allows clients and their Supports to understand more completely what is happening in the brain and why food is necessary to help keep the brain fully functioning.
- Glial cells tuck in and around neurons. They have multiple essential roles:[182]
  - ○ Adapt the chemical environment between neurons.
  - ○ Sculpt the physical connection.
  - ○ Provide structural assistance to neurons.
  - ○ Aid in serving nutrient needs so neurons can function well.
- Figures A13.1 and A13.2 show a neuron and how a specific glial cells connects with a neuron.

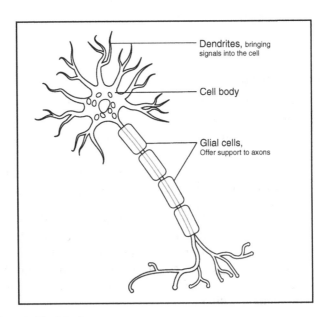

**Figure A13.1** Neuron with glial cells

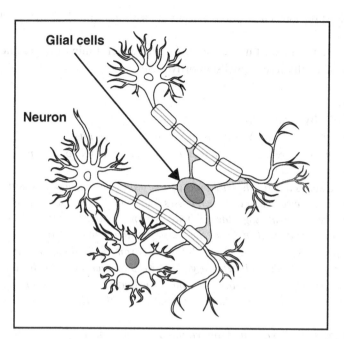

**Figure A13.2** Glial cell

Key Point: The brain uses speedy neurons to communicate thoughts, feelings, perceptions, and sensations that impact actions. This requires a lot of glucose (energy from food) and support to fire effectively.

## Clinician Checklist
⇒ Have the three rounds memorized, do not read them. Be playful.
⇒ Draw upon client and/or Support answers; let them ID their solutions.
⇒ Be prepared to look at the clients and/or Supports directly and state the key points (do not read them).

## Experiential Activity Instructions
### Rules
1. This is a game-like activity that creates a circuit of neurons helping you experience what is happening as messages travel through a brain circuit.
2. The clinician should memorize the steps to be more fluid and fun, not make it formal by reading each step.
3. There are three rounds, one demonstrating a healthy circuit, one showing the need for assistance, and one a malnourished circuit.
4. Participants are asked to take paper and wad it up into balls and pile them at one side of the room.

5. Direct half of the participants to create a line, with one end close to the pile of paper wads.
6. The paper wads represent neurochemicals, such as serotonin or dopamine.
7. The other half will serve as glial supportive cells.

## Steps and *Scripts*
## Round 1: Healthy Brain Circuit

1. *This is a "neuron game." You are neurons creating a circuit.*
2. *The wads of paper are the chemical messages, such as serotonin or dopamine that you pass along to communicate.*
3. *The first person is a dendrite, who picks up one wad at a time and passes it onto the next person, who is the cell body who then passes it onto the next person who is the axon. The dendrite takes in the message, the cell body uses energy to determine if the message will continue, and the axon then passes the message onto the next neuron.*
4. *The first person keeps passing the wads to the neuron cell person, one after the other, even if another part of the circuit gets clogged up. Keep the neurochemicals flowing!*
5. *The fourth person, and every fourth person in the line, uses their arms to create a circle, or hoop. The axon persons are to throw the wadded balls through the hoop. The hoop is the synapse.*
6. *Note: the persons who are the axons cannot put your hands over or into the hoop; you are to be beside the hoop and try to throw the balls through it.*
7. *The next person, who is the dendrite of the next neuron, is to catch the balls and pass them onto the cell body.*
8. *This process continues to the end of the circuit.*
9. *If any wads of paper fall on the floor, the axons and dendrites are <u>NOT</u> to pick them up. Leave them.*
10. *Okay, 'Go!'*

## Round 2: Glial Support

1. Ask participants to pick up the paper wads and return them to the initial pile.
2. Instruct the other half of participants to come and stand on both sides of the neuron circuit.
3. *You are glial cells. You support the synaptic hoop to make better connections. If you are standing by the hoop, pick up the serotonin or dopamine (wads of paper) from the floor and throw them through the synaptic hoop to increase the message and aid in nutrient assistance.* Additional people playing glial cells are to help catch the wads of paper that come through the hoop and hand them onto the dendrite.
4. *When I say "GO," the dendrite by the circuit pile begins again and the flow of the neurotransmitters continues through the circuit.*
5. *This time, you are experiencing how the brain has created its own support system to ensure better brain communication through its circuits, with the assistance of the glial cells.*
6. *Does everyone know their role? Okay, "GO!"*
7. The clinician facilitates the game in action as the circuit people are having fun passing the wads of paper through the neuron and synaptic hoops *and* the glial people are picking up the dropped wads and throwing them through the hoops.

8. After all the wads are passed through, the clinician asks the following questions:

   a. *Persons who are in the circuit, what was it like to have the glia people assisting you to get the serotonin or dopamine transmitted?*

   b. *Dendrite person who collected the balls when they came through the hoops, what was that like for you to collect the additional serotonin or dopamine coming through the hoop with the help of the glial cells?*

9. Clinician points out:

   a. *The glial cells helped compensate by creating a structure to collect the lost wads and send them back across the synapses.*

   b. *However, if there is only one person collecting the wads (serotonin or dopamine), then it becomes impossible to collect all of the wads of paper, so the brain instantly grows more openings (ion channels) in the dendrites to have more sites (or people) collecting the neurotransmitters.*

   c. *This process is how healthy brain circuits function to transmit their messages. The brain adjusts and adapts instantly to meet increased amounts of neurotransmitters and draws continuously on its glial cells to ensure all are functionally well.*

   d. *AND, it takes enough nutrients (glucose or energy) to keep this circuit running well.*

## Round 3: Underfed Neuron Circuit

1. Instruct participants to return the paper wads to the original pile.

2. Inform the participants: *"Now let's experience what the brain experiences when there are not enough nutrients or glucose to keep the circuits functioning well."*

3. Instruct the circuit of participants to move the wads of paper, the serotonin or dopamine, very slowly, having some gaps when nothing is being sent through. When the axon person throws the paper wad into the hoop, it is to be done slowly, so more may miss the hoop, because there is not enough force.

4. Glia people are instructed to continue their same roles.

5. *Everyone ready? Okay, "GO!"*

6. The clinician watches and coaches the paper wads to go slower and slower until the circuit has nothing to use.

7. The clinician then stops the activity and while all are still standing, asks them the following questions:

   a. *"What was it like as a circuit with its glia to receive so little dopamine or serotonin?"*

   b. *"Could you send your message adequately?"*

   c. *"What were your experiences or observations in this neuron activity?"*

8. The clinician integrates the answers as summarizing key points.

## Discussion Prompts

- Neurons need food. If denied, thoughts become rigid and actions diminish.
- Axons' shell-like coating is made from fats. If a person does not eat enough fats, the axon coating withers away preventing the electrochemical signals from passing through.

- Axons run from the brain and spinal cord to the ends of one's arms, legs, and every area of the body to coordinate body sensations and responses.
- Sensory neurons that carry information about, for example, touch and pain are afferent neurons. They send signals from the outside or body area to the brain. Efferent neurons send responses of what to do from the brain to the body area needing to respond.

## How to Treat to These Traits

1. After experiencing the neuron activity, anorexia nervosa clients consistently respond that they realize the importance of the role of food at a neuron level and the need for Support persons, who are their "glial" support.
2. The brain cannot function without food and assistance, and neither can AN clients.

Key Points
- The brain uses speedy neurons as highways of circuits to transmit thoughts, feelings, and actions.
- Brian circuits need energy and support to function adequately.
- Food restriction and not eating are sure ways to diminish functional thoughts and actions.
- The brain adjusts instantly by creating extra dendrites to take in increases of neurochemicals coming across synapses IF it receives enough energy.

## Homework

- Clients eat their complete meal plan.

## Clinician Notes

_____

_____

_____

_____

# Appendix 14 Brain Wave: TBT-S Neurobiological Experiential Activity

Laura Hill

## Neurobiological and Trait Targets
- Brain circuit responses
- Altered interoception
- Altered ventral striatal response

## Objectives
- Bring the brain to life. Experience and identify brain circuits and areas of the brain related to ED symptoms metaphorically and playfully.
- Clients identify their own neurobiological responses that impact their ED actions and thoughts and share with their Supports.

## Who Is Involved?
- Clients who have ED and/or Support persons.
- This is a face-to-face group activity for a minimum of eight people with no upper limits.

## Materials and Time Needed
- A type of food that can be easily passed around, e.g., a banana, apple, or orange.
- Room space for all persons in the group to spread out in a circle.
- Brain Wave Cards.
- 45 minutes.

## What Does the Research Say?
- Eating disorders are brain and biologically based illnesses (a core TBT-S principle).
- Brain circuits are altered in those who have AN, including the reward circuit (e.g., nucleus accumbens), the cognitive circuit (e.g., dorsolateral prefrontal cortex, caudate), and the salience or interoceptive circuit (e.g., insula). Disruptions in these circuits contribute to altered reward sensitivity, decision-making, inhibitory control, body image perceptions, and interoception (i.e., one's experience of internal physiological sensations, like hunger).
- Millions of brain circuits fire simultaneously to communicate thoughts, feelings, actions, perceptions, and sensations. This activity is a metaphor using a single circuit to represent many.

---

A variation of this activity is in the electronic text, Hill, L. (2017). *"A Brain-Based Approach to Eating Disorders"* at www.BrainBasedEatingDisorders.org

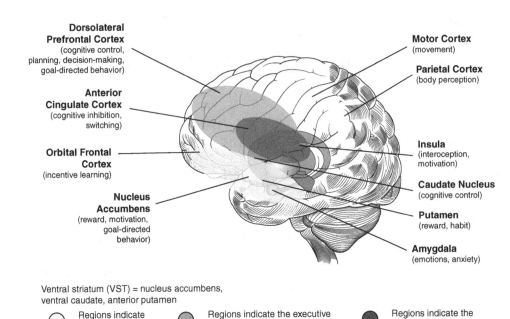

**Figure A14.1** Areas of the brain involved in eating

**Table A14.1** Brain Wave cards

| Brain wave card | Area of brain | Brain functions related to ED |
| --- | --- | --- |
| Card 1 | Thalamus | A central gateway in the brain controlling the flow of bodily messages to other brain areas. (Starting point/home base) |
| Card 2 | Insula | Receives and interprets body sensation signals such as hunger, fullness, taste, and pain to guide motivated behavior. |
| Card 3 | Amygdala | The panic center and source of emotional expressions. |
| Card 4 | Nucleus accumbens | A place where reward signals fire pleasure to affirm decisions, motivate actions, and offer satisfaction, e.g., from eating. |
| Card 5 | Orbitofrontal cortex | Takes messages from areas 2–4 to promote learning based on rewarding contingencies, also involved in impulse control. |
| Card 6 | Caudate | Performs cognitive evaluation to inform decision-making. |
| Card 7 | Anterior cingulate cortex | Involved in inhibitory control, error monitoring, and set shifting |
| Card 8 | Dorsolateral prefrontal cortex | Decision-making, planning, anticipation, set shifting, executive functioning |
| Card 9 | Parietal cortex | Body perception |

Key Point: The brain fires differently in those who have ED compared with those who do not, via altered brain circuits contributing to AN symptoms.

## Experiential Activity Instructions
### Steps
<u>Game Rules:</u> Clinician gives the following instructions (*script* in italics):

1. Describe the neurobiological points outlined earlier prior to the brain wave activity
2. Have nine participants stand in a circle. (Additional participants will be asked to be with persons holding cards 8 and 9.)
3. A type of food will be passed around a circle (such as a banana). Each time it is passed around the circle, it a metaphor for how different areas of the brain respond one bite (or round) by bite.
4. *Now that you have begun to learn about brain areas related to eating, this activity takes that information a step further by having you EXPERIENCE brain areas and give voice to the neurochemical messages, metaphorically for those who do (1) NOT have an ED, (2) RESTRICT, and (3) BINGE eat.*
5. *I am going to assign each of you to a brain area and remind you of its function by giving you a card. You are to follow the instructions on your card when it is your turn.*
6. Hand out the brain wave cards 1–9 stating one of the brain area functions.
7. *Please read the message on your card. When the banana is handed to you, please say the message out loud to the "rest" of the brain.*
8. There will be three sets of cards, played out in three rounds.

   *Round 1 is for those who don't have an ED.*

   *Round 2 is for those with AN who restrict.*

   *Round 3 is for those who binge eat.*

9. The Thalamus person 1, Card 1 is the only card that the person says nothing but simply passes the food on representing the relay function of the thalamus.

## The Brain Wave Rounds

### Round 1: Brain Wave for Those Who Do NOT Have an Eating Disorder. Set 1 of the Xards

1. When all clients/Supports have their cards, and have memorized their message, the clinician gives a banana (or other piece of food) to the thalamus, Card 1 to begin.
2. *Let's begin.* The round starts at the thalamus with each person saying the message on the card then passing the banana to the next brain area.
3. After Card 9, the clinician directs that the banana is to continue around the brain for round two, or bite 2 of the banana. *Script: Another round for another bite of the banana.*
4. A third round begins with the clinician saying, *Keep going, another bite of banana is being eaten.*

### Group Discussion for Round 1
- At the end of the third round, the clinician says, *Okay. Three bites have been taken from the banana.*

- *For those of you in the group who do not have an eating disorder (Supports), is this in any way similar to how your brain responds when you eat a food you like? If there are no persons in group without eating disorders, the clinician could say, This is similar to brain responses when a person does not have an ED.*

## Round 2: Brain Wave for Those Who Restrict with AN. Set 2 of the Cards

1. The second group of cards is handed out.
2. *On this set of cards are the messages from the brain areas when a person has AN.*
3. *Note that there are instructions on your card. The first time everyone is to say the message in a regular voice volume, so everyone hears what the message is saying.*
4. *For the second and third rounds, the volume of the messages is to change. Some of you will whisper or simply mouth the words, while others are to shout the words; some of you are instructed to say the words over and over.*
5. *Okay, let's begin. Thalamus, pass the banana on.*
6. Round 1 with an even volume, so everyone hears the messages.
7. Rounds 2 and 3 the volumes change to reflect altered brain circuit responses, and cards 8 and 9, say their loud message repeatedly.

Group Discussion for Round 2

- The clinician stops the activity after the third round and asks, *For those of you who have AN, is this in any way similar to what you experience? How is it different from your experience?*
- *Supports, did you know this is what it is like for your loved ones? Are there any questions you want to ask the clients?*

## Round 3: Brain Wave for Those Who Binge Eat. Set 3 of the Cards

1. The third group of cards is passed around. The clinician says, *This set of cards have possible brain response messages of those who binge eat.*
2. *Follow the instructions. Again, the volume of the brain areas reflects the intensity of circuit responses.*
3. *The first round, everyone speaks at a normal volume, so everyone hears the messages. The second-round volumes reflect circuit responses when binge eating.*
4. *Thalamus, are you ready? Okay, let's begin.*
5. The clinician is to have the banana passed faster and faster as the volume increases as it passes around each time through the dorsolateral prefrontal cortex (DLPFC) and back to the insula.

## Group Discussion for Round 3

1. *Clients who binge eat, is this round similar to your experience? How is it different from your experience?*
2. *Script: Supports, did you know this is what it is like for your loved ones? Are there any questions you want to ask the clients?*
3. Handout the "Brain Wave Handout."
4. Have clients fill in the boxes describing how their own brain responds.

If they are uncertain of their own experience, or if the area is not relevant to them, have them leave it blank.

## Group Summary Discussion

* *Please take your personal Brain-Wave Handout and describe your brain responses to your Supports. Supports ask questions if you need clarification. Clients, you are the experts of this illness. Your answers should be based on what you experience. If you don't have an answer, simply say that.*
* The larger group comes back together. The clinician asks the clients and Supports, *What did you learn from one another? What have you learned from this activity?*

## How to Treat to These Traits

1. After experiencing the brain wave activity, clients consistently respond that they no longer feel guilt and self-blame and shame for their ED symptoms, having experienced biological underpinnings.
2. The activity shifts the paradigm from the problem client to begin experiential problem solving via TBT-S activities.

---

**Key Points and Notes for Clinician**
* When brain circuits are altered, they can alter thoughts, body perception, feelings, and decisions.
* Many clients with AN and other EDs have altered neuro-signals, disrupting the ability to know what to do.
* The point of demonstrating altered neurocircuits is not about teaching mindful exercises to "awaken" sensations. It is about teaching what is poorly functioning and identifying ways to compensate.

---

## Homework

* None

## Clinician Checklist

⇒ Memorize the neurobiological points and grid that describe brain circuits involved in eating and eating disorders.
⇒ Refer to Figure A14.1 to show the location in the brain of areas and their functions.
⇒ Print the three sets of brain wave cards.
⇒ Print the Client Brain-Wave Handout.
⇒ Be playful.
⇒ At the end, be prepared to look at the clients and/or Supports directly and state the key points (do not read them).

## Clinician Notes

_____
_____
_____
_____

# Anorexia Nervosa: What is true for me?

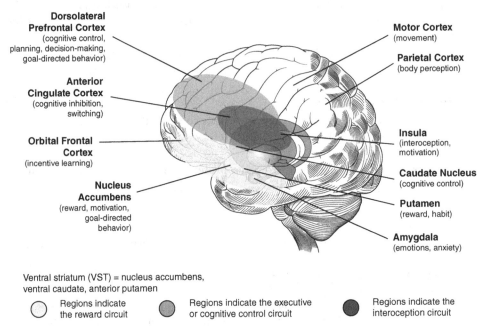

Ventral striatum (VST) = nucleus accumbens,
ventral caudate, anterior putamen

○ Regions indicate the reward circuit

◐ Regions indicate the executive or cognitive control circuit

● Regions indicate the interoception circuit

**Figure A14.2** Areas of the brain involved in eating

**Table A14.2** Brain responses for AN: What's true for me?

| Area of brain | Brain functions | Average brain interpretations to foods for those with anorexia nervosa[1] | What is true for me? |
|---|---|---|---|
| Insula | Body sensations, e.g., hunger, pain, taste signals | I'm not hungry or full, or sense much pain | _____ |
| Amygdala | Fear, emotional responses | I'm worried or afraid | _____ |
| Nucleus accumbens or ventral striatum | Pleasure/reward: is this better than my expectation; punishment: less than expectation | Yuck, I sense little to no pleasure | _____ |
| Orbitofrontal cortex | Impulse control and associative learning based on rewarding or negative contingencies | "Whoa" to new foods or experiences | _____ |
| Caudate area | Weighing pros and cons | It is not easy for me to know if a decision is good or bad? | _____ |

**Table A14.2** (cont.)

| Area of brain | Brain functions | Average brain interpretations to foods for those with anorexia nervosa[1] | What is true for me? |
|---|---|---|---|
| Anterior cingulate cortex | Inhibition, error monitoring, and cognitive control | Don't eat it. | _____ |
| Dorsolateral prefrontal cortex | Decision-making, planning, anticipation | What do I do? What do I do? | _____ |
| Parietal | Seeing one's body within surrounding space | I look huge | _____ |

# Binge eating: What is true for me?

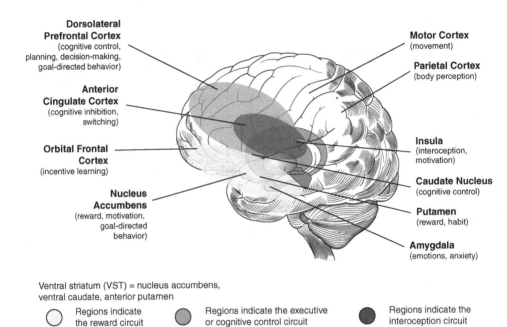

**Figure A14.3** Areas of the brain involved in eating

**Table A14.3** Brain responses for binge eating: What's true for me?

| Area of brain | Brain functions | Average brain interpretations to foods for those who binge eat | What is true for me |
|---|---|---|---|
| Insula | Hunger, pain, taste signals | (first round): That tastes delicious! (second round) Where's the taste? I'm not hungry. | _____ |
| Nucleus accumbens or ventral striatum | Pleasure/Reward: better than my expectation Punishment: less than expectation | I'm NOT satisfied | _____ |
| Orbitofrontal cortex | Impulse control and associative learning based on rewarding or negative contingencies | More food NOW | _____ |
| Caudate area | Weighing pros and cons | That's good. How about chocolate | _____ |
| Anterior cingulate cortex | Inhibition, error monitoring, and cognitive control | Eat it! | _____ |
| Dorsolateral prefrontal cortex | Decision-making, planning, anticipation | I need more! I need more! | _____ |

## Round 1: Brainwave for persons without an eating disorder.

### Instructions

- Brain wave sheets are printed on full-size pages.
- Each page is given to a different person. If there are additional people, they are assigned to be grouped together with the Dorsolateral Prefrontal Cortex and the Parietal.
- Ask people to stand in a circle in the order the pages are passed out.
- Ask participants to read the words in quotations on their sheet when they are given the banana.
- After they say their "brain response," they pass the banana to the next person.
- The clinician has the participants pass the banana around three times.
- Each time is equal to one bite.
- The clinician says as the banana begins the first round, *This is similar to how the brain responds when you take a bite of banana and you (1) do not have an eating disorder, (2) have anorexia nervosa, (3) binge eat.*
- Note: The binge eating cards apply to (1) AN; subtype binge, (2) Binge eating for those with bulimia nervosa, and
  (3) binge eating disorder.

  o The amygdala and parietal areas do not have a common response and are left out of this round.

# Brain Wave
## of those who
## **do not have**
## **an eating disorder**

# RELAY STATION

## THALAMUS

(Nothing said, message passed onto brain areas)

2

# "I'm Hungry!"

## INSULA

(Interoception: Taste, Hunger, Fullness, Motivation)

3

# "I'm calm."

## AMYGDALA

(Emotions: Calm-Panic, Fear)

4

# "YUM"

# NUCLEUS ACCUMBENS

(Reward, Motivation, Pleasure)

5

# "A-OK."

## ORBITOFRONTAL CORTEX (OFC)

(Incentive Learning/Inhibition and/or Impulse Control)

6

# "It's good."

## CAUDATE

(Weighs Pros/Cons, Merges Thoughts with Feelings)

7

# "EAT IT."

## ANTERIOR CINGULATE CORTEX (ACC)

### (Mediates Decisions, Shifts Thoughts)

8

# "I'll have another bite."

## DORSOLATERAL PREFRONTAL CORTEX (DLPFC)

(Executive Planning, Decision-Making, Anticipation)

9

# "I look OK"

## PARIETAL CORTEX

(Body Perception)

10

# Brain Wave

for persons

## with anorexia nervosa

1

# RELAY STATION

## THALAMUS

(Nothing said, message passed onto brain areas)

2

# "I'm NOT hungry!"

**(After first time around,** whisper this message**)**

## INSULA

(Interoception: Taste, Hunger, Fullness, Motivation)

3

# "I'm worried. I'm afraid."

**(After first time around, YELL this message)**

## AMYGDALA
(Emotions: Calm-Panic, Fear)

4

# "Yuck!"

**(After first time around,** whisper this message**)**

# NUCLEUS ACCUMBENS

(Reward, Motivation, Pleasure)

5

# "Whoa."

**(After first time around, GET LOUDER with this message)**

# ORBITOFRONTAL CORTEX (OFC)

(Incentive Learning/Inhibition and/or Impulse Control)

6

# "It's bad!"

**(After first time around, GET LOUDER with this message)**

## Caudate

(Weighs Pros/Cons, Merges Thoughts with Feelings)

7

# "DON'T EAT IT!"

**(After first time around, YELL this message)**

## ANTERIOR CINGULATE CORTEX (ACC)

(Mediates Decisions,
Shifts Thoughts)

8

# "What do I do? What do I do? What do I do?"

**(After first time around, GET LOUDER and say repeatedly)**

## DORSOLATERAL PREFRONTAL CORTEX (DLPFC)

(Executive: Planning, Decision-Making, and Anticipation)

9

# "I LOOK HUGE!"

**(After first time around, GET LOUDER and say it repeatedly)**

## PARIETAL CORTEX

(Body Perception, Body Image)

10

# Brain Wave

for person with

## binge eating disorder
## or
## binge portion of bulimia
## nervosa

1

# RELAY STATION

## THALAMUS

(Nothing said, message passed onto brain areas)

2

The first time, blissfully say

# "That tastes delicious!"

**(After the first time,** whisper**)**
"Where's the taste?
I'm not hungry."

## INSULA

(Interoception: Taste, Hunger,
Fullness, Motivation)

3

# "That was wonderful!"

(After the first time whisper)

# "Where's the pleasure?"

## NUCLEUS ACCUMBENS
(Reward, Motivation, Pleasure)

4

# "More!"

## ORBITOFRONTAL CORTEX (OFC)

(Incentive Learning/Inhibition and/or Impulse Control)

5

# That's good! How about adding chocolate?

## Caudate

(Weighs Pros/Cons, Merges Thoughts with Feelings)

6

# "EAT IT!"

## (After the first time, get LOUDER with this message)

# ANTERIOR CINGULATE CORTEX (ACC)

## (Mediates Decisions, Shifts Thoughts)

7

# "I need more!
# I need MORE!
# I NEED MORE!"

**(After the first time, get LOUDER and say it repeatedly)**

# DORSOLATERAL PREFRONTAL CORTEX (DLPFC)

(Executive: Planning, Decision-Making, Anticipation)

8

# Appendix 15  Anxiety Wave: TBT-S Problem-Solving Experiential Activity

Laura Hill

## Neurobiological and Trait Targets
- Anxiety
- The tendency to be physically active

## Objectives
- Identify each client's ED symptoms when anxiety is low compared with when anxiety is high.
- Identify responses clients need from Supports when anxiety is low and high.

## Who Is Involved?
- Clinician and one or more clients and preferably Support persons.
- This could be a virtual or face-to-face activity.
- Professor and students.

## Materials and Time Needed
- Anxiety Wave Handout: Client Symptoms.
- Anxiety Wave Handout: Support Responses.
- 30–45 minutes.

## What Does the Research Say?
- Anxiety is a complex trait.
  - Trait anxiety is a genetically induced tendency to be anxious in varying levels throughout life.
  - State anxiety is a response to specific situations.
- Persons with AN have a genetic tendency to have high trait anxiety.[167] (See "Ten Biological Facts on Anorexia Nervosa," Appendix 1).
- Anxiety can be experienced cognitively (e.g., anxious thoughts, worry, obsessions), physiologically (e.g., stomachache, nausea, difficulty breathing, racing heart), emotionally (e.g., fear, panic, agitation, increased vigilance, decreased emotional state), and/or in anticipation (fear of upcoming event).
- Concentration diminishes as anxiety increases. When anxiety is high for a person with AN, the body resorts to fighting (such as by turning inward and making oneself vomit) or freezing (such as not eating) or fleeing (such as avoiding food). Heart rate increases and breathing becomes shallow.

---

A variation of this activity is in the electronic text called *A Brain-Based Approach to Eating Disorders* at www .BrainBasedEatingDisorders.org

- The tendency to be physically active is a trait.
  - The brain integrates sensory information from the external world (e.g., visual cortex, somatosensory and perceptual processing in the parietal cortex) or internal body states (e.g., insula) with cognitive and emotional evaluation (e.g., prefrontal cortex, limbic circuit) to produce a motor response (via the cerebellum, basal ganglia, and motor cortex).
  - Active movement serves to meet one's goals (e.g., how to get through the gauntlet).
  - Learning occurs through repeated action. This practiced behavior modifies the brain to develop more efficient pathways to assist the behavior.
- Brain areas responsible for movement are interconnected with cognition (circuits through dorsolateral prefrontal cortex, caudate), emotions (limbic area including amygdala) and perceptions (parietal). See Figures A15.1 and A15.2.

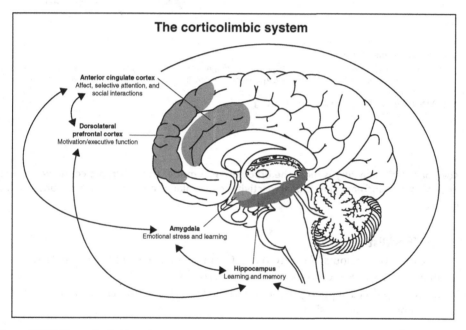

**Figure A15.1** The corticolimbic system

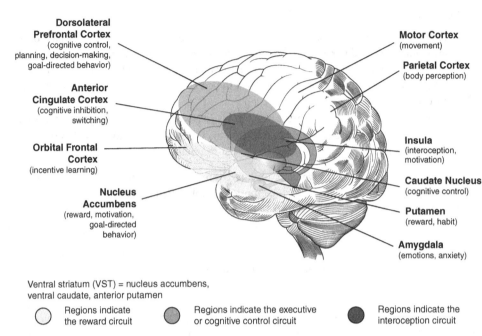

**Figure A15.2** Areas of the brain involved in eating

---

Key Point: When anxiety is high, the brain enters a mode which disrupts cognitive control (thoughts) and increases emotional reactivity (panic, alarm) and behavioral response (fight, flight).

## Clinician Checklist

⇒ Have the two handouts "Anxiety Wave: Client Expressions" and "Anxiety Wave: Support Responses" copied or emailed for virtual session.

⇒ Have client select a Support person with whom to do this activity face-to-face or virtually, or via phone during session.

## Experiential Activity Instructions

### Rules

1. This activity is used when the clinician wants clients to address their trait anxiety responses.

2. It helps clients to identify

   a. their own expressions when anxiety is low and high

   b. what they need from their Supports

   c. the opportunity to communicate their needs with their Supports

3. It uses two Anxiety Wave Handouts, "Anxiety Wave: Client Expressions" and "Anxiety Wave: Support Responses."

4. The clinician has the option to share the brain's and body's responses to anxiety before having clients complete the handouts.

## Steps and *Scripts*

1. Give clients the two Anxiety Wave handouts, "Anxiety Wave: Client Expressions" and "Anxiety Wave: Support Responses." Figures A15.3 and A15.4.
2. Begin with "Anxiety Wave: Client Expressions."

   a. Instruct clients to identify what their anxiety looks like when it is low and when it is high. They can choose from options on the right side of the page or use their own descriptions.
   b. Ask the client to share their responses.
   c. *Notice that when your anxiety is high, your expressions are nonverbal and are either an action, such as binge eating or self-induced vomiting, or frozen action, such as not eating.*
   d. *The brain is not able to help you talk when anxiety is high.*
   e. *Your Supports need to know this.*
   f. *When anxiety is low, it is easier to talk with others.*

3. Instruct the client(s) to fill out "Anxiety Wave: Support Responses."
4. Tell the client(s) to share with their Support(s) the responses they identified that would help at high and low levels of anxiety.
5. Ask the Support(s), *Do you have any comments on what the client shared/wrote? Do you see any expressions on the list that you have observed your loved one (e.g., roommate) doing? Clarify with the client what level of anxiety they have when they express it.*
6. To the client, *Can you allow yourself to accept what you need from your Support when your anxiety is high? It is hard to accept assistance because you are a highly competent person. But all of us need assistance at times.*
7. To the Support, *The client has shared what they need from you when their anxiety is high and low. Offer the assistance in spite of negativity, even if anxiety is high.*

## Discussion Prompts

• Anxiety may be experienced as a continuous "noise," an endless litany of self-blame, body hatred, or anger from eating or eating too much.
• Many clients report that their anxiety surges so fast that they are unable to experience their responses when anxiety is at moderate levels. Is that true for you?
• What expressions did the client(s) describe about themselves at low and high levels of anxiety?
• When anxiety is high, a person is often unable to be verbal. Anxiety is instead expressed via actions, such as purging or freezing.
• When anxiety is low, a person is able to talk, interact, and think through actions.
• Anxiety can be motivating and productive at low levels. It can be an irritant to motivate a person to do a productive action, such as finish an assignment at school or work.

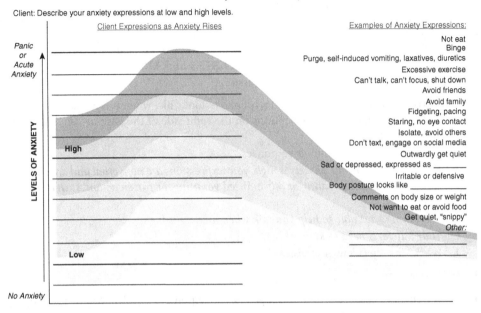

**Figure A15.3** Anxiety wave symptoms

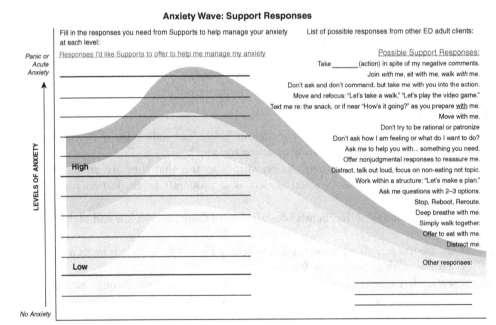

**Figure A15.4** Anxiety wave responses

## How to Treat to These Traits

- Have the Supports choose responses that are a good fit to their temperament.
- Have clients identify their own anxiety expression and what is needed from Supports. Give the client and Support the opportunity to practice while in session. The clinician is providing the needed structure for the client to move forward in learning how to better manage their anxiety trait.

### Key Points

- Adult clients cannot talk through what they need when anxiety is high.
- After experimenting, clients can tell Supports what they need for assistance, reducing Supports' guessing and exhaustion.
- "When anxiety is up, Shut up." (A father's comment after completing the handout.)

## Homework

- Ask Supports to practice the identified response they would most like to try on, over the next week.
- Ask clients to discuss their difficulty in allowing their Supports to offer their assistance, and then practice humbly accepting it.

## Clinician Notes

_____
_____
_____
_____
_____
_____

A variation of this activity is in the electronic text called *A Brain-Based Approach to Eating Disorders* at www.BrainBasedEatingDisorders.org

# Appendix 16 Anxiety Brain Sculpt: TBT-S Problem-Solving Experiential Activity

Stephanie Knatz Peck

### Neurobiological and Trait Targets
- Anxiety (including anticipatory anxiety)

### Objectives
- Describe and highlight the experience of anxiety surrounding mealtimes.
- Provide an opportunity for Supports to learn about anxiety through experience.
- Facilitate opportunities to discuss anxiety management strategies including

   ○ Distraction/redirection
   ○ Strategies for Supports.

### Who Is Involved?
- ≥ 6 participants (ideally Supports and Clients).

### Materials and Time Needed
- 45–60 minutes.
- A group room large enough to accommodate 5–20 participants.
- Post-It notes.
- Wireless headphones and music.

### What Does the Research Say?
- Approximately 75 percent of people with anorexia nervosa also suffer from at least one anxiety disorder.[189]
- A significant number of people with AN also experience heightened anxiety around mealtimes (before, during, and after meals), which leads to food avoidance, restriction, and other eating disorder behaviors.
- Research suggests that the natural dopamine release associated with food intake leads to anxiety in those with AN (versus pleasure for those without AN).

Key Point: The experience of anxiety and anxiety disorders plays a role in food restriction and avoidance in AN. For people with AN who experience anxiety, the brain has miscoded food as dangerous and something to be avoided. This uncomfortable experience can lead to extreme food avoidance and restriction.

### Clinician Checklist
⇒ Completed experiential activity.
⇒ Orchestrated group discussion using Activity Discussion Points.

⇒ Provided psychoeducation and review on skills (see Trait Profile Checklist, Appendix 2).

⇒ Assigned homework.

## Experiential Activity Instructions

This group activity is designed to create a representational version of anxiety. Clients are asked to describe thoughts, feelings, and sensations that they experience (1) before, (2) during, and (3) after eating. Each group member then volunteers to represent each of these experiences. Each member plays the role of the thought, feeling, or sensation by verbalizing it out loud while standing in a line. Volunteers are then asked to walk down the line while each group member plays out their part.

### Activity Aims

1. To facilitate client and Support reflection and awareness on thoughts, feelings, and sensations associated with eating.
2. To highlight how these combined experiences are overwhelming and contribute to anxiety and food restriction.
3. To provide a platform for creative problem solving on ways to manage anxiety, for both clients and Supports.

## Steps and Scripts (scripts in italics)

1. Each client in the group is asked to write down a goal they would like to practice/achieve for the next meal. Each goal is written on a small post-it notepaper.
2. Clients are then asked to stick their post-it note goal to the wall on one side of the room.
3. The facilitator then leads the clients to the opposite end of the room. (The room should be cleared of chairs and other obstacles so that there is room to walk from one end to the other. Clients and Supports can remain standing during this activity.)
4. The facilitator explains that they are going to help the clients build a "brain sculpture," meaning a representation of what happens inside their brain surrounding mealtimes.

   *For this activity, we would like to hear about all the experiences that make it challenging for you to meet your goal. Your goal is on the opposite end of the room, and we want to know about some of the experiences that you must get through to make it to your goal. I want you to imagine that there is an imaginary line between where you are standing and your goal. These are all of the experiences you face before, during, and after a meal. For this exercise, we are going to imagine that this line is divided into three parts – before, during, and after a meal. We're going to ask you to tell us a little bit about any thoughts, feelings, sensations, or any other inner experiences you have during these times.*

5. The facilitator asks one client to participate in the exercise by sharing about their experience and chooses one of the time frames to start with (before, during, or after).

   *Alternatively, the facilitator can have all clients share and build a shared brain sculpture. This is a good modification when the group members are reluctant, or when there is a benefit in highlighting similarities.

   *Let's start with after meals. What are some of the things you experience after you eat?*

6. Once the client shares an experience, a group member is assigned to play that part.

*Ex. Client A said that she has the thought "Why did I eat that?" Support B, can you please play that part? For now, just remember your line.*

7. Continue to facilitate the client sharing about all of their experiences at each time frame until it is complete, assigning parts to other group members after each experience is shared. (There should be at least a two–three inner experiences shared for each time frame.) The facilitator should ensure they are capturing an array of inner experiences, including a variety of thoughts, feelings, and body sensations.

8. Once the brain sculpt is complete, the facilitator asks the client to ensure that it is accurate by having each group member play their role.

   *Now that we are done, let's check that this is accurate for you. Group members, we are going to ask you to each play your part.*

   At this point, the facilitator acts as the "conductor" and prompts the group to each act/say their part in unison. They then check in with the client to ensure its accuracy, and whether anything should be modified. The facilitator should ask specifically about volume, intensity, and tone so that the client has an opportunity to remark on the intensity and quality of these experiences. Generally, the brain sculpt will sound like an orchestra of many voices talking at the same time. The majority of clients will agree that this is accurate for them, which highlights the intrusive and overwhelming nature of anxiety and the "mind chatter" that many with AN experience. However, it is also fine to change anything that the client requests, including having each part play out sequentially, versus in unison.

9. The client is asked whether they would like any of their Supports to "walk through" the brain sculpt to gain an understanding of their experience. Supports are also invited to walk through.

   At this point, all participants should be in two single-file lines facing each other. There should be enough room between them for any volunteers to walk through, as though walking through a narrow tunnel, which mimics the intrusive nature of anxiety.

10. ***Practicing Commonly Prescribed Skills.*** The volunteer is then asked to brainstorm things that would help make the experience less aversive. It is important to allow the participant to throw out any ideas, which can further allow the clinician to elaborate on the nature of anxiety and limitations in lessening it and/or making it go away. For example, if the volunteer asks that the thoughts be "quieter," the clinician can highlight that unfortunately, aside from medications, we don't have the brain tools to "turn the thoughts down."

11. ***Practicing Thought-Challenging.*** The facilitator provides an opportunity to see if thought-challenging is effective within the exercise. Many clients with AN have received cognitive-behavioral therapy (CBT) or have been asked to practice challenging thoughts or using positive affirmations. While this can be helpful in certain situations, often these are not effective strategies for managing heightened anxiety.

    a. The facilitator asks that someone stand next to one of the volunteers playing a thought.

    b. The new volunteer practices thought-challenging by arguing or attempting to debate the thought.

    c. The volunteer repeats walking through the anxiety tunnel.

d. The facilitator highlights that the thought-challenging simply added more noise rather than reducing anxiety.

12. ***Practicing Distraction/Re-Attending Attention.*** The facilitator provides an experience of practicing distraction. To do this, the clinician asks the volunteer to put on headphones and plays music as the volunteer walks through the anxiety tunnel. The volunteer is asked to comment on the helpfulness of the music. The facilitator should highlight the following:

a. The music gave the person something else to focus on rather than the thoughts.
b. *And yet*, the music didn't completely drown out the noise of the anxiety.

13. This exercise can be repeated with other clients if the facilitator wants to highlight each individual's personal brain sculpture. (This does not need to be done since all will have had the experience of participating and the post-activity discussion focuses on each client highlighting personal similarities and differences.)

## Important Points to Highlight

- *After Meal Time Frame.* Many clients will say that this is the most challenging time frame. During the exercise, facilitators should highlight the research (see "What Does the Research Say?") that some people with AN may experience the natural dopamine release associated with food intake as anxiety provoking instead of as pleasurable (like people without AN). The clinician should also highlight that this experience of distress after meals is how and why people with AN learn to avoid food and can lead to pre-meal anxiety and avoidance (in the before meal time frame). This is a natural response because our brain learns to avoid things that are aversive.

- *Before Meal Time Frame.* Per the earlier information, sometimes it is useful to move directly from the after meal time frame to discussing experiences that occur before the meal. This way, facilitators can make the connection that the anxiety and urges to avoid that often occur before eating are related to past experiences of distress. Thus, anticipatory anxiety and avoidance are natural, learned brain responses. Many with AN experience anticipatory anxiety characterized by excessive thoughts and worry about the food or eating or its outcome. This anticipatory anxiety can often result in heightened inhibition around food, making it difficult for a client to get started.

- *During Meal Time Frame.* Some with AN will note that anxiety is lower during this time period, and fewer unpleasant experiences are occurring during eating compared with before and after eating. If true, it is important to highlight because it suggests that the primary points where skills and intervention are necessary are surrounding the meal. It is also important to facilitate any sharing of body sensations, including fullness. If the client shares experiences such as fullness, the clinician can note that there are alterations in brain circuitry interpreting hunger and fullness that can cause fullness to be mis-signaled, similar to a car having a broken gas gauge.

## Discussion Prompts

Once the game is over, the facilitator leads a group discussion so that each client and Support can share their experiences and insights from the exercise. An effective way to do this is to break the group up into smaller mixed groups to allow group members to share and get feedback. The questions that follow are examples of ways to facilitate group discussion. The purpose is to elicit feedback from clients about the experiences surrounding eating that make it challenging to eat. The discussion is also important to allow clients to highlight skills and strategies to manage the experience, and to advise Supports on effective assistance strategies. Each client should provide direction for how they would like Supports to assist with anxiety around mealtimes.

- *What parts of this exercise do you relate to (for clients)?* At the end of the discussion, each client is asked to share how this exercise related to their experiences with eating. Which period surrounding meals is most challenging for you (before, during, after)?
- *What can help you effectively navigate this? What skills do you need to use?* Clients are asked to share what kinds of tools they can use to navigate these experiences.
- *Supports, what did you learn from this exercise?*
- *Clients, what can supports do to help surrounding meals?*

## How to Treat to These Traits:

- *Distraction/Re-Attending Attention.* Anxiety is biologically designed to get and hold one's attention. When intense, it can be challenging if not impossible to "ignore it" or "talk it down." Instead, many clients benefit from learning to redirect their attention to another activity or topic. Activities must straddle the delicate line of being both simple and yet engaging. Common examples include iPhone games, table games, adult coloring, and gentle movement. Supports can learn to assist with distraction activities by ensuring neutral topics of conversation while eating and facilitating the use of distraction techniques.
- *Structure and Routine.* Routines are known to be anxiety reducing. People with AN often have high uncertainty intolerance. Uncertainty can create anxiety. Establishing and sticking with clear structure and routine surrounding meals (set mealtimes, set meals and snacks, and distraction routines) can reduce anxiety. Supports can learn to facilitate and uphold structure and tolerate client's need for these features.
- *Support Skills*
  - *Clear Directives versus Open-Ended Questions.* When anxiety is present, it is difficult to make decisions, and it can be helpful to have someone provide clear and decisive directions. In the presence of anxiety, Supports can learn to make directive statements (versus using open-ended questions) to assist a client with redirecting their attention to another topic.
  - *Responding to Rumination and Perseveration: Validate and Redirect.* Perseveration occurs when a client repeats the same topic question. Rumination can occur silently but refers to the internal mental dwelling on a topic or experience. Both of these features occur with anxiety and can be common in AN. It can be to seek assurance about a topic (e.g., Am I fat?) or can occur because a client is having an intense thought or experience. Supports can learn to avoid inadvertently worsening anxiety by engaging with a client on these topics. Supports should avoid asking additional questions or trying to reason a client out of their experience, both of which can make rumination and perseveration worse. Instead, Supports should learn to validate and redirect. For example, a Support can say, "*It sounds like you are stuck on that question. I've already given you an answer, so let's take a walk and talk about the show we want to watch tonight.*"

## Homework

- **Clients and Supports:** Practice using the skills discussed as helpful around meals for the remainder of the day.

## Clinician Notes

_____
_____
_____
_____
_____
_____

# Appendix 17 Wire–Re-wire: TBT-S Problem-Solving Experiential Activity

Laura Hill

## Neurobiological and Trait Targets
- Neuroplasticity
- Brain capacity for compensation

## Objectives
- Experience how the brain wires and re-wires circuits.
- Experience what it takes for circuits to become habitual.
- Identify each client's traits that helped them shift dominant ED tendencies to productive expressions.

## Who Is Involved?
- Clinician and clients with ED and/or Supports.
- Students in classroom.
- This could be a virtual individual or group activity, as well as face-to-face.
- Two or more players.

## Materials and Time Needed
- Large spools of string or yarn. One spool per dyad.
- 20 minutes.

## What Does the Research Say?
- The brain creates circuits (wires) when a neuron transmits to an adjacent neuron, which transmits to an adjacent neuron, repeating this pattern to communicate information. Neurons that fire together, wire together.
- Each circuit passes through and connects various brain areas working together to perform a task.
- Neurons in distinct brain areas may be faulty, altering the signals as the circuit passes through, and decreasing the performance of the relevant task (e.g., thoughts or actions). For example, the insula may have altered, lower signals that impact circuits passing through, decreasing hunger or fullness signals for those with AN.
- Brain circuits vary in length and direction for every task, thought, feeling, and perceptional experience. They are expansive electrochemical connections.

---

A variation of this activity is in the electronic text, Hill, L. (2017). "*A Brain-Based Approach to Eating Disorders*" at www.BrainBasedEatingDisorders.org

○ It may take millions of circuits combined to sense, feel, think, and respond to a single task the first time it is experienced.

○ For example, the moment a person sees something, a circuit carries signals in the eye to the back of the brain, the visual cortex, which is connected to a number of other circuits specialized to perceive and register what is seen, identify the spatial context of the image, identify the object meaning, create a memory of the image, and generate thoughts and feelings about the image in order to respond.

• The brain prunes its circuits as it streamlines responses.

• The more that actions are repeated, the more they become automatic, or habitual.

• When an action shifts, different neurons fire together. This shifts or builds new circuits (like highways) to transmit (re-wire) signals throughout the brain to perform the new action or set of thoughts.

• Each time the brain re-wires new highways of transmission, it is creating a new action, or thought, or perception, etc.

• Each time the same action is repeated, the faster the brain refines and prunes by eliminating unnecessary neurons, keeping those that can replicate the action without as much thought. *This process is the development of skills and habits.*

• See Figure A17.1 to identify areas of the brain involved in eating that wire and re-wire as actions and thoughts change.

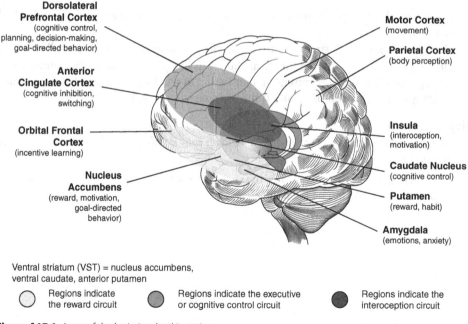

Ventral striatum (VST) = nucleus accumbens, ventral caudate, anterior putamen

**Figure A17.1** Areas of the brain involved in eating

> **Key Points**
> - The brain combines neurons to create a circuit or "wire."
> - When thoughts, perceptions, and actions change, brain circuits adjust and create new circuits to adapt. The brain re-wires,
> - Habits form after a new action is practiced repeatedly and becomes automatic.

## Clinician Checklist

⇒ Have large balls of string or yarn prepared.
⇒ If it is a virtual activity, ask clients to have a ball of string or skein of yarn ready.
⇒ Memorize or prepare the steps, do not read them.
⇒ Memorize and share the key points while looking directly at the clients and/or Supports to increase impact.

## Experiential Activity Instructions

### Rules

1. This activity provides clients and/or Supports a metaphorical experience of the brain wiring an activity and then re-wiring a new activity.
   a. It demonstrates that clients need to think in detail when identifying new actions to replace ED symptoms for new habits to be formed.
   b. When clients are not specific in identifying desired goals, the brain is unable to wire specific actions to form productive habits.
2. Divide into dyads virtually or face-to-face (this could be clinician and client in individual sessions).
3. Give each dyad a ball of string or yarn or ask virtual clients to hold up their ball of string.
4. Once a person begins to wind the string, they must keep moving or wiring continuously throughout the activity, representing that the act of winding *is* the act of brain circuits sending signals through the brain. If the winding stops, brain action stops.

### Steps and Scripts

1. The clinician instructs: "*One person is to hold up your hands (the holder) with about a foot of space between them.*"
   - If there are Supports and clients, the client is to wind the string (the winder) and the Support person is to be the holder.

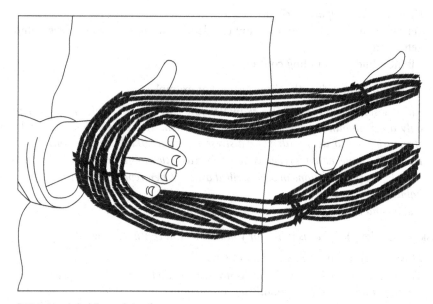

**Figure A17.2** Hands holding a skein of yarn

## Round 1: Wire

Instruct the client to wind the string from one of the holder's hands over the other in a circular fashion, repeatedly. See Figure A17.2.

2.  After a few rounds of yarn being wound around the person's hands, ask the winder, *What is it like to wind the string around your partner's hand? Don't stop winding while you answer.*

    - Some winders say it is awkward.
    - Others may say it is not that hard.
    - Let each winder share their experience to recognize the varied responses when doing something new.

3.  While the winding is taking place, ask the winders to identify out loud one of their eating disorder behaviors. For example,

    - Restricting.
    - Binge eating.
    - Purging (Note: this needs to be clarified. Have each client identify if this means vomiting, laxatives, excessive exercise, etc.).

4.  The clinician repeats the ED symptom in an objective and factual voice tone.

    - Keep the pace moving forward, so there is not more attention given to any one symptom.

5.  If the winder stops winding, the clinician simply says, *"Keep winding."*

6.  While the winding continues, ask the participants:

    - *How would you define a rule?*
    - *How would you define a ritual?*

- *How do rules compare to rituals?*
- Let the clients build upon one another's definitions, reflecting and developing their definitions.
- All the while, the winding continues.

7. The clinician summarizes the three terms. For example:

- *Rule: A set of conditions. For example, you may create a rule that you can eat only a set amount of food. If the rule is broken, you may decide on a rule to structure how to deal with your distress or anger, like "I must vomit!"*
- *Habit: The same action is repeated until it needs little attention and becomes automatic.*
- *Ritual: A series of actions in a prescribed order. When repeated the ritual may become habitual.*
- *Habits and rituals can be productive or destructive.*

8. Ask the winder(s), *What is it like for you now as you continue to wind?*

- Most report it is now easy and automatic.
- *This is similar to what it is like for you when you do ED symptoms repeatedly. You are creating a habit and then ritualizing your actions.*

9. The clinician shares, *You have been winding for about 10 minutes now. Note the size of your bundle of string, as you continue to wind.*

- *The string represents brain circuits that are your ED symptoms wired into a brain pathway.*
- *What do you imagine your brain circuit pathway looks like after 10 weeks instead of 10 minutes? 10 months? 10 years?*

## Round 2: Re-Wire

1. While the holder continues to hold the bundle of string, the clinician says to the winder:

   a. *I would like each of the winders to identify a specific action that you could do tonight to reroute yourself away from a ritualized ED symptom.*
   b. *Make it a simple action, because it must compete with your automatic ED ritual that doesn't demand you to think about it.*
   c. *For example, if your ED symptom takes three steps, then try to identify a set of actions that takes three steps or less, such as, self-induced vomiting requires you to (1) go to the location where you vomit, (2) hold back your hair or open the toilet lid, and (3) vomit.*
   d. *What would a three-step productive action be?* (Clients may identify initiating a text and responding two times or walking out of the house with a significant other and walking in one direction and returning.)

2. Clients should be specific in identifying the rerouted actions. For example, exactly what is done and the name of the person(s) they *do* the action with (if relevant).

3. Provide the winder a little time to identify a rerouting action(s) with their partner(s).

4. The clinician asks the winders to share their ideas. The clinician and other clients help each client to be as specific as possible. The clinician then instructs:
   a. *You are beginning to rewire a new circuit of actions.*
   b. *IF the action is completed by you (the winder) alone, then you may say, "After dinner I am typing my paper while playing music I like in my room."*
   c. The clinician instructs the winder to re-wire their plan into action by moving the string from one of the hands of the holder to a new location on the winder. For example, if the client plans to walk to a different room (the wire goes around the winder's leg to represent walking) and type my paper (the string goes to one of the winder's hands) and play music while typing (the string goes to a side object, such as near chair).

5. Once the new route is identified, the clinician shares, *Now that you have identified this specific reroute of re-wiring your actions, repeat the new cycle, or circuit, by saying each step out loud as you wind the string to the next location, re-wiring the new circuit repeatedly to initiate a new habit.*

6. *When forming new habits that become ritualized, you stop focusing on the action(s). They have become automatic, productive rituals to replace ED rituals.*

7. If another person is included in the alternate set of actions, the clinician instructs the winder to
   a. *Identify who is involved and go from one hand of the holder to a hand of another person. It takes more energy to include others, so you need to reach out and wire them into your script.*
   b. For example, the winder may say I'll ask my friend Jill to call me at 6 p.m. and talk with me while I get food out and prepare dinner to keep me from avoiding the meal.
   c. The clinician and other clients help the winder to be as specific as possible, so the brain knows what to do and when in order to re-wire new actions. There is not a magic formula of how to rewire. It is metaphorical. Clients and their Supports become quite creative with rewiring.
   d. *Take the wire from one of the holder's hands and wire it to another person, who is Jill, then back to yourself, such as a hand that is getting food out of the cupboard, and then include an object to wind in a plate and silverware, and then back to Jill repeatedly. Say each thing you are doing out loud as you re-wire so you can hear yourself instruct yourself in preparation of the action you will be doing tonight.*
   e. *Keep rewiring the new circuit, saying the actions over and over just as your brain would consciously focus on managing new actions.*

## Discussion Prompts

- *Can you see yourself clearly doing this new set of actions tonight? Is there anyone you need to text now to prepare to include them? Please do that now.*
- *What is it like for you to include others in the alternative set of actions?*
- *Can the new actions you identified be a rule for you tonight?*
- *How many times would you need to repeat these actions to make them a habit?*
- *When might this new habit become a ritual for you?*
- *Note: if the action varies, it takes new and different circuits.*

- *If you do a different set of actions every night, for seven nights, it would require seven sets of different re-wirings. How long would each set of actions take to each become a habit?*
- *If you do the same set of actions every night, how long would it take to become a habit?*
- *You have a new set of actions that need to become habitual to compete with the huge, bundled ED ritual. The brain needs easy repetitive productive actions to compete with ED symptoms.*
- *If your new set of actions work with some of your traits, it will become easier to re-wire.*
- *Any new action feels similar to what you felt when you began to wire your ED symptom into place. The more you practice new actions, the more habitualized, easier, and ritualized they become, whether productive or destructive.*
- *The brain will automatically return to the default ED actions if it is not consciously directed to re-wire a new action, moment by moment.*

## How to Treat to These Traits

1. The re-wiring of activities may not provide as much relief as an ED symptom.
2. Re-wiring can bring some relief as your body and brain become healthier over time and the actions are congruent with your traits and overall temperament.

   a. For example, if you plan to take actions that require you to interact with lots of people, and you have an introverted trait, then the plan will take more energy and you will be less motivated to do the action because it is counter to how you respond naturally (temperamentally) with others.

   b. If the planned activity is to interact with one or a few people, then it is more congruent with your introverted trait, and it will become ritualized more easily.

**Key Points**
- **The brain is continuously wiring.**
- **Clients have the ability to re-wire their brains, developing new productive habits and rituals.**
- **Clients have the control to re-wire themselves in the present moment, re-wiring second by second as the circuit/string moves along.**
- **The more re-wired actions are congruent with client traits, the easier it is to develop new rituals naturally.**

## Homework

- Practice the new re-wire circuit of actions tonight and over the next two weeks.

## Clinician Notes

_____

_____

_____

_____

# Appendix 18  Stop, Reboot, Reroute: TBT-S Problem-Solving Experiential Activity

Laura Hill

## Neurobiological and Trait Targets
- Tendency to be physically active
- Impulsivity
- Determination
- Attentive/focused

## Objective
- Experience an action to interrupt impulsive reactions.

## Who Is Involved?
- Clinician and one or more clients and/or Supports.
- This could be a virtual or face-to-face activity.
- Students in a classroom.

## Materials and Time Needed
- No materials.
- 10 minutes.

## What Does the Research Say?
- The tendency to be physically active is a trait.

   ○ The brain is structured to utilize *actions before* cognitive solutions can be identified in unexpected new situations.
   ○ The brain integrates sensory information from the external world (e.g., visual cortex, somatosensory and perceptual processing in the parietal cortex) or internal body state (e.g., insula) with cognitive and emotional evaluation (e.g., prefrontal cortex, limbic circuit) to produce a motor response (via the cerebellum, basal ganglia and motor cortex).
   ○ Motor responses can be goal directed (i.e., intentional) or automatic (i.e., impulsive, habit).

- Impulsivity is a trait that is often related to high-intensity or thrill-seeking activities.

   ○ Impulsivity is associated with reduced activation in brain circuits involved in self-regulatory and inhibitory control areas such as the anterior cingulate cortex (ACC) and prefrontal cortex (PFC).

---

A variation of this activity is in the electronic text called, Hill, L. (2017). "*A Brain-Based Approach to Eating Disorders*" at www.BrainBasedEatingDisorders.org

○ Most research approaches impulsivity as reckless or destructive with a need for intense effort to control or the expectation to eliminate impulsivity. However, a trait cannot be eliminated.

○ Many traits, including impulsivity, can be productive. By working *with* the impulsive urge, a person could shift the impulse to be productive. For example, impulsively speaking out for someone who is being falsely criticized.

○ A person with AN could practice using their impulsive trait to help them step into a healthy situation they want themselves to do before anxiety rises up.

- Determination and/or attentive/focused traits are associated with greater cognitive control (opposite end of the spectrum from impulsivity). However, like all traits, they can be used destructively to drive the client toward an ED symptom (e.g., calorie counting) or productively to propel them from the symptom (e.g., adhering to meal plan).

> **Key Point: What seems problematic in one's temperament may serve as the foundation for solutions.**

## Clinician Checklist

⇒ Have the client take the Trait Profile Checklist prior to this activity.
⇒ Learn the game rules.
⇒ Enter the situation playfully.

## Experiential Activity Instructions

### Rules

1. This activity is one where a participant(s) moves around the room while three commands are stated out loud by the clinician. Then the participant says the commands themselves out loud to practice changing directions from going toward a harmful action to walking away, redirecting a destructive/harmful impulse to a productive response.

2. When a client is moving toward a place that can result in a destructive outcome, say out loud, "Stop" (and the person stops), reboot (the person turns around 180°), and reroute (walk forward) and keep walking in the new direction until away from the destructive location.

   a. For example, this can be applied if a client was walking toward a toilet to self-induce vomiting, or toward the kitchen to binge eat.

## Steps and Scripts

1. If the client has identified an impulsive trait, the clinician says, *How has your impulsive trait been expressed recently?* (The client may respond via purging.) *What type of purging do you do impulsively?* (For example, the client may impulsively purchase and then impulsively take laxatives or diuretics or impulsively self-induce vomiting.)

2. *Have you ever used your impulsive trait productively? How?*

3. *Let's try on using your impulsive trait with a tool that sets a structure to redirect your destructive impulse to a different less destructive and possibly more productive response, and see how it fits for you.*

4. *Please stand up and walk forward. I'm going to say, "Stop," then "Reboot," then "Reroute." You are to stop, then turn around 180° and then walk in a new direction.*
5. *After you do it once, I want you to do it again, and you say it out loud while you do it.*
6. *I will try on the tool with you. I'll say the words the first time, and then you lead the tool three times.*

## Discussion Prompt

- Identify a target impulse that is destructive.
- Would this be a tool you could readily utilize to respond to destructive impulses?
- Describe an example of what you would do to apply this tool whether walking or driving or texting.
- Impulsivity is a trait that consists of spontaneous intense responses.
- Identify times when an impulsive response would be helpful.
- Identify actions clients want to move/walk toward. Point out that walking away from a destructive action is productive, even if you are not walking toward something.
- Determination is a powerful trait that pushes the impulse and pushes an action forward to do something more productive and less destructive.
- Focused attention can guide the way out of a problem situation.

### Key Points
- **Impulsive destructive actions can be shifted to impulsive productive actions.**
- **Action, determination, and focused attention are powerful traits that push an impulse forward or backward.**

## Homework
- Practice the activity at least three times a day for the next week.

## Clinician Notes

_____

_____

_____

_____

# Appendix 19 Landmine: TBT-S Problem-Solving Experiential Activity

Laura Hill

## Neurobiological and Trait Targets

These traits could work *against* the client in this situation:

- Altered interoception
- Altered reward response
- Difficulty trusting decisions
- Harm avoidance

These traits could work *for* the client in this situation:

- Determination
- Anxiety
- High achieving
- Attentive/focused

## Objectives

- Experience how to work around and through ED symptoms when faced with unexpected triggers.
- Experience what it takes to successfully manage ED triggers when brain sensations and decision-making are "blinded."
- Identify each client's traits that helped them shift dominant ED tendencies to productive expressions.

## Who Is Involved?

- Clinician and clients who have ED and/or Supports.
- Students in a classroom.
- This is a face-to-face group activity that needs a minimum of six people.

## Materials and Time Needed

- Several objects put on the floor, such as sheets of paper, books, pencils.
- 45 minutes.

---

A variation of this activity is in the electronic text called Hill, L. (2017). "*A Brain-Based Approach to Eating Disorders*" at www.BrainBasedEatingDisorders.org

- Enough room space for all players to line up in two rows (about 4 feet, or a little over one meter, apart) facing one another around the objects on the floor.

## What Does the Research Say?

- *Interoception* is one's ability to accurately experience internal physical sensations, e.g., hunger, pain, fullness, touch. The insula is the hub for interoception. For those with ED, the insula transmits altered signals causing aberrations in one's ability to sense physical sensations accurately, such as hunger, fullness, and pain signals. Without accurate signaling, individuals are "blinded" from experiencing useful body-related guidance. See Figures A19.1, A19.2 and A19.3.

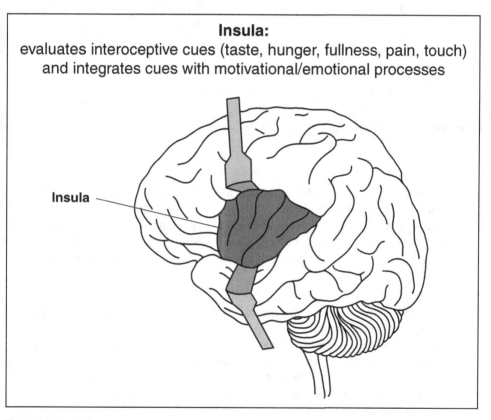

**Figure A19.1** Insula

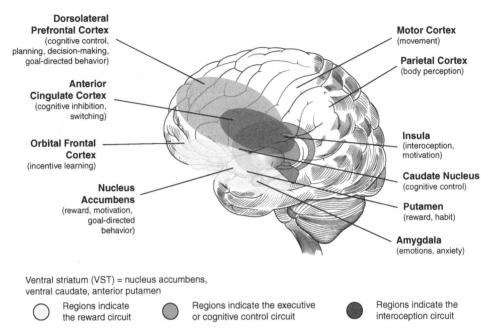

**Figure A19.2** Areas of the brain involved in eating

- The *ventral striatum* signals dopamine which is experienced as pleasure to confirm decisions and increase motivation.
- Persons with AN have reduced ventral striatal reward response to food, suggesting little to no pleasure when eating, or a lack of pleasure to affirm decisions or to motivate a person to act. These weakened circuit responses "blind" the person to trust their decisions.
- The tendency to be physically active is a trait.
  - The brain is structured to utilize *actions before* cognitive solutions can be identified in unexpected new situations.
  - The brain integrates sensory information from the external world (e.g., visual cortex, somatosensory and perceptual processing in the parietal cortex) or internal body state (e.g., insula) with cognitive and emotional evaluation (e.g., prefrontal cortex, limbic circuit) to produce a motor response (via the cerebellum, basal ganglia, and motor cortex).
  - Physical activity serves to help solve the problem, by moving the person through the event allowing clients to cognitively recognizing their own productive solutions around the eating disorder triggers.

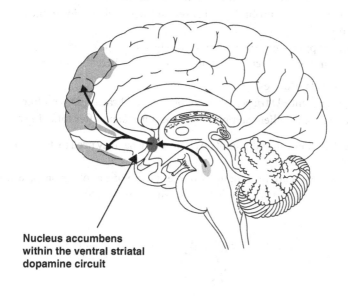

**Reward (limbic) Circuit:**
identifies and valuates rewarding or emotionally significant stimuli and generates emotional response

Nucleus accumbens
within the ventral striatal
dopamine circuit

**Figure A19.3** Reward circuit

Key Point: The ED brain has altered neurocircuit responses "blinding" motivation and sensations that inform one's ability to know what to do and contributes to ED symptoms.

## Clinician Checklist

⇒ Have clients complete the Trait Profile Checklist prior to this game (Appendix 2).
⇒ Practice sharing the neurobiological research outlined earlier that sets the foundation for this activity.
⇒ Memorize "key points" to share with players at the end.
⇒ Memorize the steps to allow fluency and fun. Do not read each step.
⇒ Orchestrate group discussion.

## Experiential Activity Instructions

### Rules

1. The landmine game metaphorically enacts the difficulty of getting over and around ED triggers (landmines) that when stepped on explode and cause the person to go backward (ED symptom). The game also allows clients with ED to actively experiment to discover

exactly what it takes to get through the landmines (such as drawing upon Supports and their own productive traits).

2. The goal of the game is to get around the landmines to the other side – while "blinded" (with eyes closed).

3. Instruct clients and/or Supports to form two lines, about 4 feet (4 meters) apart, facing each other. The space between the lines is the "landmine field."

4. The clinician reviews the neurobiological bases outlined earlier prior to the activity or in a former session.

5. All clients and/or Supports are asked to bring objects, such as pieces of paper, wads of paper, books, or pencils and scatter them randomly on the floor where the activity will take place.

   • The objects are landmines.
   • Landmines represent ED triggers that can blow up and cause ED symptoms.
   • ED symptoms are the client stepping backward five steps after touching a landmine.

6. Clients explore what they can and cannot do alone, and what they need to do to win the game. See Figure A19.4.

7. Clients and/or Supports are to stand in two lines facing one another on each side of the objects. It does not matter who stands next to whom. If needed, a player could sit.

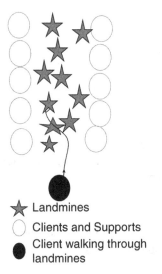

★ Landmines
◯ Clients and Supports
● Client walking through landmines

**Figure A19.4** Landmine sketch, client solo, uncompleted meal

8. This activity works with the brain's natural tendency to utilize actions to identify solutions in order to create a cognitive plan.

## Steps and Scripts

1. The clinician asks the clients and/or Supports to set up the landmine field and stand on both sides facing each other.

2. The clinician identifies a client to come to one end of the landmines. The first client should be one who is motivated to participate.

3. *The goal of this game is to get to the other side without touching a landmine.*
4. *The objects are landmines or eating disorder triggers. If you step on one, it triggers an explosion of an ED symptom.*
5. *IF you touch a landmine, you are to step backwards 5 steps just as an ED symptom takes you backwards.*
6. *As you have begun to learn, your ED symptoms tend to be caused by altered brain circuits that diminish your ability to sense body signals, such as hunger, fullness, or pain.*
7. *These alterations blind your ability to trust your decisions, triggering ED symptoms.*
8. *Hence when entering unexpected, highly triggering situations, you are blind to clearly know what to do. To reflect your brain responses, when you go through the landmine, you are to have your eyes closed.*
9. *I'm going to describe a difficult situation for you to get through.*
10. *Your friends have just told you that they want you to join them now to go to a restaurant. You have never been there; you do not know the menu to help you plan what to eat. You have no time to look at menu online before you leave.*

   a. The clinician asks the identified client, *What are you thinking at this moment?* (Not feeling but thinking).
   b. The clinician takes 3–4 of the client's thoughts and assigns each "thought" to one or more persons standing in the two lines.
   c. The clinician states to the client, *When you get to the other end of this passage of landmines you will have ordered, eaten and completed the meal. You will have won the game.*

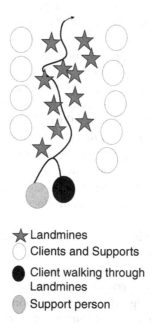

★ Landmines
◯ Clients and Supports
● Client walking through Landmines
◉ Support person

**Figure A19.5** Landmine sketch, with Support, completed meal

d. To the players in the two lines: *When I say "go," all of you standing on the sides are to begin saying your assigned thoughts loudly and repeatedly.*

e. To the client: *When I say go, begin walking with your eyes closed toward the other side. Just in case you have begun to memorize where the landmines are (which is a good idea!) I am going to move them again after you close your eyes.*

f. *If you step on or touch a landmine, then I'll say "Stop!" All thoughts become quiet and you back up 5 steps. If you touch another landmine, you go back 5 more steps.*

g. *"Stop" means thoughts become quiet just like when doing an ED symptom, such as purging.*

h. *Everyone ready? Now close your eyes and . . . begin!*

11. Clients have never gotten through the landmine field without stepping on landmines.

12. <u>The clinician does not offer suggestions.</u> The clinician provides the structure and establishes a playful setting for the client to experiment problem solutions.

13. When the client takes 5 steps backward, the clinician immediately prompts:

a. *Okay, now move forward. GO!*

b. Use few words, and simple commands, in a playful way. The client can begin to integrate those words into their own mind to move forward after ED symptoms are expressed outside of treatment.

14. Allow the client to experiment getting through the landmines up to three times. After stepping back the third time –

15. The clinician asks, *What do you need to <u>do</u> to get through the landmines?*

a. Nearly 100 percent of the time the adult client says something like, "I need Support."

b. The clinician asks, *Who do you choose to ask for Support*? The client still has eyes closed and chooses a Support person. If the person is not present, the clinician assigns a person to represent the identified Support person.

c. *Tell the Support person what you need them to do to help you through.*

d. The client explains to the Support person what to do. The clinician asks the Support person, *Do you understand? If so, Okay, GO!*

e. Note: A client's initial instructions to Supports tend to be minimal assistance. Clients figure out themselves, via active experimentation, what type and how much assistance are actually needed to get through the difficult situation.

f. The client begins walking forward through the landmines with the Support doing what the client has asked for guidance. See Figure A19.5.

g. Many times the client still steps on a landmine.

h. If the client steps on a landmine, the clinician says in the same instructive voice to the client, *Okay, step back 5 steps.* The Support does not help since ED symptoms are expressed alone.

i. Supports often express guilt at this point. The clinician does not step back to process the comment but remains focused on the action to move forward.

j. The clinician asks the client, *Is there anything more you need from your Support or is the assistance you are getting what you need?*

k. Clients tend to be increasingly detailed. Instructions range from "hold my hand and guide me with your voice and hand movements," to the Support picking up the client's foot and putting it over the landmine, to the client asking the Support to carry the client over the landmines.

16. Change arrangements of the landmines and repeat steps 10–15 for each client.

   a. Note: While it seems that each subsequent client will go right to the bottom line and ask for Support persons for assistance, that response almost never happens among SE-AN clients. Each adult client is convinced they can get through the landmines on their own until they personally experience the landmines, try repeatedly and fail.

   b. Since it is a game and the atmosphere is fun, the opportunity to change responses carries less guilt that their attempt was not perfect the first time.

   c. Note: Each subsequent adult client tends to ask the minimal amount of assistance until they experience themselves that they need more assistance and have to ask for it.

## Discussion Prompts

1. While still standing on the other side of the landmine field after the client has won the game, the clinician asks the client any or all of the following questions:

   - *Was that in any way similar to what you experience when you try to go through a new and difficult situation?*
   - *What was walking through the landmines alone like for you?*
   - *What was it like moving forward compared to backward?*
   - *What did it take for you to win?* Clients usually state, "Supports were needed."
   - *Which of your traits did you use to get yourself through the landmines?* Refer them to their Trait Profile Checklist for them to identify their own productively used traits (e.g., determination, persistence, anxious energy, focus).
   - *What does success feel like, having made it through?* Often clients report, exhausting, hard, difficult, and distressing.

2. The clinician asks the Supports any or all of the following questions:

   - *What was this experience like for you?*
   - *What helped you?*
   - *What observations do you have of what the client did to get through?*
   - *If the client is experiencing something new tonight or this week, what will you do?*
   - Check with the client to see if the Support's response is acceptable. Clarify if the client needs to ask for assistance from the Support, or when the client needs the Support to step in and offer identified assistance.

3. The clinician asks the other clients and Supports:

   - *What did you observe from the client and Support getting through the landmines?*
   - *What were your observations and insights as you said the client's inner thoughts out loud repeatedly?*

4. Client and Support actions are now clarified to help solve the problem of who does what in new and difficult situations.

## How to Treat to These Traits

1. Clinicians should draw upon the client's own solutions from this activity and their own traits used to get through the landmines.

2. Clinicians could affirm clients' altered interoception and altered ventral striatal responses are blinding their ability to sense fundamental signals that are necessary to know what to do, yet they identified how to compensate by recognizing what they need and when and how they need to ask for assistance.

3. Explain the brain is able to re-wire new actions for all ages each time the client repeatedly acts on their newly identified solutions.

4. Clients may benefit by going to the same restaurant and ordering the same meal a few times to practice how to get through the meal better each time. Eventually clients may be able to go to that restaurant without Supports, having practiced enough times how to maneuver around the landmines.

5. Clinicians work with the clients to identify which of their productive traits from the client Trait Profile Checklist they used to help them through these highly triggered experiences. For example:

   a. Anxiety combined with determination

   b. High achievement and or attentive/focused traits to motivate and push forward

---

**Key Points**
- Clients can intentionally use their own productive traits as assets to move forward.
- A structured game can provide SE-AN clients with a means to identify when and how to ask for assistance that offers Supports specific instructions to help their loved ones maneuver around new ED triggers.
- Successfully getting over ED symptoms is hard. It takes focus, assistance, and practice.

---

## Homework
- Clients practice, practice, practice their identified solutions.
- Clients utilize their productive traits and their Supports.
- Supports practice what the client instructed them to do to assist through difficult new situations.

## Clinician Notes

_____

_____

_____

_____

# Appendix 20 Social Gauntlet: TBT-S Problem-Solving Experiential Activity

Laura Hill

## Neurobiological and Trait Targets
- A tendency to be physically active
- Persistence and determination
- Altered set shifting

## Objectives
- Experience passing through multiple and continuous social messages on body image, weight, etc.
- Experience how each person successfully manages through continuous negative social body image messages.
- Identify each client's traits that helped them successfully manage social body and weight pressures.

## Who Is Involved?
- Clinician and a minimum of six clients and/or Supports.
- Students in classroom setting.
- This is a face-to-face group activity.

## Materials and Time Needed
- No materials.
- 10–15 minutes.

## What Does the Research Say?
- The tendency to be physically active is a trait.
  - The brain is structured to utilize *actions before* cognitive solutions can be identified in unexpected new situations.
  - The brain integrates sensory information from the external world (e.g., visual cortex, somatosensory and perceptual processing in the parietal cortex) or internal body state (e.g., insula) with cognitive and emotional evaluation (e.g., prefrontal cortex, limbic circuit) to produce a motor response (via the cerebellum, basal ganglia, and motor cortex). Movement/actions serve to help meet one's goals (e.g., how to get through the gauntlet).
  - Learning is enhanced by repeating the same movements. This practiced behavior modifies the brain to develop more efficient pathways to respond.

---

A variation of this activity is in the electronic text called Hill, L. (2017). "*A Brain-Based Approach to Eating Disorders*" at www.BrainBasedEatingDisorders.org

- Determination and persistence are traits that can propel a person forward to health or backward into relapse.
  ○ Persistence enhances vigilance and assertive-like actions that can work for the client when intentionally expressed, such as by moving toward a specific daily goal. It works against the client when left unmanaged, contributing to persistent maladaptive thoughts and ED symptoms.
  ○ Persistence is also related to motor activity and the ability to continue an action.
- Set shifting is one's ability to shift thoughts and actions from one topic to another with ease. The cognitive circuit (including the dorsolateral prefrontal cortex and anterior cingulate) is involved in set shifting.
  ○ Research shows that individuals with AN have difficulty shifting thoughts and behaviors. This manifests as perseverative or repetitive thoughts and actions that are sometimes described as being "stuck in set." Difficulty with set shifting is associated with altered frontal-striatal activation.
  ○ External prompts may be needed to interrupt stuck thoughts, such as by asking the client a question or touching one's arm to redirect rigid focus.

Figure A20.1 shows the dorsolateral prefrontal cortex and anterior cingulate cortex involved in cognitive set shifting.

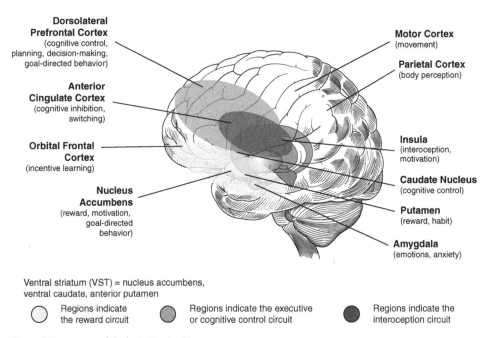

**Figure A20.1** Areas of the brain involved in eating

---

**Key Point: Movement and persistence can serve to push through seemingly impossible tasks, one step at a time.**

## Clinician Checklist

⇒ Know game rules and approach the structured treatment intervention in a playful manner.

⇒ Create two lines about 3 feet (or one meter) apart for clients to walk between. The space serves as the "plank" for clients to walk through during the game.

## Experiential Activity Instructions

### Rules

1. This is a game that uses the medieval platform of a gauntlet as a means to experiment how to get to the other side without being pushed off the plank.

2. A gauntlet was a plank or tunnel-like path surrounded by harsh objects, such as axes and mallets swinging or people flailing sticks and weapons. A person who had broken the law was to "run the gauntlet." If an object knocked him off, or if beaten down, he was guilty. If he was able to maneuver through the gauntlet, he was freed. See Figure A20.2.

3. This activity is a metaphor for daily client experiences running a "social gauntlet" of messages that demonize size, shape, personal identity, or race and ethnicity, via texts, Instagram, Facebook, etc. How does one get through the social gauntlet on a daily basis?

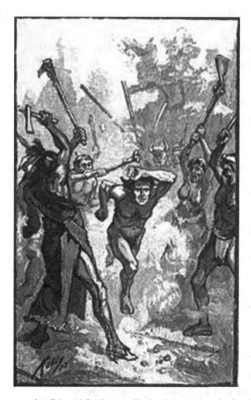

**Figure A20.2** Running the gauntlet. Edward Eggleston, Elizabeth Eggleston Seelye, *Tecumseh and the Shawnee Prophet*, 1878.

4. Players are instructed to form two lines, about 3 feet (one meter) apart. One or more players are assigned to say a social message repeatedly, such as, "I look huge" or "Too fat!" Everyone is assigned a social message. The same message is said by multiple people.

   a. As players say the social message words assigned, and stand in the two lines facing one another, they are to move forward and backward one-two steps randomly (not in order).

   b. This is the metaphor that negative and harmful social messages "attack" or bump a person off track randomly throughout each day.

   c. The players moving back and forth represents the gauntlet of weapons attacking the person along the path.

5. A person is chosen to come to one end and run the social gauntlet to see if and how they can get through the social, negative messages of the day.

   a. Note: Many with AN and other EDs have a competitive trait and want to "win" by getting through, in spite of inhibition or avoidant traits.

6. Every client is to run the social gauntlet, since no one gets to avoid the social negative messages in most days.

## Steps and Scripts

1. Clinician asks, *Does anyone know what it means to "run the gauntlet"?*
2. Clinician reflects client answers to formulate a playful definition.
3. The clinician then explains the game rules for a social gauntlet as a metaphor for the medieval game.
4. Clients and/or Supports line up in two lines facing one another, with their negative social words assigned, prepared to move back and forth. The clinician could say,

   a. *Now that each of you has a social message to say repeatedly, you are to repeatedly move forward and backward 1–2 steps as you say the messages.*

   b. *This enacts the weapons beating the person who is running the gauntlet. You are getting in the client's way with negative messages, interrupting and potentially getting the person off course.*

   c. *Winning means the client figures out how to maneuver around the pressures and messages of the social system during one episode of time.*

5. The clinician chooses a client to run the gauntlet first, instructing the client to stand at one end of the gauntlet.
6. *Your goal is to get to the other side. You must stay inside the gauntlet because you face these messages every day, so it is time you face them head on. Do what you need to do to get through.*
7. After each person runs the gauntlet, ask the discussion questions listed next.
8. Summarize with the key point, *"When in doubt, keep moving!"*

## Discussion Prompts

- (Directed at each client after they have finished running the gauntlet:

  o *What did it take for you to get through the gauntlet?* (Common answers are focus, determination, or just kept moving to get through.)

  o *What was it like for you to run the gauntlet?* (Not how did you feel.)

- ○ *What traits of yours got you through?*
- ○ *What did those in the gauntlet observe that the client did to get through the gauntlet?*
- ○ *How do you see yourself using your solutions that you just played out, from the moment you leave today when faced with ongoing social messages?*
- Summarize the key points (share them, do not read them).
- A key point is that an intense interaction requires focus. Focusing intentionally can guide one through uncomfortable situations.
- What would clients like their Supports to do to help them interrupt or refocus their thoughts or actions?

## How to Treat to These Traits

- Identify what traits each client drew upon to run the gauntlet. The client's temperament can be a source for solutions.
- If clients are aware of their constructive traits, they can continue to practice those traits productively (see Trait Profile Checklist, Appendix 2).
- Since clients with ED tend to have problems with set shifting, this can be used to their advantage by identifying specific targets upon which to focus daily, shifting their thoughts to work for them instead of against themselves – for example, getting a work assignment completed.
- Intentional action increases focus.
- A playful activity gives clients the opportunity to experience their traits in action and clarifies *how* they utilized their own traits to solve the problem.
- Identify circumstances in the day when social messages increase for the client (for example, when texting, or viewing Instagram or Snapshot, or on Facebook).
  - ○ Identify two of the things you did and now want to do when in those social messaging circumstances.
  - ○ What two traits do you want to utilize to get through without being "pulled down" by negative messages?

### Key Points
- When in doubt, keep moving.
- Movement/action can push one through difficult situations, and shift thoughts in the process.
- Persistence can empower a person to intentionally push through social messages.

## Homework

- Practice using your two identified traits in each social messaging situation over the next week.
- Use the same methods you used to move through the gauntlet when you are social messaging over the next week.

## Clinician Notes

_____
_____
_____
_____

# Appendix 21  Charades: TBT-S  Problem-Solving Experiential Activity

Laura Hill

## Neurobiological and Trait Targets
- The tendency to be physically active
- Learning through practice

## Objectives
- Actively demonstrate and practice all of the tools in the TBT-S toolbox.
- Identify TBT-S tools when demonstrated.

## Who Is Involved?
- Clinician and clients with ED and/or Supports.
- This could be a virtual individual or group activity, as well as face-to-face.
- Two or more players.
- Students in educational settings.

## Materials and Time Needed
- A list of tools/skills the clinician wants clients and/or Supports to practice with enough copies for each client and/or Support. (See list example at end of this activity.)
- Each tool is cut into separate tool labels.
- Optional: the list is copied onto magnetic paper, allowing it to stick to the refrigerator.
- Note: if this is a virtual group session, the clients and/or Supports do the cutting after making their own list from their toolbox, or after the clinician emails a list of the tools/skills identified.
- 20 minutes.

## What Does the Research Say?
- The tendency to be physically active is a trait and a way to behaviorally expresses thoughts, feelings, perceptions, and needs.
- Physical activity and movement cause neurons to fire together. With practice, these neurons that fire together wire together. This is the brain basis for learning.
- Practicing a new skill or behavior, rather than talking about it, is the most effective way to re-wire the brain to turn skills into habits.

> ### Key Points
> - Movement, or activity, is a core trait that behaviorally expresses thoughts and feelings.
> - When the same actions are repeated, habits are formed as the brain shifts from reliance on goal-directed circuits to habit circuits.
> - The brain efficiently and quickly wires productive and destructive habits into place.

## Clinician Checklist

⇒ Have copies of the list of TBT-S and/or other tools/skills prepared, or have the client generate the list.

⇒ If face-to-face, the list could be copied onto magnetic paper for clients and/or Supports to put on their refrigerators.

⇒ Cut each tool/skill into separate rectangles (referred to as tool labels).

⇒ Learn the game rules so you do not have to read the steps and lead in a playful manner.

## Experiential Activity Instructions
### Rules

1. Charades is a game of pantomime where a player "acts out" a word or phrase without speaking, while the other player(s) try to guess what the word/phrase is. The goal is to be the first player to guess the word or phrase.

2. This TBT-S activity is a variation of Charades. The purpose of this version is to provide a fun way for clients to practice tools/skills playfully, while other clients and/or Supports can become increasingly aware of different tools/skills that could be used to manage ED symptoms and to observe how others act them out, while guessing what the tool is.

3. Disseminate a set of tool labels to each player.

4. Have each player lay the tool labels out on a table face up. This allows the players to choose which tool they want to act out. Observers use the face up tool labels to identify what is being acted out.

5. In this version, every client and/or Support receives the paper (or magnet) tool labels instead of the leader being the only one who sees the tool.

6. The clinician chooses the first person to play. That person chooses one of the tool labels that is face up, without others seeing and begins to act out the tool/or skill.

7. The first to guess the tool is the next person to act out a tool.

8. Once a tool has been acted out, everyone turns that label face down, so that it cannot be chosen again.

9. The game continues until all tools/skills are played.

10. The clients and/or Supports then turn all tools face up again.

   a. Each chooses three tools they want to practice over the next two weeks.

   b. If the tools are printed on magnet paper, the clients and Supports are encouraged to take them home and put them on the refrigerator, arranged so the top tools are easy to see from the others.

## Steps and Scripts

1. The clinician asks, *"Who has played Charades?"* Identify a player who answers in the affirmative, to explain the game rules. (This encourages clients to take the lead immediately.)

2. *This activity is a variation of Charades.*

   a. *The goal of this TBT-S version of Charades is similar in that clients and/or Supports identify a word, in this case it is a tool/skill, and the others guess what the tool is as the person acts it out. In this case, a word is not acted out; the actual tool is acted out to show how it can be applied.*

  b. *The rules of this version are adjusted so you can in fact speak out loud when enacting the tool or skill (such as active listening) and you can recruit another person to assist if that is how the tool is applied.*
  c. *In this version, everyone gets the tool labels. Lay them out, <u>face up</u>.*

2. Disseminate the tool/skills printed and cut in tool labels.

  a. *The designated person chooses one of the tools and acts it out.*
  b. *The other players are to guess what the tool is.*
  c. *The person who guesses first is the next to enact a tool. The label of the tool acted out is then turned face down by everyone so that it is not chosen again.*
  d. *The game ends after every tool is played and all labels are face down.*

3. After the last tool is played, the clinician says, *Now turn all the tool labels face up again.*

  a. *Choose three tools you need to practice for the next two weeks.*
  b. *By repeatedly practicing the same tool, it will begin to become a habit after a couple of weeks.*

## Discussion Prompts

• When do you plan to use one of your top three tools this week?
• Was there a way one of the clients played out the tool that you had not considered?
• Which of your traits enable you to use the traits you identified (if the clients have taken the Trait Profile Checklist)? The more the tools you choose that align with the clients' traits, the more natural it will be to apply them.

## How to Treat to These Traits

1. Activity helps integrate thoughts and memory[139] and diminish inhibition. Activity is the core of this game.
2. By playfully enacting the tools, they are less "work" and have been "tried on" to see which ones "fit" better than others. Fit means congruent to one's traits.

> ### Key Points and Notes for Clinician
> • Client tools are critical skills that need to be "tried on" and practiced to reduce ED symptoms.
> • How and when to apply tools/skills can be broadened by watching others' actions.

## Homework

• Practice the top three identified tools/skills for the next two weeks.

## Clinician Notes

_____
_____
_____
_____

# Appendix 22 What Will You Do? TBT-S Problem-Solving Experiential Activity

Stephanie Knatz Peck and Laura Hill

## Neurobiological and Trait Targets

- Decision-making
- Anxiety
- Attention to detail (low central cohesion)

## Objectives

- Explore "what to do" in upcoming difficult situations by requesting ideas from other clients.
- Plan how to incorporate one's own traits when exploring new actions.
- Practice asking for help.

## Who Is Involved?

- Clients.
- Supports.
- This is a group activity that could be offered virtually, face-to-face or in a classroom.

## Materials and Time Needed

- Enough pieces of paper, or post-it notes for each person to write a note to each member in the assigned group.
- Pencils/pens for each group member.
- Container to hold the paper.
- This activity takes 1 to 1½ hours.

## What Does the Research Say?

- Due to altered neural circuit responses in the ventral striatal, limbic, and prefrontal cortex areas, clients with AN often have difficulty trusting their decisions.
- Reward signals in the ventral striatum tend to over-fire (in individuals who engage in binge eating) and tend to under-fire (in individuals with restricting-type AN), which makes it difficult for the client to experience confidence when making a decision. Altered reward signaling may leave the client uncertain about whether a decision is a good one or a bad one. The client can think through a decision cognitively but tends to not have an internal cue that confirms a decision. This decreases certainty and increases doubt in the decision.
- Temperament traits may influence altered neural circuit function and decision-making.

A variation of this activity is in the electronic text, Hill, L. (2017). "*A Brain-Based Approach to Eating Disorders*" at www.BrainBasedEatingDisorders.org

○ If the client has a perfectionistic trait and is unable to sense a reward response, the need to know the "right" response may be heighted, along with a fear of making errors.

○ If the client has an inhibited trait, decisions may be delayed or avoided to prevent making mistakes or taking erroneous actions.

> **Key Points**
> - **Persons with AN experience altered brain circuit responses that cause a tendency to mistrust decisions.**
> - **Relying on trusted others for help is an effective way of compensating for difficulty in trusting one's decisions.**

## Clinician Checklist

⇒ Have paper and pencils/pens for all group members.

⇒ Divide the group in half.

⇒ If the group is larger than 10 persons, divide the group into three units.

## Experiential Activity Instructions

### Rules

1. This game is about learning to ask others for help and developing a plan of action to offset uncertainty around decision-making.
2. The activity is played out after the TBT-S Toolbox, the Trait Profile Checklist, SE-AN or YA Behavioral Agreement, and neurobiological psychoeducation have been shared and practiced.
3. The group is divided in half.
4. Each group member is directed to ask a question to a member of the other group, related to unresolved questions or concerns about what to do when outside of treatment. For example how will X-person handle lunch when at work?
5. Each group member writes a question to each member of the other group. For example each person in group A asks a question directed to each person in group B.
6. The questions that each group member poses could be the same question for each person, different questions for each person, or a combination of both.
7. Ensure that each member has enough pieces of paper to write each member in the assigned subgroup a question.
8. If the game is played virtually, questions are typed and sent to the clinician.

### Steps and Scripts

1. Post the list of subgroup members for all to see (clients and optional Supports).
2. Have the *core statement*, "What would you do?" posted for all to see.
3. The clinician gives the following game instructions:
   a. *A TBT-S tool is to ask others for help. In this game, you are asking for ideas from others in the group.*
   b. **Write a question for each person in the other subgroup, asking how that person may approach, or respond to, an issue or concern that you have.**

c. *The question may be about how or when a person would use a TBT-S tool or, you may feel uncertain about how to approach a situation. Ask a person who you think might have a solution.*

d. *Write the person's name. to whom you are directing your question, at the top of your note. You do not need to sign your own name as the questioner.*

4. Allow about 10 minutes for the participants to write their questions.
5. Have the group members email the clinician the questions, if they are participating virtually. If face-to-face, have a group member gather the pieces of paper from the other participants.
6. If face-to-face, the clients and/or Supports sit in a circle and pass the basket of questions. A question is taken out and read by one participant at a time.

a. *For example, Jane, let's start with you. Please take a slip of paper from the basket. State who the question is directed to and read the question aloud for all participants to hear.*

b. *Then the person to whom the question is directed offers an answer based on what they have learned in treatment, practiced in treatment, wants to try on, or based on what has been successful for the person in the past.*

c. *If the person has no idea of what to say, they can ask for help from another person.*

7. The clinician follows up on most questions after a group member answers them, by asking, *What traits are required to carry out that recommended response?*
8. One by one, persons ask a question. Go around the group multiple times until either all questions have been asked or the allotted time has been used up.

## Discussion Prompts

- The clinician makes the point that each person's answers may help everyone in the group.
- The person answering should share a response that is true for themselves not what they think should be.
- The suggested answers may be a good fit for some clients more than others, based on each client's temperament profile of traits.
- SE-AN clients are experts. They have temperament resources to draw upon and experiences that can point to what works and what does not work.

## How to Treat to These Traits

- The clinician stresses that traits are central in implementing the suggested answers.
- Encourage group members to explore suggested client solutions that have a good fit with their own temperaments.

## Homework

- Each client is to try on the client and/or Support recommendations to their questions if the recommendations are congruent with the client's own temperament.

## Clinician Notes

# Appendix 23 Expert Client Advice: TBT-S Problem-Solving Experiential Activity

Stephanie Knatz Peck and Laura Hill

### Neurobiological and Trait Targets
- Attention to detail
- Intelligent and high achieving

### Objective
- To provide a structure for each adult client with AN to convey their expertise to increase understanding among Supports.

### Who Is Involved?
- This is a group activity.
- Supports and adult clients with AN.
- This could be a virtual or face-to-face activity.

### Materials and Time Needed
- No materials.
- About 45 minutes to one hour for a group of eight clients and Supports.

### What Does the Research Say?
- Persons with SE-AN report pride in their achievements in spite of the chronicity of their illness.[181]
- AN is associated with increased years of education.[170] This is related to high achievement and potential ability to articulate thoughts and feelings.
- Persons with AN have enhanced attention to details allowing them to describe things in detail.

> **Key Point:** AN adult clients are intelligent and experts in knowing their own symptoms, allowing them to describe their experiences to help others understand AN.

### Clinician Checklist
⇒ Anxiety Wave Experiential Activity needs to be completed prior to this activity. The handouts Anxiety Wave Symptoms and Anxiety Wave Responses should be completed prior to this activity.

---

A variation of this activity is in the electronic text: Hill, L. (2017). "*A Brain-Based Approach to Eating Disorders*" at www.BrainBasedEatingDisorders.org

⇒ Clinicians assign each client to a different client's Support(s), matching Support(s) who could relate with that specific client.

⇒ Prepare an assignment list for the whole group showing which adult client is matched with which Support(s).

⇒ Send (if virtual) or hand out the completed Anxiety Wave Response worksheet, written by the client of the Support person with whom the newly assigned client will be working. The Supports in the group should also have a copy of their own loved ones' worksheets.

## Experiential Activity Instructions
### Rules

1. The purpose of this activity is to provide an opportunity and structure for Supports to practice responses recommended by their loved one, while being coached by clients who are not their loved ones. Unrelated clients are more likely to be objective and understanding.
2. Adult clients are introduced as experts on AN.
3. Assign a client to another client's Support(s).
4. The activity is over when all the response recommendations on the Anxiety Wave Responses Worksheet have been practiced within each subgroup.

### Steps and Scripts

1. The clinician assigns client/Support(s) combinations. Some clients may have more than one Support. If there are multiple Supports for the same client, they should be grouped together with the assigned new client to hear the same feedback and advice simultaneously.
2. The assignment list is posted virtually, or on a board if face-to-face.
3. The clinician disseminates (or emails if virtual session) each client's Anxiety Wave Response worksheet to the newly assigned client and Support(s).
   Client A → Trains Support(s) of Client B → Using the Anxiety Wave Response worksheet of Client B.
4. The clinician asks clients to sit with their assigned Supports or virtually creates subgroupings of assigned participants.
5. The clinician offers the following instructions: *Supports, your loved one has listed responses that you could do, that would help them when their anxiety is high, and when their anxiety is low. You have been assigned to an "outside" ED expert who is going to coach you on how to offer these responses. You are to practice with your assigned coach to refine your responses. Ask questions of the ED expert who will offer answers drawing from their own experiences. If the ED expert does not have an answer, call upon the clinician for back up assistance. Please practice at least two recommended responses for both high and low anxiety. Okay, let's begin.*
6. The clinician is to rearrange the subgroup so that each client is with their own Support(s).
7. The clinician instructs: *Now that Supports have been coached by ED experts, Supports, it is time to rejoin your own loved one and practice two of the responses that your loved one has recommended when their anxiety is high, and two responses when anxiety is low.*

## Discussion Prompts

- At the end of the exercise, the clinician instructs clients to use the "critique tool" with their own Support(s) responses. Clients:

  o What Support responses helped?
  o What Support responses didn't help?
  o What do you want Supports to do differently?

- Directed to all clients and Supports, which of your own traits did you need to draw upon to respond as needed?

## How to Treat to These Traits

- Experiment.
- Adjust based on feedback.
- Practice.

## Homework

- Supports are to practice new responses with their loved ones when their anxiety is increasing.

## Clinician Notes

_____
_____
_____
_____

# Appendix 24 Communicating and Listening: Young Adult TBT-S Experiential Activity Addressing Family Relationships

Stephanie Knatz Peck

## Neurobiological and Trait Targets
- Anxiety
- Agreeable, cooperative
- Conscientious

## Objectives
- Practice assertive communication and effective listening.
- Facilitate discussion and feedback between clients and parents to improve their relationship in the recovery process.
- Negotiate and describe an effective recovery relationship through the YA Behavioral Agreement.

## Who Is Involved?
- Clients and parents.

## Materials and Time Needed
- Paper/writing utensils.
- 60 minutes.
- This activity could be implemented virtually or face-to-face, client/parent outpatient to group settings in all levels of care.
- This activity could be implemented in a client/parent or group therapy setting.

## What Does the Research Say?
- Improving communication between clients and parents is a dimension of the individual and family healing relationship that reduces anxiety.
- Research evaluating skills training for carers of people with AN suggests that improving communication reduces distress, caregiving burden, and difficulties associated with eating disorder symptoms.
- Clients of parents who received intervention that focused on improved communication held positive attitudes toward the interventions. Intervening on communication may also improve outcomes for adults with AN.
- Clients' and parents' productive traits, such as conscientiousness and agreeableness/cooperativeness are underlying triggers or prompts that carry them through this process.

> **Key Point:** Effective communication between clients and parents is important to negotiate to have an effective recovery relationship.

## Clinician Checklist

⇒ Teach assertiveness and validation.

⇒ Assign individuals or group members to identify a request of their loved ones that is related to recovery and to write it using the "DEARMAN" format.

⇒ Assign group members to practice assertiveness and validation by sharing their DEARMAN script.

⇒ Facilitate discussion and feedback.

## Experiential Activity Instructions

### DEARMAN (Assertiveness Skill)

- DEARMAN is a Dialectical Behavior Therapy skill from the Interpersonal Effectiveness module. DEARMAN is an assertiveness skill that is applied by asking for something or asserting "no."
- It is intended to teach individuals how to find a balance between meeting their needs and preserving important relationships.
- DEARMAN is one method of teaching assertiveness that is effective for AN because it is highly structured.
- DEARMAN is an acronym where each letter represents a different aspect of assertiveness.
- It provides a structured method for individuals to practice assertiveness.
- The individual or group learns about each aspect of the DEARMAN skill and its rationale:
  - ○ <u>D</u>escribe the problem. (Provide a background of the issue or situation, answering the five Ws.)
  - ○ <u>E</u>xpress the importance of the need. (Express how the person would feel if this request was met.)
  - ○ <u>A</u>ssert one's need. (Clearly and simply make the request.)
  - ○ <u>R</u>einforce the need. (How this will benefit the other party?)
  - ○ <u>M</u>indfulness. (Practice staying focused on one topic.)
  - ○ <u>A</u>ct confident. (Express needs with confidence.)
  - ○ <u>N</u>egotiate. (Learn specific tools to negotiate, like asking questions such as, *"What would you need in order to grant me this request?"* or *"If this isn't possible, what would be possible?"*)

### Validation Skill

- Validation is explained to the individual or group as the reciprocal skill to DEARMAN for the person hearing/receiving the communicated statements.
- Discuss and practice the purpose of validation and how to express validation.

### Steps

1. Review the importance of assertiveness and validation in effective communication.

2. Clinicians teach the **DEARMAN and Validation skills** to the individual client/parent or group using client-chosen examples. (20–30 minutes)
3. **Construct a DEARMAN:** each participant is asked to reflect on something they would like to ask of their loved ones, or a specific request related to recovery, and use the DEARMAN format to frame the request.
4. If in a group format, each group member who is not directly involved in the DEARMAN exchange is assigned to be an observer. Observers are to intervene when necessary by providing suggestions and assistance to ensure success. Clinicians instruct observers to interrupt ineffective interactions and encourage if the speaker is effective. The client/parent speakers are encouraged to access their observers for help and can pause to seek advice during the DEARMAN interactions. Observers are instructed to provide feedback and constructive criticism at the end of each DEARMAN to both the presenter and the person practicing validation.
5. Practice using DEARMAN and Validation as two skills for Effective Communication:
   a. Each person practices making a request or asserting a need using the DEARMAN.
   b. Client(s) is(are) encouraged to use their script as little or as much as needed, with responses ranging from reading the script to simply holding it in their lap for reference.
   c. The parent(s) is(are) instructed to respond by using validation.
   d. If in a group setting, other family/group members provide feedback to one another after the exercise
   e. If in a group setting, the exercise is repeated until all clients have practiced DEARMAN and all parents have practiced Validation.

## Discussion Prompts and Scripts (scripts in italics)

- After the activity, seek client/parent feedback on the communication interactions. Ask clients/parents:
  - *What was it like to hear your loved one communicate in this way?*
  - *How did their way of talking change your impressions?*
- If in a group format, ask observers:
  - *What went well? Anything you think could have been communicated differently?*

## Homework

- Practice expressing assertiveness and validation skills.

## Clinician Notes

_____

_____

_____

_____

# Appendix 25 Family Circuits: Young Adult TBT-S Experiential Activity Addressing Communication and Family Structure

Stephanie Knatz Peck

## Neurobiological and Trait Targets
- Anxiety
- Agreeable, cooperative
- Conscientious

## Objectives
- Define and review interaction patterns surrounding recovery.
- Develop and practice new patterns of communication to facilitate recovery.

## Who Is Involved?
- YA clients and parents.
- This is a group activity for clients and/or parents in outpatient through higher levels of care.
- This activity could be implemented virtually or face-to-face.

## Materials and Time Needed
- Posterboard paper.
- Writing utensils.
- One hour.

## What Does the Research Say?
- Improving communication between clients and parents is a dimension of the individual and family healing relationship that reduces anxiety.
- Research evaluating skills training for carers of people with AN suggests that improving communication reduces distress, caregiving burden, and difficulties associated with eating disorder symptoms.
- Clients of parents who received intervention that focused on improved communication held positive attitudes toward the interventions. Intervening on communication may also improve outcomes for adults with AN.
- Clients' and parents' productive traits, such as conscientiousness and agreeableness/cooperativeness, are underlying triggers or prompts that carry them through this process.

> Key Point: Effective communication between clients and parents decreases anxiety and facilitates collaborative progress toward recovery.

## Clinician Checklist

⇒  Introduce the family circuit activity.
⇒  Assign families to draw their family circuits.
⇒  Assign families to rescript their circuits.
⇒  Facilitate practice of new circuits.

## Experiential Activity Instructions

### Rules

1. "Patterns of interaction" are interpersonal circuits where the action of one person leads to a specific response from the other person, which then influences the following response of the initial person. This continues until a series of actions is completed. It is referred to as "circuits" to denote the process the brain uses to code repeated sequential actions that become automatic, or interpersonally routine (habit).
2. This activity is intended to assist families in reflecting on circuits of interaction surrounding recovery.
3. Clients and parents are to observe and disrupt cycles of ineffective communication.
4. Parents are asked to reflect on automatic negative interactive cycles they have with their loved ones that have become automatic.
5. The nature of circuits implies that there is no clear instigator. There is no one at fault; rather, these cycles can start if any of the actions along the circuit is instigated.
6. Once circuits are clarified, client-parent teams are asked to rescript a new circuit of interaction that they want to repeatedly practice in treatment and at home to establish a new circuit for recovery.

### Steps and Scripts

1. Families work together in this exercise. It is ideal to have families work together; however, if they are not at the point where they can do so productively, the clinician can offer the activity as a mixed-family exercise and have each client comment on their family circuit with a member of another family before sharing with the group at large.
2. Introduction: The clinician provides a description of interactive circuits, and how it parallels brain circuit development.

   ○  *In this exercise, you will examine the patterns of relating and communicating that you frequently find yourselves in with your family members.*
   ○  *Families develop cycles or "circuits" of communication where one person's action leads to another family member's response, which leads to the first person reacting and so forth.*
   ○  *Often these cycles of communication become so practiced that they become automatic and habitual. Because of this, they become encoded in your brain, and become habitual.*
   ○  *Identify your circuit of communication that currently occurs. Is it helping or hindering recovery?*
   ○  *A new helpful circuit will be practiced to "re-wire" your interactions to move toward recovery.*

3. Drawing Family Circuits:
   a. Clinician assigns clients to work with their parents.
   b. Families are given instructions to write/draw out their existing family circuits.
   c. Clinicians demonstrate a simple method to do this by connecting actions in a sequence using arrows in either a circular direction or in a straight line. They draw their family circuit in whatever way makes sense to them.
   d. Actions are to be described followed by reactions, followed by the next typical action/reaction, etc.
   e. Once the circuit is complete, clients and parents are instructed to draw a new family circuit of new actions that the clients and parents think would be more productive and help move toward recovery. (See Case Example.)
      o *In this exercise, work together to identify one or more family circuits that occur between you and your family member that is unhelpful.*
      o *Clients, you can choose one, or each family member can identify one circuit to work one.*
      o *Draw the circuit out, connecting actions of each family member to reflect how they are connected and what reactions they trigger.*
      o *Then, draw a new family circuit with that details a circuit you would like to practice together that could become automatic interactions toward recovery.*

4. Role Play Practice
   a. Once the unhelpful and desired circuits are complete, each client/parent demonstrates to the group the negative family circuit and then demonstrates practicing the new productive family circuit.
   b. Practice the new family circuit repeatedly during subsequent sessions in treatment to help establish a productive habit.
   c. Practice allows participants to experience the positive effects of productive communication styles and provide each other with positive feedback to reinforce new interactions.

## Family Circuit: Case Example
### Unhelpful Family Circuit
Client feels anxious about a meal → Starts to ask her mom about the contents of the meal and how much is in it → Mom feels anxious and worried → Mom tries to make client less anxious by answering her questions → Client keeps asking questions, feels more anxious → Dad feels frustrated and forcefully tells client to stop asking questions and provides unhelpful facts in an unemotional tone → Client feels guilty and anxious.

### Productive Re-Wired Family Circuit
Client feels anxious about a meal → Starts to ask her mom about the contents of the meal and how much is in it → Mom feels anxious and worried → Mom and dad BOTH remain calm and gently redirect client to go play the piano while she waits for the meal.

## Discussion Prompts

- Once families have outlined their new circuits, the clinician facilitate a discussion to elicit feedback on family members' experiences. Prompt questions include the following:
  - ○ *What was it like to practice doing (action) differently?*
  - ○ *What surprised you about the new circuit?*
  - ○ *How did your action change the way your family member responded?*
  - ○ *How did that feel compared with the unhelpful circuit?*
  - ○ *How did you feel when family member XX did (action) differently?*
  - ○ *How did that change your reactions?*

## How to Treat to These Traits

- Communication and our perception of the way others communicate are impacted by our traits.
- Clients with AN may be more sensitive, anxious, or experience things differently because of their trait profile.
- This exercise allows for family members to get feedback on the client's needs and to learn to communicate in ways that are helpful to the client's temperament.

## Homework

- Practice interrupting old circuits.
- Practice rewired circuit skills.

## Clinician Notes

_____

_____

_____

_____

# Appendix 26 Family Wise Mind: Young Adult TBT-S Experiential Activity Addressing Communication and Family Relationships

Stephanie Knatz Peck

## Neurobiological and Trait Targets
- Anxiety
- Agreeable, cooperative
- Conscientious

## Objectives
- To explore trait expressions that impact family relationships and communication.
- To facilitate reflection and feedback from clients and Supports regarding effective communication and assistance.

## Who Is Involved?
- Young adult clients and parents.
- These are single client/parent or client and/or parents group activities in outpatient through higher levels of care.
- This activity could be implemented virtually or face-to-face.

## Materials and Time Needed
- No materials needed.
- 60 minutes.

## What Does the Research Say?
- Improving communication between clients and parents is a dimension of individual and family healing relationships that reduces anxiety.
- Research evaluating skills training for carers of people with AN suggests that improving communication reduces distress, caregiving burden, and difficulties associated with eating disorder symptoms.
- Clients of parents who received intervention that focused on improved communication held positive attitudes toward the interventions. Intervening on communication may also improve outcomes for adults with AN.
- Clients' and parents' productive traits, such as conscientiousness and agreeableness/ cooperativeness are underlying triggers or prompts that carry them through this process.

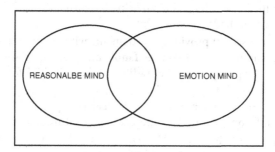

**Figure A26.1** Wise Mind dialectical model

> **Key Point:** Effective communication between clients and parents decreases anxiety and facilitates collaborative progress toward recovery.

## Clinician Checklist
⇒ Review emotion, reasonableness, and wise mind.
⇒ Lead activity to facilitate self-reflection and feedback to parents.
⇒ Facilitate client/parent feedback and discussion.

## Experiential Activity Instructions
### Rules
1. Dialectical behavior therapy (DBT) skills are taught and actively practiced in the young adult 5-day, 40-hour program that has been studied. Skills are taught to both clients and their parents in a multi-family format. The exercises outlined in this appendix draw from traditional DBT skills.
2. Briefly review, Emotion Mind, Rational Mind, and WISE MIND (refer to the Dialectical Behavioral Skills Training Manual).

### Wise Mind Overview
1. Wise Mind is a dialectic behavior therapy exercise on a "Mindfulness Skill" that teaches about two states of mind, **Emotional Mind** and **Rational Mind.**
2. Emotional Mind refers to the state in which people are guided by emotion. This state of mind is characterized by flexibility, spontaneity, creativity, and other characteristics that come when people access emotion.
3. Rational Mind refers to the state of mind that is guided by reason and logic. This state of mind is characterized by factual and linear thinking.
4. These two states of mind are presented within the dialectical model.
5. DBT suggests that two seemingly opposite states of mind can be integrated (see Figure A26.1). Their synthesis, the place where the two states of mind are integrated is referred to as *Wise Mind.*
6. Wise Mind is described in DBT as an inner, intuitive place where Reasonable Mind and Emotional Mind overlap. In this state of mind, an individual can access information from their emotions/feelings, *and* logic/reason to make decisions.

7. When teaching the Wise Mind skill, participants learn about the three states of mind and practice to attain the Wise Mind skill.
8. This exercise is focused on providing participants with skillful ways to navigate communication and interactions among family members. DBT skills are briefly taught and explained to the group using the traditional didactic DBT format (approximately 15–20 minutes of teaching).
9. In keeping with the philosophy of TBT-S "learn-by-practice" model, these skills are practiced and applied through the exercises outlined in this appendix.
10. A brief description of the WISE MIND skill is outlined. Clinicians are recommended to consult the DBT Clinician Manual for more information about WISE MIND.

## Steps and Scripts

1. Present WISE MIND diagram and provide descriptions of Emotion Mind, Rational Mind, and Wise Mind.
2. Use questions to facilitate discussion and understanding:

    a. *Think of someone you would describe as "emotional." What characteristics come to mind?* (Clinician writes characteristics in the emotion mind sphere.)
    b. *Think of someone you would describe as "rational." What characteristics come to mind?* (Clinician writes characteristics in the rational mind sphere.)
    c. Highlight pros and cons of each. Ask about situations and jobs where Emotion Mind and/or Rational Mind are helpful.

3. Review Wise Mind as the third state of mind, the synthesis of the two dimensions.
4. YA clients are instructed to move without using any verbal explanation in the following two steps.
5. *Self-reflection*: After the three states of mind are described, ask participants to self-reflect on their dominant state of mind overall.

    a. The clinician draws an imaginary line that spans the length of the treatment room, or virtually in space, with extreme Emotional Mind on one side and Rational Mind on the other side, with Wise Mind in the middle.
    b. Participants are then asked to place themselves (if face-to-face) or identify where they are on the virtual line.
    c. Each participant describes why they are at their specified location on the line.

6. Perspective sharing

    a. Clients are instructed to move their parents to the place they perceive them to be on the dialectical spectrum.
    b. Clients are instructed to move their parents to the state of mind that predominates in most ED-related interactions.
    c. Clients share their perspective on how this affects their own state of mind (i.e., what state of mind this pushes them into).
    d. Clients are then instructed to move their parents to the place along the spectrum where they think it would be most effective to provide assistance.

7. Each client shares why they placed their parent in the specific location. Parents are instructed to listen. This allows parents to gain perspective on how their interactive styles are perceived by their loved ones.

## Discussion Prompts
### Interfamily Feedback
- Clinician directs clients and parents to meet together. Clients are instructed to provide feedback to their parents where along the spectrum it is most helpful for them to be.
- Provide clear examples of what they could do to practice actions that reflect that spectrum location.

## How to Treat to These Traits
- Reviewing the three states of mind provides a way for group members to discuss the way their perceptions are shaped and how their dominant approaches reflect problems and communication.
- A person's mind-state tendency can be closely tied to temperament and personality.
- This exercise provides an opportunity for clients and parents to gain awareness of their innate tendencies.

## Homework
- Supports: Practice responses that express the state of mind suggested by the client.

## Clinician Notes

_____
_____
_____
_____

# Appendix 27 Young Adult Behavioral Agreement (YA BA)

Stephanie Knatz Peck

---

### Young Adult Behavioral Agreement (YA BA)

Developed by Stephanie Knatz Peck

**Objective:** To restore_____'s health and well-being, prevent higher level of care, prevent weight loss, and return to life goals. Help client to be free from eating disorder and enjoy a healthy, active life.

#### Meal and Snacks Commitments

☐ Eat 3 meals and\_\_\_\_snacks every day following the schedule below:

    ☐ Breakfast at\_\_\_\_AM.
    ☐ AM Snack at\_\_\_\_AM.
    ☐ Lunch at\_\_\_\_PM.
    ☐ PM Snack at\_\_\_\_PM.
    ☐ Dinner at\_\_\_\_PM.
    ☐ Evening Snack at \_\_\_\_PM.

☐ Complete 100% of meals and snacks.

☐ SUPPLEMENTING: Supplement drinks (or bars) will be used if meal/snack is not completed.

    ☐ If more than 50% but less than 100%, 1 supplement will be consumed.
    ☐ If less than 50%, 2 supplements will be consumed.

☐ Meals follow the USDA plate model. Examples that could be default meals:

| BREAKFAST EXAMPLES | | |
|---|---|---|
| | | |

| LUNCH EXAMPLES | | |
|---|---|---|
| | | |

| DINNER EXAMPLES | | |
|---|---|---|
| | | |

1

☐ Snacks will be based on approved snack list. Default snacks include:

    _____        _____
    _____        _____
    _____        _____

☐ Meals will be eaten in____minutes and snacks will be eaten in____minutes.

☐ I will remain in the presence of a Support for 60 minutes following meals and snacks to avoid purging.

☐ Bathroom visits will be supervised by a Support.

☐ Support persons,_____and_____will remain informed of meal plan and any changes.

☐ Supports will attend the following regular appointments: _____
_____

☐ Supports will be present for the following meals and snacks regularly:

    ☐ Breakfast at____AM.
    ☐ AM Snack at____AM.
    ☐ Lunch at____PM.
    ☐ PM Snack at____PM.
    ☐ Dinner at____PM.
    ☐ Evening Snack at____PM.

☐ When Supports are not present, I commit to:

    ☐ Having meals with others who can assist me (Name:_____).
    ☐ Reporting back to Supports by: (describe how you will keep them updated).
    ☐ Video chatting during meals and snacks (list which ones).
    ☐ _____
    ☐ _____

☐ When Supports are present, will:

    ☐ "Check off" that my meal/snacks meet dietary requirements.
    ☐ Assist with distractions.
    ☐ Provide the following feedback if I am having difficulty initiating/completing my meal: Discuss and write strategies you would like your Support to use.
    _____

    ☐ Provide the following feedback if I am engaging in any ED behaviors during meals/snacks:

    _____
    _____

## PRIVILEGES

**Daily**

☐ Every day that I am able to follow my energy plan, I/my Support person will allow myself the following privilege:_____.
(reward/privilege)

**Weekly**

☐ For every week that I am able to follow my energy plan, I/my Support person will allow myself the following privilege:_____.

(reward/privilege)

**Long Term**

☐ If I am able to follow my energy plan for_____, then I/my Support person will allow

(time frame, weeks, months, or specific time marker)

_____.

(reward/privilege)

## CONSEQUENCES

**Daily**

☐ If I miss/fail to complete a meal/snack, then I commit to giving up:_____.

**Weekly**

☐ If I miss/fail to complete_____# of meals/snack, over a week-long period, then I commit to giving up:_____.

**Long Term**

☐ If I am unable to follow my energy plan for____consecutive weeks, then I will commit to:

　☐ Increasing treatment/enrolling in a higher level of care.

　☐ Increasing supervision around meals (describe plan below).

_____

_____

_____

### Meal and Snacks: Support Persons' Commitments

☐ Support persons,_____and_____will remain informed of meal plan and any changes.

☐ Supports will attend the following regular appointments:

_____

☐ Supports will be present for the following meals and snacks regularly:

　☐ Breakfast at____AM.

　☐ AM Snack at____AM.

　☐ Lunch at____PM.

　☐ PM Snack at____PM.

　☐ Dinner at____PM.

　☐ Evening Snack at____PM.

☐ When Supports are not present, I commit to:

　☐ Having meals with others who can assist me (Name:_____).

　☐ Reporting back to Supports by: (describe how you will keep them updated).

　☐ Video chatting during meals and snacks (list which ones).

3

☐ When Supports are present, they will:

    ☐ "Check off" that my meals/snacks meet dietary requirements.
    ☐ Assist with distractions.
    ☐ Provide the following feedback if I am having difficulty initiating/completing my meal:
    (Discuss and write out statements and other strategies you would like your Support to use.)

    _____

    _____

    _____

    ☐ Provide the following feedback if I am engaging in any ED behaviors during meals/snacks:

    _____

    _____

    _____

**PRIVILEGES TO BE NEGOTIATED WITH SUPPORTS** (Optional)

☐ For every **day** that_____follows the meal plan, I agree to_____.

☐ For every **week** (7 consecutive days) that_____follows the meal plan, I agree to _____.

☐ Once_____follows the meal plan for_____consecutive weeks, I agree to _____

**Commitments to Increase Involvement of Support Persons**

☐ If I miss/fail to complete a meal, then I commit to:

    ☐ Letting the following Supports know:_____.
    ☐ Supplementing/replacing missed meals/snack in the presence of_____.
    ☐ Completing the next day of meals with a Support person.

☐ If I miss/fail to complete____# meals/snacks over a 1-week period, then I commit to:

    ☐ Increasing meal/snack assistance (presence of Support persons at meals) to:

    _____

    until I am regularly completing meals/snacks again.
    ☐ Treatment will be increased by_____.
    ☐ All meals and snacks will be completed at home for____days.
    ☐ _____
    ☐ _____

**Long-Term Goal**

☐ My long-term goal is to:

    ☐ Return to college.
    ☐ Live independently.
    ☐ _____

☐ In order to know that I am ready to take this on, I must be able to consistently meet my meal plan for___consecutive months.

☐ **Supports:** In order for me to assist in this long-term goal, I would expect to see my loved one_____ meeting their meal plan for___consecutive months.

---

### Commitment to a Strong Body and Healthy Weight

☐ I commit to meeting/maintaining the treatment team's weight recommendations.

☐ I will be weighed once a week by_____.

☐ *For weight restoration:* I commit to increasing my energy plan per the treatment team's recommendations if my weight is not increasing at the recommended rate.

☐ My Support persons will be informed of:

    ☐ My weight at all vitals checks and weigh-ins.

    ☐ My weight and vitals every___weeks.

    ☐ My weight IF:

        ☐ I fall below my recommended range.

        ☐ I lose 2 lbs. in two consecutive weeks.

        ☐ I am failing to gain the recommended weight over 2 consecutive weeks.

### Privileges

☐ For every week that I achieve my weight goal, I will allow myself to:_____

☐ *SUPPORTS(Optional):* For every week that my loved one meets their weight goal, I agree to:

### Long-Term Goal

☐ I can begin to pursue my long-term goal once I achieve my weight goal and maintain it for ___consecutive months.

☐ *SUPPORTS:* In order to assist my loved one in pursuing their long-term goal, I expect them to achieve weight goal and maintain it for___consecutive months.

### Consequences

☐ If I fall below my recommended weight range and am not able to restore it after 2 weeks.

☐ If I lose 2 lbs. over 2 consecutive weeks.

☐ If weight restoring: If I fail to restore weight for 2 consecutive weeks.

**THEN:**

    ☐ Increase meal/snack assistance (presence of Support persons at meals) with:_____ until I am regularly completing meals/snacks again.

    ☐ Treatment will be increased by_____.

    ☐ I will enroll in a higher level of care.

    ☐ All meals and snacks will be completed at home for___days.

5

### Physical Activity

☐   I commit to following the movement and physical activity plan recommended by the treatment team.

☐   The physical activity plan is:

_____

### Eating Disorder Behaviors

I commit to abstaining from engaging in eating disorder behaviors including:

☐   excessive exercise (exercise beyond what is recommended) and/or secretive exercise
☐   restricting
☐   binging
☐   purging
☐   calorie counting
☐   measuring
☐   hiding food
☐   cutting food into small pieces
☐   micro-biting
☐   restricting food groups/specific food types
☐   social media and internet use related to food, shape, and weight
☐   negotiating
☐   lying
☐   self-harm

☐  If I engage in an ED behavior, I commit to:

    ☐   Informing my Support person.

    ☐   Coming up with a plan for preventing further behaviors and sharing it with my Support.

    ☐

    ☐

☐  *SUPPORTS:* If my loved one confides in me about an ED behavior, I commit to:

    ☐   Responding nonjudgmentally.

    ☐   Assisting them with a plan to prevent further behaviors.

    ☐   Validate and use reflective questioning to assist in coming up with a plan.

### Long-Term Goal

☐  I can begin to pursue my long-term goal once I am abstinent from_____for

_____                                           (ED behavior)
(time period)

☐  *SUPPORTS:* In order to support my their in pursuing their long-term goal, I would like to see abstinence from_____for_____.
                      (ED behavior)      (time period)

6

# Appendix 28  Severe-and-Enduring Anorexia Nervosa (SE-AN) Behavioral Agreement

Laura Hill

---

**Preparation for SE-AN Adult Behavioral Agreement**
for Anorexia Nervosa Ages 18–60+
**Worksheet 1**
**Temperament Based Therapy with Support (TBT-S)**

Written by (Client name): _____

My Diagnoses 1:_____Diagnosis 2:_____
 Diagnosis 3:_____Diagnosis 4:_____

**Support** is critical for my recovery. To make myself stronger and my treatment more successful, I am willing to enter into the following agreement with the following person(s) to be my "Support":

Support person 1:  _____

Support person 2:  _____

Support person 3:  _____

Support person 4:  _____

<u>Identify the errors, or what is not true for me in the sentences below.
Change any word(s), phrases, or sentence to make the statements true for me.</u>

I recognize that I can be my own worst enemy. In my desire to become stronger physically, psychologically, and interpersonally, I at times sabotage my own efforts in moving forward. While I may want myself to improve, I at times block myself from progress and push others away who want to help me.

## I agree to be honest (Client)

Truth is essential. If I am not honest with myself and others, trust is lost. If I am to recover, then honesty is the first step.

- [ ] I agree to share the full truth, even if it makes "ED" angry. Honesty keeps me accountable to myself and others.
- [ ] I recognize that honesty is a skill that needs to be practiced. If I am not honest, then I will share the truth with the person via text, email, phone, or face-to-face.
- [ ] I can be honest one day at a time.

## I agree to offer interpersonal respect (Client)

Interpersonal respect can sometimes be difficult to manage while in the midst of eating disorder noise and anxiety. (Check what you are *willing to try* to offer.)

- [ ] I agree to take responsibility for my actions and to act kindly and show respect for others in and outside of treatment.
- [ ] If I am not taking responsibility and/or am not respectful, I agree to apologize to the person(s).

1

---

## My (Client) Warning Signs or Red Flags Include:

I need to help my Supports know what I do when relapsing into ED thoughts, feelings, and behaviors:

☐ Eat longer than others, or delay eating snacks and meals.
☐ Change my attire (i.e., wearing baggier clothes).
☐ Be more argumentative about food/eating/treatment/recovery.
☐ Avoid reaching out for help or to my Support.
☐ Direct my anger and negative emotions onto Supports.
☐ Increase my social withdrawal and isolation or avoid previously enjoyed activities.
☐ Increase my negative body comments.

## Support Person(s) Strengths:

S-1 S-2 S-3 S-4 (Support numbers are names indicated above)

☐☐☐☐ Listens: Reflects back what they hear with no judgment
Willing to practice new tools
Models and owns their own emotions
(e.g., this is scary for me, I am exhausted, and I am determined.)

☐☐☐☐ Willingness to try/learn
Able to be accountable
Is logical

☐☐☐☐ Won't give up
Keeps an open mind
Problem solves
Other_____

## I agree to do/not do the following (Supports):

S1 S2 S3 S4

☐☐☐☐ Encourage the balanced meal plan and the Behavioral Agreement. (Do)
Instead of judging, ask questions by starting with, "Can you help me understand ...?" or "I don't understand ..." (Do)

☐☐☐☐ Offer 2–3 options to help my loved one with decisions. (Do)
Active Listening: Rephrase what you heard your loved one say without adding your own judgment. (Do)

☐☐☐☐ Refrain from endorsing "diets." (Not do)
Other things that are *bothersome* to the client: _____

☐☐☐☐ Other things that are *helpful* to the client: _____

2

# Goals and Objectives
## SE-AN Behavioral Agreement
### Worksheet 2
### Temperament Based Therapy with Support (TBT-S)

Name _____ Date: _____

**Goal 1:** Identify my strengths and weakness: My temperament
**Goal 2:** Commit to my meal and movement plans.
**Goal 3:** Reduce my eating disorder symptoms.

---

**Goal 1:** Identify my strengths and weakness: My temperament

My temperament is the biological foundation of who I am, my natural tendencies that influence my thoughts, feelings, and behaviors. When I express my traits productively, they are my strengths. When I express them destructively, they are my weaknesses. How I express my traits is up to me and it takes work.

**Be true to who _I am_:**

1.   Take  the "Trait Profile Checklist."

2.   Identify and practice tools from the "TBT-S Toolbox" to reshape destructive traits and reduce my ED symptoms.

**Goal 2:** Commit to my meal and movement plans.

_Biologically, Food is Medicine._ Food is the fuel or energy fundamental to life. For me, food is medicine with uncomfortable side effects. However, I need to eat prescribed meals and snacks each day as my medication for physical and mental strength. I will probably experience higher anxiety when eating certain foods, increasing irritability and distorted thoughts. My thoughts may become "noisy" and negative, making it harder for me to interact with others. These "side effects of food" can keep me from eating or trigger me to binge eat. In spite of these biological reactions, I can better manage my "medication side effects" by choosing from the options below.

## Check the options I could do to manage my meal and exercise plan:

☐    Develop a meal plan with a dietitian, virtually or face-to-face.

   ☐ a. Due to my temperament, inform the dietitian that the meal plan should

   i. Be practical, with foods easy to buy at my grocery,
   ii. Have clear portion sizes, and
   iii. Allow food combinations that can be easily prepared and repeatedly practiced.

1

    ☐  b.  Include identified Supports whom I want to eat with at times_____, _____.

    ☐  c.  Supports have a copy of the meal plan.

☐  Identify a strengthening movement plan with my dietitian or my medical professional to develop stronger muscles and body strength.

    ☐  a.  Include identified Supports to do active movement together_____,_____.

    ☐  b.  Supports have a copy of the movement plan.

☐  Due to my temperament, I agree to **not eat "intuitively"** when in new eating situations. at this time.

## Check the options I could use to manage my meal plan

Eat 100% of ☐ Breakfast  ☐ AM Snack  ☐ Lunch  ☐ PM Snack  ☐ Dinner  ☐ Evening Snack

☐  Create a Plan A or default meal and snack. It becomes the meal /snack to eat when stressed.

☐  Take my default meal and snack with me when I leave home.

☐  Exercise or do my movement plan IF I eat/drink 100% of prescribed foods within the past 24 hours.

☐  Go to the grocery alone to purchase foods/drinks in my meal plan.

☐  Keep accurate food logs via, e.g., app_____or using form_____.

☐  Keep accurate movement logs via e.g., app_____or using form_____.

☐  Drink liquid supplements if I cannot eat the food in the prescribed doses, e.g., Boost, Ensure, electrolyte beverages, milk, juice

☐  Drink_____oz of fluid per day (non-caffeinated).

☐  Eat within 1½ hours of getting up and every 3–4 hours.

☐  Text, Skype, or virtually be with_____following_____meal(s).

☐  Set phone alarms for meals/snacks and other reminders.

☐  Use the tools I identified in my TBT-S Toolbox.

☐  Ask_____to shop for my groceries at this time.

☐  Eat at least 1 protein, 1 carb, 1 EF (fat) per meal/snack.

☐  If there are bowel movement problems, talk with medical clinician about supplemental medication.

☐  **Use my productive traits, from my Trait Profile Checklist,** to help me manage my food and movement plans. List 3 of my productive traits that will help me eat my meal plan.

_____, _____, _____

☐  Ask my Supports to offer a couple of options when discussing what to eat at a restaurant, instead of open-ended questions, e.g., "What do you want to eat?"

☐  Ask my Supports to have foods for my default meal on hand. If I am having a stressful day, that is what I'll eat.

☐  Ask my Supports to buy the foods on my meal plan when they are going to the store, instead of my going to the grocery myself.

☐  Ask a Support to go with me to the grocery to get the foods I need. Identify when I will do this_____.

☐  Ask a Support to eat together in person or via face time (ID when and where)_____.

☐  Ask a Support to text or FaceTime me to offer assistance before or after eating. If so, identify when_____.

☐  Inform my Supports if the dietitian adjusts my food or movement plan.

Other:_____

2

**Repairs:** If I don't meet my Meal and Movement Plans:

☐ Text_____(Support) while eating next meal face-to-face or remotely.

☐ Eat or drink missed servings (carbs, pros, and endurance fuels) within 24 hours of the day they are missed, in the form of smoothie, bar, liquid supplement, etc.

☐ If I delay eating, ask_____to text me at set time and talk while I eat.

☐ Have my dietitian or_____monitor my food logs.

☐ Return to the Plan A default or backup meal plan.

☐ If I am unable to eat all my "medicine" more than 3 times a week, I will seek more structure by either setting up more structure with my Supports_____or enter a higher level of treatment_____

☐ Other:_____

## Goal 3: Reduce my eating disorder symptoms.

### Check all ED symptoms that are true for me:

☐ Fasting or restricting

☐ Binge eating

☐ Self-induced vomiting

☐ Cutting or self-mutilating

☐ Weighing myself more than_____

☐ Body checking to self-monitor

☐ Chewing and spitting

☐ Excessive alcohol, marijuana, or smoking (circle one(s) relevant)

☐ Other_____

☐ Hiding or stealing food

☐ Excessive exercising

☐ Laxative abuse

☐ Abusing alcohol or drugs

☐ Using diet pills

☐ Delaying eating

☐ Isolating > 4 hrs. a day.

### Who: I need to work with the following to help reduce my eating disorder symptoms (virtually or face-to-face)

☐ Myself using my productive traits

☐ Supports to know what is being planned and to learn the tools to apply

☐ My clinician

☐ My medical professional

☐ My dietitian

### Ways I could reduce or eliminate ED symptoms

☐ Use my productive traits (Trait Profile Checklist), to help me manage ED symptoms.

☐ Combine 2–3 tools from the TBT-S Toolbox to divert, interrupt or reshape ED symptoms.

☐ Use my_____ and _____ productive traits to help me push forward.

☐ Have my weight monitored (if relevant) by _____.

☐ Agree to have my vitals monitored (if relevant) by _____.

☐ Not exercise until I have eaten 100% of my meal plan in the last 24 hours with no purging, e.g., vomiting or laxatives.

☐ IF I am of legal age and IF it is legal in my state or country, I can use marijuana within the limit identified by my medical professional and IF I have no addiction trait.

☐ I agree to not drink alcohol due to urges it triggers.

☐ Ask my Supports to learn the following tools from my Toolbox to help me practice new skills to shift my destructive traits and reduce my symptoms.
_____, _____, _____

☐ Describe my symptoms to my Supports so they know what to look for.

☐ Clarify when it helps and when it does *not* help for my Supports to offer assistance.

☐ Inform my Supports that it may take multiple tools from the Toolbox to help me manage

☐ _____symptom and_____symptom.

☐ Inform Supports that if they become afraid and uncertain of what to do, they have my permission to request time with my therapist and me to discuss the issue together.

☐ Other_____

## Repair: If I do an ED symptom:

☐ If I self-induce vomit or take more laxatives than recommended, then immediately drink an electrolyte beverage (16 oz minimum).

☐ If I do ED symptoms more than two times a week, I understand more structure is needed. This may mean I need more assistance at work, home, or school to help me or more treatment during the week.

☐ I agree to return to work or school only when the following conditions are met.
1. _____
2. _____
3. _____

☐ If I body check, I will take down the mirror (or cover it) and use a "distract" tool: (see TBT-S Toolbox)_____.

☐ If I use laxatives or self-induce vomiting, I will replace the meal eliminated with an equal amount of liquid supplement or foods.

☐ If I restrict, I agree to refer back to my meal plan and eat the carbs, proteins, or endurance foods (fats) to make up the difference.

☐ If I cannot repair restriction or over-exercise, or other ED behaviors by myself, I agree to a higher level of care.

☐ If I do not follow my meal plan, I will do NO exercise for the following 24 hours.

☐ If I purge in any way, I must eat 100% of my meal plan for 2 days and with no additional movement/exercise, and then I could continue with my movement plan.

☐ Do movement with_____(Supports).

☐ Share the ED symptom with_____Support(s) to hold myself accountable.

☐ Agree to have more assistance during_____(time of day).

☐ Text/zoom/Skype/FaceTime_____(Support) to share time with me during the vulnerable time.

☐ Take three tools (from TBT-S Toolbox) with me to distract or reroute from destructive actions for a specific vulnerable time period.

☐ When I return home, I will enter my home *after* I identify 1–2 tools that can help me reroute from a destructive action.

☐ Other: _____

"Always bear in mind that your own resolution to succeed is more important than any one thing." —Abraham Lincoln

# SE-AN Adult Behavioral Agreement Summary
## Worksheet 3
### Temperament Based Therapy with Support (TBT-S)

Name _____ Date: _____

## My Problem:

ED symptoms I express are:

_____

_____

### I agree to commit to: (draw from my responses in Worksheet 1)

Honesty by doing: _____

Interpersonal respect by doing: _____

## Three of my "Red Flags" are:

1. _____

2. _____

3. _____

## My Supports

## Three things my Supports agree to do are:

1. _____

2. _____

3. _____

## Two things I want my Supports to do to help me to reduce my ED symptoms are: (draw from Worksheets 1 and 2)

1. _____

2. _____

## Two tools I would like my Supports use are: (draw from TBT-S Toolbox)

1. _____

2. _____

1

**Goal 1:** (Drawing from **Worksheet 2, my "Trait Profile Checklist and TBT-S Toolbox**):
<u>Be True to Who I Am: Draw upon my own Temperament or Traits:</u>

Three traits I express productively that I can draw upon to help manage my symptoms are:

    1. _____

    2. _____

    3. _____

Two of my current destructive traits that I express without thinking and want to reshape are:

    1. _____

    2. _____

**Goal 2:** Commit to my meal and movement plans.

I have a meal plan identified with the dietitian_____:

Three ways I plan to complete my meal plan each day are: (from Worksheet 2)

    1. _____

    2. _____

    3. _____

Three of my productive traits that I can draw upon to complete my meal plan are: (Trait Profile Checklist)

    1. _____

    2. _____

    3. _____

Two Supports who can help me carry out my plan to eat are:

    1. _____

    2. _____

Two things I want my Supports to do help me with the meal plan are: (draw from Worksheet 2)

    1. _____

    2. _____

2

**Repairs:** Two things I will do if I do not complete my meal plan: (Worksheet 2)

1. _____

2. _____

What action that I identified in my meal and movement plan is nonnegotiable? (Worksheet 2)

_____

## Goal 3: Reduce my Eating Disorder Symptoms:

I plan to use the following 3 methods to reduce my ED symptoms: (Worksheet 2 and Toolbox)

1. _____

2. _____

3. _____

Three of my productive traits that I can use to reduce my ED symptoms are: (Trait Profile Checklist)

1. _____

2. _____

3. _____

Two Support persons who can help me reduce my ED symptoms are:

1. _____

2. _____

Two things I need my Supports to do to help me reduce my ED symptoms are: (Worksheet 2)

1. _____

2. _____

**Repairs:** When I Do an ED symptoms I will make one of the following two repairs: (Worksheet 2)

1. _____

2. _____

## Living with purpose:

By the time I am_____years old, I will live my life with more purpose by doing
Or, I will be upset with myself if I am not doing_____by the time I am____years old:

_____

Client notes: _____

_____

"The best way to predict your future is to create it." — Abraham Lincoln

3

# Glossary

**Amygdala** Almond-shaped cluster of nuclei located deep within the temporal lobe of the brain that processes emotions. Considered the "panic station."

**Anorexia nervosa** A biologically based illness with brain circuit alterations and with common traits. Characterized by extremely low weight, fear of weight gain, body image disturbance, and at times binge eating and purging.

**Anterior cingulate cortex** The frontal (anterior) part of the cingulate cortex. The ventral (lower) aspect functions to integrate emotional reactions with thoughts and movement, contributing to emotional learning and automatic responses; the dorsal (upper) aspect is involved in conflict monitoring and inhibitory control.

**Anxiety** Persons with AN tend to inherit trait anxiety, a disposition that tends to judge things as threatening, versus state anxiety (situational anxiety).

**Basal ganglia** A group of nuclei that are primarily responsible for action selection and motor control and also influence emotion, thoughts, and perceptions, located at the base of the brain. It includes the thalamus, caudate, putamen, and nucleus accumbens.

**Behavioral Agreement** The TBT-S core document providing a structure for adults with AN and Supports to complete a strategic plan of who does what, when, where, and how in working together to move forward toward recovery. There are two versions, YA and SE-AN Behavioral Agreements.

**Behaviors** TBT-S advocates that clinicians not use "behaviors" as a free-standing word when referring to ED behaviors, because it is behaviors that are also the healing actions necessary for recovery. Clinicians are recommended to use an adjective to describe what kind of behavior is being addressed, so that it does not psychologically eliminate the very source of the solution, action.

**Binge eating disorder** One type of eating disorder with neurobiological alterations and characterized by uncontrollable binge eating once a week or more with no compensatory actions taken for weight or body concerns.

**Biological reductionism** Reducing causation to biological precursors and ignoring the significant impact of environmental or psychological influences.

**Bulimia nervosa** One type of eating disorder with neurobiological alterations and characterized by uncontrollable binge eating once a week or more with compensatory purgative behaviors.

**Caudate nucleus** A region of the dorsal striatum that is part of the cognitive neurocircuitry and is involved in cognitive evaluation and appraisal of stimuli, goal-directed behavior, and learning.

**Central coherence or cohesion** A person's ability to see the "big picture" or derive overall meaning from integrating many details.

**Cerebellum** A lobe at the base of the brain that controls coordination of movement and other complex actions such as posture, balance, and bodily movements.

**Character** A person's outward expressions of temperament, emotions, thoughts, feelings, the nature side of nature/nurture.

**Circuits** Connections of neurons that pass neurochemical and electrical messages throughout the brain. It is the brain's communication system, the "train tracks" along which all brain messages pass.

**Clinicians** In this book, the term used to refer to therapists, psychologists, social workers, counselors, and other mental health care workers.

**Cognitive circuit** Brain circuits that signal cognitive or thought-related executive functions such as planning, decision-making, inhibitory control, and set shifting.

**Cognitive control** Using one's thoughts to establish goals or plans to direct or control one's actions and emotions. Also referred to as executive control.

**Cortico-limbic system** Neural system that involves the prefrontal cortex and the ventral striatal region in the anterior (front) of the brain that processes a broad range of cognitive and behavioral functions such as decision-making, planning, motor control, and emotional regulation.

**Decision-making** From a neurobiological perspective, decision-making refers to choice behavior based on evaluation of outcomes, such as reward signals and interoceptive sensations. For many with AN, altered reward and interoceptive circuit function is thought to contribute to difficulty making and/or trusting decisions.

**Destructive trait expressions** All traits are expressions on a continuum. For the purpose of this book, destructive trait expressions are responses that cause harm to one's self or others, such as an impulsive trait expression that manifests as purging.

**Dialectic** The ability to view issues from varying perspectives, including acknowledging that opposite viewpoints may both be true. Using the word "and" instead of "but" allows varying perspectives to coexist.

**Dopamine** A neurotransmitter in the brain associated with the experience of, and learning from, reward.

**Dorsal** The "upper area," for example, of the brain.

**Dorsolateral prefrontal cortex** The upper (dorsal) and side (lateral) area of the prefrontal cortex that is the newest evolved brain area of humans and is involved in executive functions.

**Electrochemical signals** Charged electrical currents in neurons carrying brain messages throughout the brain and body to send and receive signals. The signals are electrical because it is the fastest method to transmit signals allowing the body to respond quickly to stimuli.

**Endurance fuels** A literal biological reference to fats. Fats burn longer than other macronutrients and have many functional purposes in the body and brain.

**Energy** A literal meaning of a calorie and all food intake.

**Executive control** See "Cognitive control."

**Executive functioning** Higher-order cognitive functions including decision-making, planning, task switching, inhibitory control.

**Experiential activities** For the purpose of this book, this refers to activities that are used therapeutically to explore a situation to better understand it and try on solutions for healthy change. TBT-S uses interactive games and other activities to experience the situation more fully for problem resolution.

**5-Day TBT-S Program** The TBT-S format studied in open trials. Adults with AN and their Supports attend this temperament based approach interactively for 40 hours in 1 week.

Qualitative and quantitative outcomes are measured.

**Food is medicine** A medical perspective of food, and if applied literally, foods are "prescribed" and "dosed" for those with severe-and-enduring AN who may be unable neurobiologically to sense the amount needed and decide on what and when to eat.

**Fuel** A literal reference to food.

**Genes** The basic unit of heredity made up of DNA.

**Glial cells** "Support" cells to neurons. They sculpt the physical connections among neurons, provide some nutrients, hold neurons in place, and remove dead neurons.

**Gustatory cortex** A multi-brain structure responsible for the perception of taste that includes the insula and other brain areas.

**Harm avoidance** A temperament trait defined by constraint, excessive worry, and avoidance of perceived harm. It varies in intensity and can be expressed in productive or destructive ways.

**High-achieving trait** A temperament driven tendency to attain more, for example, complete higher education or run farther and faster.

**Hippocampus** A brain structure in the mid-temporal area of the limbic system that is involved in memory, including spatial and relational short- and long-term memories.

**Inhibition** A temperament trait referring to the tendency to be restrained, fearful, and/or self-conscious and/or need to be alone. It varies in intensity and can be expressed productively through destructively.

**Instrumental assistance** Tangible assistance, such as financial or travel.

**Insula** Area of the brain responsible for interoception. Tucked inside the Sylvian fissure, it transmits physical body sensations such as hunger, fullness, pain, and taste onto brain areas that register memory and decision-making. The posterior (backside) connects with motor functions.

**Intensive Outpatient Therapy Program** A level of treatment that typically averages three hours of care multiple days a week. It could be any type of treatment approach, for any diagnosis.

**Interdependence** Human relationships evolve around a central principle that the self and other are interdependent. It is a developmental evolution from dependent and independent to interdependent.

**Interoception** The ability to sense the physiological condition of the body. It includes internal physical body-state experiences, such as hunger and fullness, taste, pain, touch, heartbeat, breathing, and gastrointestinal (GI) sensations.

**Intuitive eating** An approach of eating that requires interoceptive, emotional, and rational thought. For many with severe-and-enduring AN, interoception is neurobiologically altered, reducing the ability to eat intuitively unless within highly structured settings. This book takes the approach that if a client with AN has altered interoception, then intuitive eating based on hunger and fullness cues is not recommended.

**Macronutrients** Nutrients needed in large amounts to supply the body with needed forms of energy to meet its daily needs. They include proteins, carbohydrates, and endurance fuels (fats).

**Meal plan** A dietary proposal of foods that provides sufficient macronutrients and minerals to meet a person's daily energy requirements. For those with AN, it needs to include recommended portion sizes, timing, and potential Supports to assist in eating foods that will restore bodily health.

**Medical professionals** A person trained in medical practices, such as nurse practitioners, physicians, medical assistants, nurses, and others who are licensed to provide medical care.

**Metabolism** The process by which the body converts food and drinks into energy.

**Metric** For the purpose of this book, it means reliable rules from which change can be measured.

**Mindful eating** Intensified focus to increase awareness of food intake, bite by bite, without judgment. TBT-S does not encourage mindful eating for AN because it can intensify harmful over-monitoring of each bite. Distraction while eating helps persons with AN tolerate food and its "side effects" on the mind and body.

**Module** For the purpose of this book, distinct but interrelated units of treatment that can be used like building blocks, administered singularly or together in various combinations ranging from providing a single module in one session of a TBT-S intervention to combining several units over multiple days of intervention. All modules are developed to augment ongoing ED therapy.

**Mortality** Death rate.

**Multi-family therapy** Theoretical approach and intervention strategy that conducts therapy in groups that include more than one set of family members simultaneously. TBT-S offers a multi-family approach with Young Adult clients with AN. It could also be stated as "multi-Supports" meaning a group of people who offer assistance for those in treatment. Because Supports are primarily "family" members and family-based therapy is an established term, the YA TBT-S approach uses both multi-family and Supports.

**Neurobiological approach** For the purpose of this book, an approach that considers brain physiological, anatomical, biological, and developmental functions and their impact on eating disorders.

**Neurochemical** A neurotransmitter in the brain or other chemical substances that impact brain and nervous system responses.

**Neurodevelopment** Brain development.

**Neuroplasticity** The flexible continual and constant ability for the brain to change synaptic connections (to re-wire) throughout life, for example when learning and changing actions.

**"Noise" in the brain** Thoughts that dominate for those with eating disorders, focusing on calories, body size, weight, and shape.

**Nucleus accumbens** A region of the ventral striatum and basal ganglia, it is involved in cognitive processing of reward and reinforcement, and codes for actions that will increase future rewards.

**Obsessionality** A temperament trait (or state) that dominates one's thoughts by a persistent idea, desire, image, etc.

**Open trials** A type of clinical research that provides participants with the same intervention as opposed to comparing approaches or randomizing a control (untreated) group with a treatment group, to measure outcomes. It is an initial phase of clinical trials that addresses feasibility and acceptability of treatment before proceeding toward gold standard randomized controlled trials.

**Orbitofrontal cortex** Also known as OFC, located in the prefrontal cortex above the orbits, or eye sockets. It is involved in the cognitive processing of decision-making and intricately connected with emotion, memory, thoughts, and sensory input.

**Outpatient therapy** A level of treatment that provides one or multiple hours of treatment per week or month. It is outside of 24-hour hospital inpatient treatment. It can be individual, dyad, or group, and any type of treatment approach for any diagnosis.

**Parietal lobe** A lobe in the upper back of the brain involved in processing sensory stimuli, impacting perceptions. This includes how people experience themselves with the surrounding space.

**Partial Hospital Program** A level of care and treatment that is offered a minimum of six hours a day, multiple days a week. It could be any type of treatment for any diagnosis.

**Perfectionism** A temperament trait, common among those with AN, characterized by attempts to be flawless and having exceedingly high expectations. TBT-S places it on a continuum ranging from productive to destructive responses.

**Personality** Drawing from C. R. Cloninger's model, personality is the umbrella or overall presentation of both one's temperament or biological basis of the self and one's character, the outward expressions shaped by the environment.

**Prediction error** A mismatch between what is expected and what is experienced.

**Prefrontal cortex** The anterior (front) of the frontal lobe, involved in higher cognitive functioning, planning, personality, and social behavior.

**Productive trait expressions** All traits are expressed on a continuum. For the purpose of this book, productive trait expressions are responses that endorse health and strength to self and others. For example, an impulsive trait is productively expressed when a person impulsively offers a compliment or enters into a project that brings purpose or helps themself or others.

**Prompts** Cues to assist or encourage the clinician to address an identified topic. They are starters to initiate the discussions in this book.

**Psychoeducation** A core TBT-S method of treatment. For the purpose of this book, neurobiological research is summarized for clinicians to present findings to clients and/or Supports in an interactive discourse ranging from discussion to experiential activities.

**Punishment sensitivity** A temperament trait that focuses on internal and external negative feedback, which impacts cognitive control. Many persons with AN perceive neutral feedback to be negative. Negative feedback impacts cognitive control.

**Putamen** A region of the basal ganglia primarily involved in the modulation and coordination of movement, and also involved in reward processing.

**Randomized controlled trials** Also known as RCTs. The gold standard of treatment research methodology whereby participants are randomly assigned to different treatments to compare impact.

**Reward circuit** A network of brain circuits that mediates reward response and incentive learning and adaptation of behaviors to inform decision-making.

**Reward sensitivity** A temperament trait response that focuses on positive internal and external feedback that creates a tendency to pursue, learn from, and draw pleasure from positive feedback. Persons who binge eat are chasing internal rewarding responses, causing destructive or self-harming amounts of food intake.

**Rule bound** A temperament trait response related to altered decision-making. Common in those with AN. Rules establish structure that provides a cognitive road map to approach new stimuli or activities to compensate for the brain's altered ability to navigate via inner sensations.

**Self-critique** A TBT-S three-step tool, that identifies (1) what would I do again? (2) what would I do differently? and (3) How would I do it differently? Used in that order to analyze an action, interaction, or response to a situation. The intent is to refine and improve responses. It can be applied at anytime, anywhere for anything.

**Septo-hippocampal system** A neural pathway that adjusts excitability in processing memories and brain re-wiring or ability to flexibly change.

**Set shifting** An executive brain function that involves the ability to shift attention between one task and another.

**Skills** Skillful actions acquired via practice.

**Strength gain** A TBT-S term for weight gain, shifting focus from a number on the scale to a state of body composition with improved health state.

**Supports** The "S" of TBT-S meaning Support(s). It refers to both people (the noun) and the role they play (verb). It is capitalized throughout this book to designate its function and role in TBT-S. The word was chosen by adults with AN regarding the type of assistance they wanted and needed.

**Symptoms** Indicators of illness, many of which can be reduced or eliminated in anorexia nervosa.

**Targets** For the purpose of this book, selected aims for treatment, discussion, or client objectives.

**Temperament** Temperament is the biological basis of our personality, influenced by genetics and brain circuit development and function over one's life span. Temperament is to nature as character is to nurture.

**Temperament Based Therapy with Support** A novel treatment to augment ongoing therapies by inserting modules of temperament based interventions to address underlying triggers to mental health symptoms. It began by focusing on anorexia nervosa, the mental illness with high mortality and low long-term efficacy outcomes.

**Thalamus** An oval-shaped mass of neurons at the top of the brainstem that serves as a relay station for incoming sensory stimuli and outgoing responses.

**Tools** For the purpose of this book, simple and/or practical actions taken to manage and reduce eating disorder symptoms. A means to develop skills.

**Trait Profile Checklist** A temperament checklist developed for multiple diagnoses, including eating disorders, consisting of traits identified from multiple personality models and eating disorder research.

**Traits** Innate and genetically induced tendencies that make up a person's personality.

**Ventral** Lower aspect of the brain.

**Ventral striatum** The lower area of the striatum, that includes the nucleus accumbens.

**Virtual sessions** A form of therapy that takes place via phone, an app, or a video interchange. This option for therapy interaction has increased due to the COVID-19 pandemic and allows clients and Supports to participate in treatment from any site that provides technical connection, such as home, outside, work, or school.

**Wise mind** The overlap of emotional and rational mind-set. What may appear a paradox may have a synergistic commonality.

# References

1. Birmingham C, Su J, Hlynsky J, et al. The mortality rate from anorexia nervosa. *Int J Eat Disord.* 2005;**38**:143–6.

2. Crow S, Petersen C, Swanson S, et al. Increased mortality in bulimia nervosa and other eating disorders. *Am J Psychiatr.* 2009;**166**:1342–6.

3. Foerde K, Steinglass J. Decreased feedback learning in anorexia nervosa persists after weight restoration. *Int J Eat Disord.* 2017;**50**(4):415–23.

4. Udo T, Bitley S, Grilo C. Suicide attempts in US adults with lifetime DSM-5 eating disorders. *BMC Med.* 2019;**17**(1):120.

5. American Psychiatric Association. DSM-5 Development. www.dsm5.org/Proposed Revision/Pages/proposedrevision.aspx? rid=26; 2012.

6. Bulik C, Blake L, Austin J. Genetics of eating disorders: What the clinician needs to know. *Psychiatr Clin North Am.* 2019;**42**(1):59–73.

7. Zeeck A, Herpertz-Dahlmann B, Friederich H, et al. Psychotherapeutic treatment for anorexia nervosa: A systematic review and network meta-analysis. *Front Psychiatr.* 2018;**9**(158):1–14.

8. Hill L. Can Your Brain Cure Anorexia? A Brain-Based Approach to Eating Disorder Treatment Eating Disorders Catalogue. Carlsbad, CA: Gürze Books Publishing 2017.

9. Knatz Peck, S., Towne, T., Wierenga, C. E., Hill, L., Eisler, I., Brown, T., Han, E., Miller, M., Perry, T., & Kaye, W. (2021). Temperament-based treatment for young adults with eating disorders: acceptability and initial efficacy of an intensive, multifamily, parent-involved treatment. Journal of eating disorders, 9(1), 110. https:// doi.org/10.1186/s40337-021-00465-x

10. Rothbart M. Advances in temperament, history, concepts and measures. In Zentner M, Shiner RL (Eds.), Handbook of Temperament (p. 3). New York: Guilford Press; 2012.

11. Mervilde I, De Pauw S. Models of child temperament. In Zentner M, Shiner RL (Eds.), Handbook of Temperament (pp. 21–40). New York: Guilford Press; 2012.

12. Aron E. Temperament in psychotherapy: Reflections on clinical practice with the trait of sensitivity. In Zentner M, Shiner RL (Eds.), Handbook of Temperament (pp. 645–670). New York: Guilford Press; 2012.

13. Cole C. Infant temperament predicts personality more than 20 years later. Neuroscience News; 2020.

14. Mitchell K. Innate. Princeton, NJ: Princeton University Press; 2018.

15. Whittle S, Allen N, Lubman D, et al. The neurobiological basis of temperament: Towards a better understanding of psychopathology. *Neurosci Biobehav Rev.* 2006;**30**(4):511–25.

16. Whittle S, Yucel M, Fornito A, et al. Neuroanatomical correlates of temperament in early adolescents. *J Am Acad Child Adolesc Psychiatr.* 2008;**47**(6):682–93.

17. Yucel M, Harrison BJ, Wood S, et al. State, trait and biochemical influences on human anterior cingulate function. *Neuroimage.* 2007;**34**(4):1766–73.

18. Hettema J, Bourdon J, Sawyers C, et al. Genetic and environmental risk structure of internalizing psychopathology in youth. *Depress Anxiety.* 2020;**37**(6):540–8.

19. Tang A, Crawford H, Morales S, et al. Infant behavioral inhibition predicts personality and social outcomes three decades later. *Proc Natl Acad Sci USA.* 2020;**117**(18):9800–7.

20. Kaye W, Bailer U. Understanding the neural circuitry of appetitive regulation in eating disorders. *Biol Psych.* 2011;**70**(8):704–5.

21. Kaye W, Wierenga C, Bailer U, et al. Nothing tastes as good as skinny feels: The neurobiology of anorexia nervosa. *Trends Neurosci.* 2013;**36**(2):110–20.

22. Kendler KS, MacLean C, Neale M, et al. The genetic epidemiology of bulimia nervosa. *Am J Psychiatr*. 1991;**148** (12):1627–37.

23. Walters EE, Kendler KS. Anorexia nervosa and anorexic-like syndromes in a population-based female twin sample. *Am J Psychiatr*. 1995;**152**(1):64–71.

24. Lilenfeld L, Kaye W. Genetic studies of anorexia and bulimia nervosa. In Hoek HW, Treasure JL, Katzman MA (Eds.), Neurobiology in the Treatment of Eating Disorders (pp. 169–194). Hoboken, NJ: John Wiley; 1998.

25. Strober M, Freeman R, Lampert C, et al. Controlled family study of anorexia nervosa and bulimia nervosa: Evidence of shared liability and transmission of partial syndromes. *Am J Psychiatr*. 2000;**157** (3):393–401.

26. Treasure J, Campbell I. The case for biology in the aetiology of anorexia nervosa. *Psychol Med*. 1994;**24**(1):3–8.

27. Berrettini W. Genetics of psychiatric disease. *Annu Rev Med*. 2000;**51**:465–79.

28. Bulik C, Sullivan PF, Tozzi F, et al. Prevalence, heritability and prospective risk factors for anorexia nervosa. *Arch Gen Psychiatr*. 2006;**63**(3):305–12.

29. Steinglass JE, Walsh T. Psychopharmacology of anorexia nervosa, bulimia nervosa, and binge eating disorder. In Brewerton TD (Ed.), Clinical Handbook of Eating Disorders: An Integrated Approach (pp. 489–508). New York: Marcel Dekker; 2004.

30. Anderluh MB, Tchanturia K, Rabe-Hesketh S, et al. Childhood obsessive-compulsive personality traits in adult women with eating disorders: Defining a broader eating disorder phenotype. *Am J Psychiatr*. 2003;**160**(2):242–7.

31. Stice E. Risk and maintenance factors for eating pathology: A meta-analytic review. *Pychopharmacol Bull*. 2002;**128**:825–48.

32. Lilenfeld L, Wonderlich S, Riso LP, et al. Eating disorders and personality: A methodological and empirical review. *Clin Psychol Rev*. 2006;**26**(3):299–320.

33. Bulik C, Breen G. Solving the eating disorders puzzle piece by piece. *Biol Psychiatr*. 2017;**81**(9):730–1.

34. Wadden T, Sternberg J, Letizia K, et al. Treatment of obesity by very low calorie diet, behavior therapy, and their combination: A five-year perspective. *Int J Obes*. 1989;**30**(Suppl 2):39–46.

35. Kaye W, Fudge J, Paulus M. New insights into symptoms and neurocircuit function of anorexia nervosa. *Nat Rev Neurosci*. 2009;**10**(8):573–84.

36. Kaye W, Wierenga C, Bailer U, et al. Does a shared neurobiology for foods and drugs of abuse contribute to extremes of food ingestion in anorexia and bulimia nervosa? *Biol Psychiatr*. 2013;**73**(9):836–42.

37. Kaye W, Bulik C, Thornton L, et al. Comorbidity of anxiety disorders with anorexia and bulimia nervosa. *Am J Psychiatr*. 2004;**161**(12):2215–21.

38. Cassin S, von Ranson K. Personality and eating disorders: A decade in review. *Clin Psycho Rev*. 2005;**25**(7):895–916.

39. Wagner A, Barbarich N, Frank G, et al. Personality traits after recovery from eating disorders: Do subtypes differ? *Int J Eat Disord*. 2006;**39**(4):276–84.

40. Lilenfeld L. Personality and temperament. *Curr Top Behav Neurosci*. 2011;**6**:3–9.

41. Fassino S, Piero A, Gramaglia C, et al. Clinical, psychopathological and personality correlates of interoceptive awareness in anorexia nervosa, bulimia nervosa and obesity. *Psychopathology*. 2004;**37**(4):168–74.

42. Harrison A, O'Brien N, Lopez C, et al. Sensitivity to reward and punishment in eating disorders. *Psy Res*. 2010;**177** (1–2):1–11.

43. Berner L, Crosby RD, Cao, L, et al. Temporal associations between affective instability and dysregulated eating behavior in bulimia nervosa. *J Psychiatr Res*. 2017;**92**:183–90.

44. DeGuzman M, Shott M, Yang T, et al. Association of elevated reward prediction error response with weight gain in adolescent anorexia nervosa. *Am J Psychiatr*. 2017;**174**(6):557–65.

45. Kerr K, Moseman S, Avery J, et al. Altered insula activity during visceral interoception in weight-restored patients with anorexia nervosa *Neuropsychopharmacology*. 2016;**41**(2):521–8.

46. Oberndorfer T, Frank G, Fudge J, et al. Altered insula response to sweet taste processing after recovery from anorexia and bulimia nervosa. *Am J Psychiatr*. 2013;**214**(2):132–41.

47. Wierenga C, Bischoff-Grethe A, Melrose A, et al. Hunger does not motivate reward in women remitted from anorexia nervosa. *Biol Psychiatr*. 2015;**77**(7):642–52.

48. Atiye M, Miettunen J, Raevuori-Helkamaa A. A meta-analysis of temperament in eating disorders. *Eur Eat Disord Rev*. 2015;**23**(2):89–99.

49. Steiger H, Booij L. Eating disorders, heredity and environmental activation: Getting epigenetic concepts into practice. *J Clin Med*. 2020;**9**(5):E1332.

50. Hebb D. The Organization of Behavior. New York: McGraw-Hill; 1949.

51. Kolb B. Brain Plasticity and Recovery of Function in Adulthood. Mahwah, NJ: Lawrence Erlbaum Associates; 1995.

52. Abramowitz J, Foa E, Franklin M. Exposure and ritual prevention for obsessive-compulsive disorder: Effects of intensive versus twice-weekly sessions. *J Consult Clin Psychol*. 2003;**71**(2):394–8.

53. Deacon B, Abramowitz J. A pilot study of two-day cognitive-behavioral therapy for panic disorder. *Behav Res Ther*. 2006;**44**(6):807–17.

54. Gallo K, Chan P, Buzzell B, et al. The impact of an eight-day intensive treatment for adolescent panic disorder and agoraphobia on comorbid diagnosis. *Behav Ther*. 2012;**43**:153–9.

55. Ollendick T, Ost L, Reyuterskiold L, et al. One-session treatment of specific phobias in youth: A randomized clinical trial in the United States and Sweden. *J Consult Clin Psychol*. 2009;**77**:504–16.

56. Santucci L, Ehrenreich J, Trosper S, et al. Development and preliminary evaluation of a one-week summer treatment program for separation anxiety disorder. *Cogn Behav Pract*. 2009;**16**:317–31.

57. Schmidt R, Bjork R. New conceptualizations of practice: Common principles in three paradigms suggest new concepts for training. *Psychol Sci*. 1992;**3**(4):207–17.

58. Storch E, Geffken G, Merlo L, et al. Family-based cognitive-behavioral therapy for pediatric obsessive-compulsive disorder: Comparison of intensive and weekly approaches. *J Am Acad Child Adolesc Psychiatr*. 2007;**26**:469–78.

59. Whiteside S, Jacobsen A. An uncontrolled examination of a 5-day intensive treatment for pediatric OCD. *Behav Ther*. 2010;**41**:414–22.

60. Fernandez M, Storch E, Lewin A, et al. The principles of extinction and differential reinforcement of other behaviors in the intensive cognitive-behavioral treatment of primarily obsessional pediatric OCD. *Clin Case Stud*. 2006;**12**:511–21.

61. Storch E, Merlo L, Lehmkuhl L, et al. Cognitive-behavioral therapy for obsessive-compulsive disorder: A non-randomized comparison of intensive and weekly approaches. *J Anxiety Disord*. 2008;**22**(7):1146–58.

62. Doyle P, Le Grange D, Loeb K, et al. Early response to family-based treatment for adolescent anorexia nervosa. *Int J Eat Disord*. 2010;**43**(7):659–62.

63. Bulik CM, Devlin B, Bacanu SA, et al. Significant linkage on chromosome 10p in families with bulimia nervosa. *Am J Hum Genet*. 2003;**72**(1):200–7.

64. Bulik CM, Sullivan PF, Kendler KS. Heritability of binge-eating and broadly defined bulimia nervosa. *Biol Psychiatr*. 1998;**44**(12):1210–8.

65. Duncan L, Yilma Z, Gaspar H, et al. Significant locus and metabolic genetic correlations revealed in genome wide association study of anorexia nervosa. *Am J Psychiatr*. 2017;**174**(9):850–8.

66. Hinney A, Kesselmeier M, Jall S, et al. Evidence for three genetic loci involved in

both anorexia nervosa risk and variation of body mass index. *Mol Psychiatr.* 2017;**22**(2):321–2.

67. Lock J, Le Grange D. Can family-based treatment of anorexia nervosa be manualized? *J Psychother Pract Res.* 2001;**10**(4):253–61.

68. Lock J, le Grange D. Family-based treatment of eating disorders. *Int J Eat Disord.* 2005;**37**(Suppl):S64–S7.

69. Loeb K, Le Grange D. Family-based treatment for adolescent eating disorders: Current status, new applications and future directions. *Int J Child Adolesc Health.* 2009;**2**(2):243–54.

70. Strelau J, Zawadzki B. Activity as a temperament trait. In Zentner M & Shiner RL (Eds.), Handbook of Temperament (pp. 83–104). New York: Guilford Press; 2012.

71. Eisler I, Simic M, Hodsoll J, et al. A pragmatic randomised multi-centre trial of multifamily and single family therapy for adolescent anorexia nervosa. *BMC Psychiatr.* 2016;**16**(1):422.

72. Dare C, Eisler I, Russell G, et al. Psychological therapies for adults with anorexia nervosa: Randomised controlled trial of out-patient treatments. *Br J Psychiatr.* 2001;**178**:216–21.

73. Lemmens G, Eisler I, Buysse A, et al. The effects on mood of adjunctive single family and multi-family group therapy in the treatment of hospitalised patients with major depression: An RCT and 15 months follow-up study. *Psychother Psychosom.* 2009;**78**:98–105.

74. McFarlane W. Family interventions for schizophrenia and the psychoses: A review. *Fam Process.* 2016;**55**(3):460–82.

75. Miller I, Solomon CE, Keitner G. Does adjunctive family therapy enhance recovery from bipolar I mood episodes? *J Affect Disord.* 2004;**82**(3):431–6.

76. Dimitropoulos G, Farquhar J, Freeman V, et al. Pilot study comparing multi-family therapy to single family therapy for adults with anorexia nervosa in an intensive eating disorder program. *Eur Eat Disord Rev.* 2015;**23**(4):294–303.

77. Tantillo M. A relational approach to eating disorders multifamily therapy group: Moving from difference and disconnection to mutual connection. *Families Syst Health.* 2006;**24**(1):82–102.

78. Kaye W, Wierenga C, Knatz S, et al. Temperament-based treatment for anorexia nervosa. *Eur Eat Disord Rev.* 2015;**23**(1):12–18.

79. Hill L, Peck S, Wierenga C, et al. Applying neurobiology to the treatment of adults with anorexia nervosa. *J Eat Disord.* 2016;**4**:31.

80. Crisafulli M, Von Holle A, Bulik C. Attitudes towards anorexia nervosa: The impact of framing on blame and stigma. *Int J Eat Disord.* 2008;**41**(4):333–9.

81. Wiesjahn M, Jung E, Kremser J, et al. The potential of continuum versus biogenetic beliefs in reducing stigmatization against persons with schizophrenia: An experimental study. *J Behav Ther Exp Psychiatr.* 2016;**50**:231–7.

82. Hodé Y. Psychoéducation des patients et de leurs proches dans les épisodes psychotiques [Psychoeducation of patients and their family members during episode psychosis]. *Encephale.* 2013;**39**(Suppl 2): S110–S4.

83. Farrell N, Lee A, Deacon B. Biological or psychological? Effects of eating disorder psychoeducation on self-blame and recovery expectations among symptomatic individuals. *Behav Res Ther.* 2015;**74**:32–7.

84. Lebowitz M, Ahn W. Emphasizing malleability in the biology of depression: Durable effects on perceived agency and prognostic pessimism. *Behav Res Ther.* 2015;**7**:125–30.

85. Han D, Chen S. Reducing the stigma of depression through neurobiology-based psychoeducation: A randomized controlled trial. *Psychiatr Clin Neurosci.* 2014;**68**(9):666–73.

86. Lebowitz MS, Pyun JJ, Ahn W-K. Biological explanations of generalized anxiety disorder: effects on beliefs about prognosis and responsibility. *Psychiatr Serv.* 2014;**65**(4):498–503.

87. Lebowitz M, Ahn W, Nolen-Hoeksema S. Fixable or fate? Perceptions of the biology of depression. *J Consult Clin Psychol.* 2013;**81**(3):518–27.

88. Zimmermann M, Papa A. Causal explanations of depression and treatment credibility in adults with untreated depression: Examining attribution theory. *Psychol Psychother.* 2020;**93**(3):537–54.

89. Lilenfeld LR, Kaye WH, Greeno CG, et al. A controlled family study of anorexia nervosa and bulimia nervosa: Psychiatric disorders in first-degree relatives and effects of proband comorbidity. *Arch Gen Psychiatr.* 1998;**55**(7):603–10.

90. Bulik C, Slof-Op't Landt M, van Furth E, et al. The genetics of anorexia nervosa. *Ann Rev Nutr.* 2007;**27**:263–75.

91. Watson H, Yilmaz Z, Thornton LH, et al. Genome-wide association study identifies eight risk loci and implicates metabo-psychiatric origins for anorexia nervosa. *Nat Genet.* 2019;**51**(8):1207–14.

92. Klump K, Strober M, Johnson C, et al. Personality characteristics of women before and after recovery from an eating disorder. *Psych Med.* 2004;**34**(8):1407–18.

93. Jacobs M, Roesch S, Wonderlich S, et al. Anorexia nervosa trios: Behavioral profiles of individuals with anorexia nervosa and their parents. *Psychol Med.* 2009;**39**(3):451–61.

94. Woodside DB, Bulik CM, Halmi KA, et al. Personality, perfectionism, and attitudes toward eating in parents of individuals with eating disorders. *Int J Eat Disord.* 2002;**31**(3):290–9.

95. Harrison A, Sullivan S, Tchanturia K, et al. Attentional bias, emotion recognition and emotion regulation in anorexia: State or trait? *Biol Psych.* 2010;**68**(8):755–61.

96. Klump K, Keel P, Racine S, et al. The interactive effects of estrogen and progesterone on changes in emotional eating across the menstrual cycle [Errata]. *J Abnorm Psychol.* 2013 Feb;**122**(1):137.

97. Klump K, Fowler N, Mayhall L, et al. Estrogen moderates genetic influences on binge eating during puberty: Disruption of normative processes? *J Abnorm Psychol.* 2018;**127**(5):458–70.

98. Berthoud H, Lenard N, Shin A. Food reward, hyperphagia, and obesity. *AM J Physiol Regul Integr Comp Physiol.* 2011;**300**(6):R1266–R77.

99. Cowdrey F, Park R, Harmer C, et al. Increased neural processing of rewarding and aversive food stimuli in recovered anorexia nervosa. *Biol Psych.* 2011;**70** (8):736–43.

100. Frank G, Reynolds J, Shott M, et al. Anorexia nervosa and obesity are associated with opposite brain reward response. *Neuropsychopharmacology.* 2012;**37**(9):2031–46.

101. Lock J, Garrett A, Beenhakker J, et al. Aberrant brain activation during a response inhibition task in adolescent eating disorder subtypes. *Am J Psychiatr.* 2011;**168**(1):55–64.

102. Foerde K, Steinglass J, Shohamy D, et al. Neural mechanisms supporting maladaptive food choices in anorexia nervosa. *Nat Neurosci.* 2015;**18**(11):1571–3.

103. Ehrlich S, Geisler D, Ritschel F, et al. Elevated cognitive control over reward processing in recovered female patients with anorexia nervosa. *J Psychiatr Neurosci.* 2015;**40**(5):307–15.

104. Dellava J, Thornton L, Hamer RS, et al. Childhood anxiety associated with low BMI in women with anorexia nervosa. *Behav Res Ther.* 2010;**48**(1):60–7.

105. Bischoff-Grethe A, Wierenga C, Berner L, et al. Neural hypersensitivity to pleasant touch in women remitted from anorexia nervosa. *Transl Psychiatr.* 2018;**8**(1):161.

106. Holsen L, Lawson E, Blum K, et al. Food motivation circuitry hypoactivation related to hedonic and nonhedonic aspects of hunger and satiety in women with active anorexia nervosa and weight-restored women with anorexia nervosa. *J Psychiatr Neurosci.* 2012;**37**(5):322–32.

107. Kaye W, Wierenga C, Bischoff-Grethe A, et al. Neural insensitivity to the effects of hunger in women remitted from anorexia

nervosa. *Am J Psychiatr.* 2020;**177** (7):601–10.

108. Bischoff-Grethe A, McCurdy D, Grenesko-Stevens E, et al. Altered brain response to reward and punishment in adolescents with anorexia nervosa. *Psychiatr Res.* 2013;**214** (3):331–40.

109. Frank G, Collier S, Shott M, et al. Prediction error and somatosensory insula activation in women recovered from anorexia nervosa. *J Psychiatr Neurosci.* 2016;**41**(2):304–11.

110. Roberts M, Tchanturia K, Stahl D, et al. A systematic review and meta-analysis of set-shifting ability in eating disorders. *Psychol Med.* 2007;**37**(8):1075–84.

111. Smith K, Mason T, Johnson J, et al. A systematic review of reviews of neurocognitive functioning in eating disorders: The state-of-the-literature and future directions. *Int J Eat Disord.* 2018;**51** (8):798–821.

112. Wu M, Brockmeyer T, Hartmann M, et al. Set-shifting ability across the spectrum of eating disorders and in overweight and obesity: A systematic review and meta-analysis. *Psychol Med.* 2014;**44** (16):3365–85.

113. Berner L, Romero E, Reilly EE, et al. Task-switching inefficiencies in currently ill, but not remitted anorexia nervosa. *Int J Eat Disord.* 2019;**52** (11):1316–21.

114. Decker J, Figner B, Steinglass J. On weight and waiting: Delay discounting in anorexia nervosa pretreatment and post-treatment. *Biol Psychol.* 2015;**78** (9):606–14.

115. Steward T, Mestre-Bach G, Vintro-Alcaraz C, et al. Delay discounting of reward and impulsivity in eating disorders: From anorexia nervosa to binge eating disorder. *Eur Eat Disord Rev.* 2017;**25**(6):601–6.

116. Wierenga C, Ely A, Bischoff-Grethe A, et al. Are extremes of consumption in eating disorders related to an altered balance between reward and inhibition? *Front Behav Neurosci.* 2014;**9**(8):410.

117. Brown T, Vanzhula I, Reilly E, et al. Body mistrust bridges interoceptive awareness and eating disorder symptoms. *J Abnorm Psychol.* 2020;**129**(5):445–56.

118. Strigo I, Matthews S, Simmons A, et al. Altered insula activation during pain anticipation in individuals recovered from anorexia nervosa: Evidence of interoceptive dysregulation. *Int J Eat Disord.* 2013;**46**:23–33.

119. Berner L, Simmons A, Wierenga C, et al. Altered interoceptive activation before, during, and after aversive breathing load in women remitted from anorexia nervosa. *Psychol Med.* 2018;**48**(1):142–54.

120. Oberndorfer T, Simmons A, McCurdy D, et al. Greater anterior insula activation during anticipation of food images in women recovered from anorexia nervosa versus controls. *Psychiatr Res.* 2013 **214** (2):132–41.

121. Bailer U, Narendran R, Frank W, et al. Amphetamine induced dopamine release increases anxiety in individuals recovered from anorexia nervosa. *Int J Eat Disord.* 2012;**45**(2):263–71.

122. Frank G, Bailer UF, Henry S, et al. Increased dopamine D2/D3 receptor binding after recovery from anorexia nervosa measured by positron emission tomography and [$^{11}$C]raclopride. *Biol Psychiatr.* 2005;**58**(11):908–12.

123. Wagner A, Aizenstein H, Venkatraman M, et al. Altered reward processing in women recovered from anorexia nervosa. *Am J Psychiatr.* 2007;**164**(12):1842–9.

124. Arnett J. The Oxford Handbook of Emerging Adulthood. Arnett J (Ed.). Oxford: Oxford University Press; 2015.

125. Gustavson K, Knudsen A, Nesvag R, et al. Prevalence and stability of mental disorders among young adults: Findings from a longitudinal study. *BMC Psychiatr.* 2018;**18**(1):65.

126. US Department of Health and Human Services. National Survey of Drug Use and Health (NSDUH). www.samhsa.gov/data/release/2019-national-survey-drug-use-and-health-nsduh-releases; 2019.

127. Twenge JM, Cooper AB, Joiner T, et al. Age, period, and cohort trends in mood disorder indicators and suicide-related outcomes in a nationally representative dataset, 2005–2017. *J Abnorm Psychol.* 2019;**128**(3):185–99.

128. Volpe U, Tortorella A, Manchia M, et al. Eating disorders: What age at onset? *Psychiatr Res.* 2016;**30**(238):225–7.

129. Mitrofan O, Petkova H, Janssens A, et al. Care experiences of young people with eating disorders and their parents: Qualitative study. *BJPsych Open.* 2019;**5**(1):e6.

130. Dimitropoulos G, Landers A, Freeman V, et al. Open trial of family-based treatment of anorexia nervosa for transition age youth. *J Can Acad Child Adolesc Psychiatr.* 2018;**27**(1):50–61.

131. Dimitroupoulos G, Freeman V, Allemang B, et al. Family-based treatment with transition age youth with anorexia nervosa: A qualitative summary of application in clinical practice. *J Eat Disord.* 2015;**3**(1):1–13.

132. Asen E, Scholz M. Multi-family Therapy: Concepts and Techniques. New York: Routledge; 2010.

133. Simic M, Eisler I. Multi-family therapy. In Loeb K, LeGrange D (Eds.), Family Therapy for Adolescent Eating and Weight Disorders: New Applications (pp. 110–38). New York: Routledge; 2015.

134. Linehan M. DBT Skills Training Manual (2nd ed.). New York: Guilford Press; 2015.

135. Linehan M. Dialectical Behavior Therapy in Clinical Practice. New York: Guilford Press; 2020.

136. Zuckerman M. Models of adult temperament. In Handbook of Temperament (Chapter 3). New York: Guilford Press; 2012.

137. Hill L. A brain-based approach to eating disorder treatment. www.brainbasedeatingdisorders.org/; 2017.

138. Hodgekiss A. Trying to lose weight? Try the HAND DIET: Measure food portions using just your fingers, thumbs and palm. *Daily Mail;* 2014.

139. Squire L, Kandel E. Memory, from Mind to Molecules (2nd ed.). Boulder, CO: Roberts; 2009.

140. Cross-Disorder Group of Psychiatric Genomics Consortium. Genomic relationships, novel loci, and pleiotropic mechanisms across eight psychiatric disorders. 2019.

141. Bulik C, Flatt R, Abbaspour A, et al. Reconceptualizing anorexia nervosa. *Psychiatr Clin Neurosci.* 2019;**73**(9):518–25.

142. Liu P, Peng G, Zhang N, et al. Crosstalk between the gut microbiota and the brain: An update on neuroimaging findings. *Front Neurol.* 2019;**10**:833.

143. Hubel C, Yilmaz Z, Schaumberg K, et al. Body composition in anorexia nervosa: Meta-analysis and meta-regression of cross-sectional and longitudinal studies. *Int J Eat Disord.* 2019;**52**(11):1205–23.

144. Akkermann K, Paaver M, Nordquist N, et al. Association of 5-HTT gene polymorphism, platelet MAO activity, and drive for thinness in a population-based sample of adolescent girls. *International Journal of Eating Disorders.* 2008;**41**(5):399–404.

145. Danner U, Sanders N, Smeets P, et al. Neuropsychological weaknesses in anorexia nervosa: Set-shifting, central coherence, and decision making in currently ill and recovered women. *Int J Eat Disord.* 2012;**45**(5):685–94.

146. Frank G, Kaye W. Current status of functional imaging in eating disorders. *Int J Eat Disord.* 2012;**45**(6):723–36.

147. Klump K. Puberty as a critical risk period for eating disorders: A review of human and animal studies. *Horm Behav.* 2013;**64**(2):399–410.

148. Ma R, Mikhail M, Fowler N, et al. The role of puberty and ovarian hormones in the genetic diathesis of eating disorders in females. *Child Adolesc Psychiatr Clin N Am.* 2019;**28**(4):617–28.

149. Simmons W, Avery J, Barcalow J, et al. Keeping the body in mind: Insula functional organization and functional connectivity integrate interoceptive, exteroceptive, and emotional awareness. *Hum Brain Mapp.* 2013;**34**(11):2944–58.

150. Ehrlich S, Lord A, Geisler D, et al. Reduced functional connectivity in the thalamo-insular subnetwork in patients with acute anorexia nervosa. *Hum Brain Mapp.* 2015;**36**(5):1772–81.

151. Treasure J, Zipfel S, Micali N, et al. Anorexia nervosa. *Nature Rev Dis Primers.* 2015;**1**:15074.

152. Nunn K, Frampton I, Gordon I, et al. The fault is not in her parents but in her insula – a neurobiological hypothesis of anorexia nervosa. *Eur Eat Disord Rev.* 2008;**16**(5):355–60.

153. Nunn K, Frampton I, Lask B, et al. Anorexia nervosa and the insula. *Med Hypotheses.* 2011;**76**(3):353–7.

154. Frank G, Shott M, Keffler C, et al. Extremes of eating are associated with reduced neural taste discrimination. *Int J Eat Disord.* 2016;**49**(6):603–12.

155. Szalavitz M. The currency of desire. *Sci Am Mind.* 2017;**28**:48–53.

156. Sullivan PF. Mortality in anorexia nervosa. *Am J Psychiatr.* 1995;**152**(7):1073–4.

157. Ackard D, Richter S, Egan A, et al. Poor outcome and death among youth, young adults, and midlife adults with eating disorders: An investigation of risk factors by age at assessment. *Int J Eat Disord.* 2014;**47**(7):825–35.

158. Arcelus J, Mitchell A, Wales J, et al. Mortality rates in patients with anorexia nervosa and other eating disorders. *Arch Gen Psychiatr.* 2011;**68**(7):724–31.

159. Compan V, Walsh B, Kaye W, et al. How does the brain implement adaptive decision making to eat? *J Neurosci.* 2015;**35**(41):13868–78.

160. Brainstorm Consortium. Analysis of shared heritability in common disorders of the brain. *Science.* 2018;**360**:6395.

161. Mahon P, Hildebrandt T, Burdick K. New genetic discoveries in anorexia nervosa:

Implications for the field. *Am J Pschiatr.* 2017;**174**(9):821–2.

162. Simone M, Askew A, Lust K, et al. Disparities in self-reported eating disorders and academic impairment in sexual and gender minority college students relative to their heterosexual and cisgender peers. *Int J Eat Disord.* 2020;**53**(4):513–24.

163. American Psychiatric Association. Diagnostic and Statistical Manual of Mental Disorders (DSM-V, 5th ed.). Washington, DC: American Psychiatric Association; 2013.

164. Yau W-Y, Bischoff-Grethe A, Theilmann R, et al. Alterations in white matter microstructure in women recovered from anorexia nervosa. *Int J Eat Disord.* 2013;**46**(7):701–98.

165. Stiles-Shields C, Bamford B, Lock J, et al. The effect of driven exercise on treatment outcomes for adolescents with anorexia and bulimia nervosa. *Int J Eat Disord.* 2015;**48**(8):392–6.

166. Zerwas S, Lund B, Von Holle A, et al. Factors associated with recovery from anorexia nervosa. *J Psychiatr Pract.* 2013;**47**(7):972–9.

167. Levinson C, Zerwas SC, Brosof LC, et al. Associations between dimensions of anorexia nervosa and obsessive-compulsive disorder: An examination of personality and psychological factors in patients with anorexia nervosa. *Eur Eat Disord Rev.* 2018;**27**(2):161–72.

168. Klump K, Burt S, Spanos A, et al. Age differences in genetic and environmental influences on weight and shape concerns. *Int J Eat Disord.* 2010;**43**(8):679–88.

169. Klump K, Culbert K, O'Connor S, et al. The significant effects of puberty on the genetic diathesis of binge eating in girls. *Int J Eat Disord.* 2017;**50**(8):984–9.

170. Hubel C, Gaspar H, Coleman J, et al. Genetic correlations of psychiatric traits with body composition and glycemic traits are sex- and age-dependent *Nat Commun.* 2019;**10**(1):5765.

171. McAdams C, Jeon-Slaughter H, Evans S, et al. Neural differences in self-perception

during illness and after weight-recovery in anorexia nervosa. *Soc Cogn Affect Neurosci.* 2016;**11**(11):1823–31.

172. Halmi K, Bellace D, Berthod S, et al. An examination of early childhood perfectionism across anorexia nervosa subtypes. *Int J Eat Disord.* 2012;**45**(6):800–7.

173. Esposito R, Cieri F, di Giannantonio M, et al. The role of body image and self-perception in anorexia nervosa: the neuroimaging perspective. *J Neuropsychol.* 2018;**12**(1):41–52.

174. Oberndorfer T, Kaye W, Simmons A, et al. Demand-specific alteration of medial prefrontal cortex response during an inhibition task in recovered anorexic women. *Int J Eat Disord.* 2011;**44**(1):1–8.

175. Linehan M. Cognitive-Behavioral Treatment of Borderline Personality Disorder. New York: Guilford Press; 1993.

176. Pruis T, Keel P, Janowsky J. Recovery from anorexia nervosa includes neural compensation for negative body image. *Int J Eat Disord.* 2012;**45**:919–31.

177. McCormick L, Keel P, Brumm M, et al. Implications of starvation-induced change in right dorsal anterior cingulate volume in anorexia nervosa. *Int J Eat Disord.* 2008;**41**(7):602–10.

178. Bergen A, Yeager M, Welch R, et al. Association of multiple DRD2 polymorphisms with anorexia nervosa. *Neuropsychopharmacology.* 2005;**30** (9):1703–10.

179. Frieling H, Romer K, Scholz S, et al. Epigenetic dysregulation of dopaminergic genes in eating disorders. *Int J Eat Disord.* 2010;**43**(7):577–83.

180. Richmond B, Liu Z, Shidara M. Predicting future rewards. *Science.* 2003;**301**:179–80.

181. Robinson P, Kukucska R, Guidetti G, et al. Severe and enduring anorexia nervosa (SEE-AN): A qualitative study of patients with 20+ years of anorexia nervosa. *Eur Eat Disord Rev.* 2015;**23**:318–26.

182. Banich M, Compton R. Cognitive Neuroscience. Cambridge: Cambridge University Press; 2018.

183. Gilligan C. In a Different Voice. Cambridge, MA: Harvard University Press; 1982.

184. Marek RJ, Ben-Porath DD, Federici A, Wisniewski L, Warren M. Targeting premeal anxiety in eating disordered clients and normal controls: A preliminary investigation into the use of mindful eating vs. distraction during food exposure. *International Journal of Eating Disorders* 2013;46(6):582–85.

185. Hill L. The woodburning stove: A metaphor for dietary regulation for persons with eating disorders. In Eating Disorders Treatment and Prevention, Vol. 1 (2) New York: Brunner/Mazel; 1993.

186. Kaye WH, Barbarich NC, Putnam K, Gendall KA, Fernstrom J, Fernstrom M, et al. Anxiolytic effects of acute tryptophan depletion in anorexia nervosa. *Int J Eat Disord* 2003;33:257–67.

187. Fairburn CG, Beglin SJ. *Eating Disorder Examination Questionnaire (EDE-Q)* [Database record]. APA PsycTests;1994.

188. Schebendach J, Mayer LES, Devlin MJ, Attia E, Walsh, BT. Dietary energy density and diet variety as risk factors for relapse in anorexia nervosa: A replication. *Int. J. Eat. Disord.* 2012; 45:79–84. doi: 10.1002/eat.20922

189. Gianini, LM, Walsh BT, Steinglass J, Mayer L. Long-term weight loss maintenance in obesity: Possible insights from anorexia nervosa? *International Journal of Eating Disorders,* 2017;50:341–42. doi: 10.1002/eat.22685

190. Jewell, T., Blessitt, E., Stewart, C., Simic, M., & Eisler, I. (2016). Family therapy for child and adolescent eating disorders: a critical review. Family Process, 55(3), 577–594.

# Index

Printed in the United States
by Baker & Taylor Publisher Services